TRANSFORMED STATES

Other books by Martin Halliwell

Romantic Science and the Experience of Self (1999; 2016)

Modernism and Morality (2001)
republished as *Transatlantic Modernism* (2006)

Critical Humanisms: Humanist/Anti-Humanist Dialogues (2003)
(with Andy Mousley)

Images of Idiocy: The Idiot Figure in Modern Fiction and Film (2004)

The Constant Dialogue: Reinhold Niebuhr and American Intellectual Culture (2005)

American Culture in the 1950s (2007)

American Thought and Culture in the 21st Century (2008)
(edited with Catherine Morley)

Beyond and Before: Progressive Rock since the 1960s (2011)
(expanded edition 2021, with Paul Hegarty)

Therapeutic Revolutions: Medicine, Psychiatry, and American Culture, 1945–1970 (2013)

William James and the Transatlantic Conversation (2014)
(edited with Joel Rasmussen)

Neil Young: American Traveller (2015)

Voices of Mental Health: Medicine, Politics, and American Culture, 1970–2000 (2017)

Reframing 1968: American Politics, Protest and Identity (2018)
(edited with Nick Witham)

American Health Crisis: One Hundred Years of Panic, Planning, and Politics (2021)

The Edinburgh Companion to the Politics of American Health (2022)
(edited with Sophie A. Jones)

TRANSFORMED STATES

Medicine, Biotechnology, and

American Culture, 1990–2020

MARTIN HALLIWELL

RUTGERS UNIVERSITY PRESS
New Brunswick, Camden, and Newark, New Jersey
London and Oxford

Rutgers University Press is a department of Rutgers, The State University of New Jersey, one of the leading public research universities in the nation. By publishing worldwide, it furthers the University's mission of dedication to excellence in teaching, scholarship, research, and clinical care.

Library of Congress Cataloging-in-Publication Data

Names: Halliwell, Martin, author. | Halliwell, Martin. Therapeutic
  revolutions. | Halliwell, Martin. Voices of mental health.
Title: Transformed states : medicine, biotechnology, and American culture,
  1990-2020 / Martin Halliwell.
Description: New Brunswick, New Jersey : Rutgers University Press, [2025] |
  Includes bibliographical references and index.
Identifiers: LCCN 2024004416 | ISBN 9781978817876 (cloth ; alk. paper) |
  ISBN 9781978817883 (epub) | ISBN 9781978817906 (pdf)
Subjects: MESH: Biomedical Technology—history | Politics | Culture |
  History, 20th Century | History, 21st Century | United States
Classification: LCC R859 | NLM W 82 | DDC 362.10285—dc23/eng/20240624
LC record available at https://lccn.loc.gov/2024004416

A British Cataloging-in-Publication record for this book is available from the British Library.

References to internet websites (URLs) were accurate at the time of writing. Neither the author nor Rutgers University Press is responsible for URLs that may have expired or changed since the manuscript was prepared.

♾ The paper used in this publication meets the requirements of the American National Standard for Information Sciences—Permanence of Paper for Printed Library Materials, ANSI Z39.48-1992.

rutgersuniversitypress.org

For Carl and Richard

Contents

Illustrations

Preface

Transformation is at the heart of American culture, it is the engine of business, and is at the epicenter of biotechnology as a practice of repair and enhancement. It is also embedded in the exceptionalism that has propelled the idea that the American republic is moving toward an ever perfect union, as Barack Obama reminded the electorate on the presidential campaign trail in spring 2008, when the nation was looking out on an increasingly imperfect world, not only with the global financial crisis of 2007–2008 but also glimpses of the colliding crises of economics, health, race relations, and climate change that Obama's vice-president Joe Biden evoked just over a decade later in his own successful presidential campaign.

If transformation is a basic ingredient of American life and the arc of history is moving toward "a better day" (as Obama claimed in his victory speech), then how do we account for the fragile state of the nation's health in an era of technological acceleration? To address this question *Transformed States* focuses on biotechnology, which Thomas Friedman reminds us is just one face of a "full-on societal reinvention challenge" that became "a major technological inflection point" in the 2010s.[1] Despite moves by the Obama White House to renew public trust in biotech via a National Bioeconomy Blueprint—especially in "red biotechnology" at the intersection of health care and biopharmaceuticals—Friedman worries about the pace of change.[2] These concerns echo philosopher Paul Virilio's opinion that speed can be an agent of destruction, especially when it is militarized, as the President's Council of Advisors on Science and Technology warned Obama toward the end of his presidency.[3]

We might follow Virilio in picturing postmillennial life as a state of emergency, a view that Achille Mbembe applies to biotechnology in his claim that our era is "one of plasticity, pollination, and grafts of all sorts" that "pits nature against human beings."[4] But rather than clinging to Obama's vision of progressive transformation or resigning ourselves to Virilio's and Mbembe's bleak views about the degrading colonization of human bodies, *Transformed States* pauses to explore the complex relationship between biotechnology and health at the confluence of American culture and politics.

To historicize what biophysicist Gregory Stock calls an "era of biotechnology," this book examines a thirty-year period that radically transformed American science, medicine, business, and federal policy. Since its more specific usage in the 1970s for the practice of genetic engineering, biotechnology has broadened its ambit in two main respects. On one side, it underpins a public services ethos that seeks to improve the efficacy of medicine and health care via advanced health technologies; on the other, it provides profitable platforms for venture capitalists to marketize biological entities. In its exploration of the public-private juncture of medical biotechnology, *Transformed States* is the third volume of a cultural and intellectual history that charts mental health from the combat zones of World War II to the global emergency of COVID-19. Whereas the first volume, *Therapeutic Revolutions*, examines how postwar therapy oscillated between technologies of control and the potential for self-actualization, and the second, *Voices of Mental Health*, tracks the politicization of mental health between the moon landing and the millennium, *Transformed States* takes a slight historical step back, returning to the post–Cold War 1990s as a threshold to the fourth industrial revolution of digital technologies, positioning biotechnology in dialogue with fears and fantasies about an emerging future in which health seems ever more contested.

Transformed States takes the consequential decade of the 1990s as a horizon for tracing the health implications of biotechnology via the five presidential administrations of George H. W. Bush, Bill Clinton, George W. Bush, Barack Obama, and Donald Trump, together with some early thoughts on the Biden administration in the final section and the conclusion. The role of the state is vital for understanding the post–Cold War politics of biotechnology, especially as a regulator of stem cell technology and interspecies research. Yet the politics of this book are more diffuse than *Voices of Mental Health* in its assessment of the tensions between exploratory and exploitative aspects of red biotechnology. Through the first two developmental parts of *Transformed States*, "Genetic States" and "Conscious States," and the third and fourth conceptually cumulative parts, "Dynamic States" and "Perilous States," I analyze a prism of political, biomedical, and cultural texts in order to trace the impacts of biotechnology on personal, social, and environmental health.

As a line of continuity with *Voices of Mental Health*, this is a book about the health consequences of federal legislation, biomedical endeavor, and cultural politics. However, my discussion dips beneath the federal level to assess the relationship between state-sponsored research and private-sector investment. It also moves outward to consider global biotechnologies and the governance role of the World Health Organization in valorizing biomedical interventions such as vaccines, while offering warnings about others such as genetically modified foods.[5] Across these thirty years, it is tempting to emphasize the grand biotech horizons of the post–Cold War period, the shifting expectations and tense negotiations between the market and the state in the post-9/11 years, and a recognition of biotech limitations on either side of 2020. While these contours are evident in my chapter sequence, the book's arc is conceptually and historically more complex than this sequential narrative, largely because biotech designs and applications operate on varying scales and with differing speeds and because investment in biotech start-ups during the 2010s was unprecedented.

In exploring the repercussions of what the cultural sociologist John Tomlinson calls the "unruly speed" of "contemporary globalized and telemediated societies," *Transformed States* shares with the first two volumes of the trilogy an interdisciplinary perspective on the historical, social, political, and existential determinants of mental and physical health. Whereas *Therapeutic Revolutions* is primarily a cultural history and *Voices of Mental Health* a political history, in its aim to tackle perennial yet prescient questions of identity, agency, authenticity, and responsibility, *Transformed States* adopts a more theoretical approach, linking bioethics and cognitive philosophy; posthumanist, feminist, and queer theories; disability and cultural studies; medical and environmental humanities; and the sociology and anthropology of health to assess how biotechnology spans cultural reflections, political discourses, and scientific practices. My interest in expanding conventional approaches to public health features most prominently in the ecological fourth part of *Transformed States* and develops the argument of my 2021 book *American Health Crisis* with regard to how macrolevel environmental and organizational stresses exert unhealthy—because often inequitable—pressures on vulnerable communities.

We might think of biotech transformations as those that restlessly combine innovative elements and processes in the search for agility, efficacy, or novelty, in which the new is continuously redefined as a state of becoming. This fluid immediacy often excites technophiles, but it can also be anxiety provoking, especially because access to biotechnology is so uneven between demographics and because its outcomes can generate as many worries as solutions.[6] We may view such anxieties as an inability to adapt to the present or to imagine an alternative future, but these anxious states implicate what Sherry Turkle calls "the new connectivity" of a hypertechnologized world that "helps us to manage life stresses but generates anxieties of its own."[7] In promising healthier lives, biotech breakthroughs do not evade existential and sociological questions of loss, vulnerability, and powerlessness, although these questions often are submerged in an accelerating present. So while we need to recover what Virilio calls "lateral vision" by linking the ethics, politics, and science of repair and enhancement, it is also vital to appraise the limits and possibilities of human and planetary existence because biotechnology morphs habitual ways of seeing and doing.[8]

Psychiatry tells us that anxieties about technology can be both diffuse and specific. At the diffuse level, the fourth edition of the *Diagnostic and Statistical Manual of Mental Disorders* (DSM-IV) describes "generalized anxiety disorder" as "excessive anxiety and worry (apprehensive expectation), occurring more days than not for at least 6 months, about a number of events and activities."[9] Published almost a decade later, in 2013, the DSM-5 authors were careful not to pathologize common anxieties, rearticulating the DSM-IV description of nine years earlier with the slight modification that it is generalized when "not better explained by another mental disorder," suggesting that other diagnoses need to be ruled out before reaching this one.[10] Technophobia, referring to the specific fear of advanced technology, came into usage after World War II. Now in common parlance, technophobia remains a distinctly cultural construct and does not feature in either the 1994 or the 2013 editions of the DSM, even though a DSM-5 Anxiety Work Group considered amending the diagnostic criteria for phobias to include technophobia.[11]

Technologies can trigger adverse responses such as simulator sickness in relation to virtual reality systems or the involuntary recoiling from a vaccine needle, often accompanied by primal worries about what Virilio calls "stressful claustrophobia" in a tech-saturated environment.[12] Recognizing that these fears move between general and specific, background and foreground, this book responds to Neil Postman's view that new technologies alter "the structure of our interests: the things we think *about*" and "the character of our symbols: the things we think *with*."[13]

Given that biotechnology prompts extreme responses, *Transformed States* seeks to inhabit a dynamic middle space between overoptimistic technophilia and often bleakly cynical technophobia. In an increasingly polarized national culture, what Donna Haraway calls the "great divide" seems inevitable.[14] The health space between this great divide is increasingly contested, as visualized by artists featured in the 2018 Metropolitan Museum of Art exhibition *Everything Is Connected: Art and Conspiracy*, whose work ranged from art journalism that exposed structural inequalities to work that imagined full-fledged conspiracies that implicate public health.[15] However, I argue that this intermedial space can embody a critical and regenerative set of positions that probe questions of expertise and experience and of compliance and critique without falling into agonistic thinking. This space is a mediated one—culturally, politically, and scientifically—but it is also a space of merging and emergence, where mobile elements break loose from organizational systems yet can retain their value in the face of tech saturation. Between the imperialist logic of many grand biotech projects and what Matthew Hannah calls a "conspiracy of data," I argue that this space can be socially inclusive and foster biotech agency at a local level.[16]

Informing this revitalized critical space, I expand upon two synergistic concepts: what the University of California sociologist Robert Bellah calls a "politics of imagination" and British philosopher Nikolas Rose's concept of "somatic ethics." Bellah and Rose offer pathways through this space among familiar guides to technology such as Martin Heidegger, Paul Virilio, Leon Kass, Bruno Latour, Donna Haraway, N. Kathryn Hayles, and Roberto Esposito, in conversation with other North American thinkers, writers, and public figures that feature in the book's eight chapters. Together, these diverse voices enable me to trace the biotech acceleration over three post–Cold War decades with the aim of mapping both a perspective and praxis that retain ideals whilst avoiding heroic optimism.

My objective is to discover pragmatic ways of dealing with material problems of access, inequity, and exclusion without falling into an apocalyptic stance toward global warming and viral transmissibility that entirely undercuts the heroic rhetoric of millennial biotechnologies. It is crucial that Bellah and Rose see this bioethical position as emergent rather than dominant, enabling them to recognize that the biological, neurological, and genetic fabric of human life is always in flux and to couple the healthening potential of cultural diversity and collective agency. This stance is by no means redemptive, but it is potentially restorative—or even healing—in challenging dogma, diminishing the fear of biotechnology, and propelling its goals toward care rather than conquest.

TRANSFORMED
STATES

Introduction

One of the most famous proclamations by a modern U.S. president was made eighteen months into George H. W. Bush's term in the White House. Titled "Decade of the Brain, 1990–1999," the proclamation followed a joint congressional resolution for an interagency mission that could push the human brain to the forefront of scientific and technological endeavor. By portraying the brain in this July 1990 proclamation as "the seat of human intelligence, interpreter of senses, and controller of movement" that "continues to intrigue scientists and layman alike," Bush had two primary objectives.[1] The first was to launch a grand federal program coordinated by the White House Office of Science Technology and Policy to investigate "how the brain's cells and chemicals develop, interact, and communicate with the rest of the body"; the second was to raise public awareness of the possibilities that lay ahead in the field of biotechnology for tackling neurological and mental health conditions.

On both themes, Bush's words echoed the emphasis of a joint resolution on "research, treatment and rehabilitation" that had been prompted by calls for a countrywide plan from the National Institute of Mental Health and the National Institute of Neurological Disorders and Stroke.[2] Notably, the health conditions Bush highlighted in the proclamation—"impairments of speech, language, and hearing" and Alzheimer's disease—bridged professional and personal spheres on two fronts. First, Bush's son Neil experienced reading difficulties at middle school in the late 1960s, which led the president to establish a Task Force on Literacy in 1990 and First Lady Barbara Bush to focus on literacy as her special cause. Second, rumors had circulated through the 1980s that Ronald Reagan, whom Bush served under as vice-president, was suffering from dementia. (Reagan announced that he had Alzheimer's following Bush's departure from the White House.) Delivered at "this fascinating time in the history of the world," Bush's proclamation was hopeful, future-oriented, and potentially global in scope, linking pure research to its medical application for treating conditions such as Parkinson's, epilepsy, HIV/AIDS, depression, and spinal cord injuries, as well as stroke and heart disease, about which Bush had raised awareness the previous year.[3]

It is surprising that as Bush surveyed what a 1992 Carnegie Commission report called the "wider range and greater complexity" of science and technology in a post–Cold War world, his proclamation did not refer directly to biotechnology.[4] That Decade of the Brain activities were to be co-led by the National

Academy of Sciences and the National Institutes of Health (NIH)—the budget of which increased 40 percent during Bush's presidency after lean years during the Reagan administration—meant that answers to debilitating health conditions were always likely to be technological.[5] Bush's omission of biotech was surprising because he was a keen advocate of scientific research: for example, he referred to "a new age of biotechnology" when he swore in cardiologist Bernadine Healy as the new NIH director the following summer.[6]

At that NIH ceremony in June 1991, Bush spoke of biomedical research as "key to transforming" medicine and genomic research by "building a body of knowledge that will be forever useful."[7] His comments channeled the priority of the Council on Competitiveness to keep the United States a "world leader in biotechnology" and the view of the Office of Science and Technology Policy that "biotechnical advances offer the possibility of improvements that will make a real difference in people's lives."[8] The president added a note of compassion, claiming that the "human heart" drives "the conquest of illness—including mental illness," a view that linked to the launch of the Healthy Start program geared to combating infant mortality and an annual Mental Illness Awareness Week the previous October.[9] However, Bush missed a golden chance to promote opportunities for female scientists, given that Healy was the first female NIH director and that she had announced at her Senate confirmation hearing that she planned to establish a pioneering Women's Health Initiative within a broader effort to eliminate discrimination based on genetic data.[10]

A series of symposia held at the Library of Congress over the next nine years echoed Bush's humanistic sensibility and embodied the spirit of the Decade of the Brain, as captured from the opening symposium, "Frontiers of Neuroscience," in July 1991, through to the final event, "Understanding Ourselves: The Science of Cognition," in October 1999. Sponsored by the philanthropic Dana Foundation in collaboration with the NIH, the Library of Congress program emphasized pure research in search of technological applications. However, despite its balance between ambition and pragmatism, the grand universalistic goals of the federal program and its focus on an abstracted sense of the human overshadowed a more granular analysis of the social and cultural codeterminants of health.

In addition to celebrating the research and development work of the health care industry, Bush was deeply pro-business and recognized that the revenue potential of high growth biotech platforms was "a key to the marketplace of the 21st century."[11] Bush was also wary of industry overregulation, explaining in 1992 to employees of the Michigan-based Stryker Corporation that "regulation of the healing arts and health technologies have got to respond to patients' needs and must be based on sound science, not on ideological politics or scare tactics."[12] The newly elected President Clinton echoed this message a few months later, stating that "we must free science and medicine from the grasp of politics," but it is important to note that Bush's message was a politicized one, targeted at swing-state industry workers in an election year.[13] Yet there was a specific reason why he avoided mentioning biotechnology in his 1990 proclamation: it was less because it was too technical for the electorate and more that the date was close to "a major period of disillusionment" in the biotech industry.[14]

A 1992 business report, *Biotechnology in the 1990s*, pinpoints 1988, the final full year of Reagan's presidency, as the source of this disillusionment. With the stock market "still shaken and defensive" after the crash of October 1987, San Francisco biotech corporation Genentech—"the most ballyhooed U.S. entrepreneurial start-up since Apple computer, and the flagship of the emerging biotechnology industry"—exaggerated the benefits of its heart drug TPA (tissue plasminogen activator), a potentially breakthrough protein that could dissolve blood clots as a treatment for strokes and thromboses.[15] Wary of grand claims and market fragility, Bush focused on federal programs rather than commercial biotechnology but also placed great faith in collaboration between public and private sectors—to find a cure for AIDS, for instance, even though Bush's critics argued that his response was neither sufficient nor soon enough. With this impetus, federally sponsored biomedical research prospered in the early 1990s, although research involving tissue from aborted fetuses could not be used until Congress lifted its five-year moratorium in 1993.

That same 1992 business report anticipated that the biotech industry would "sizzle in the 90s" after fizzling in the late 1980s, with investment and sales picking up in January 1991, four months after the official launch of the Human Genome Project that was to dominate NIH research over the next decade.[16] However, in contrast to the congressional Office of Technology Assessment's celebration of biotech innovation in 1991, the authors of *Biotechnology in the 1990s* recognized that it was a risky sector to enter, that the speed of start-ups typically outpace public awareness of experimental science, and that federal regulations often clash with corporate aspirations.[17] For example, this 1992 report noted that consumer protection was "fraught with issues for which there are no real answers" because "companies and regulators alike have been caught in a bind over how loose or tight regulations of biotechnology should be for different areas of application."[18] The need for vigilance is crucial if we recall Martin Heidegger's view that it is impossible to unthink technologies once they are brought into the world and that they always have unpredictable consequences.[19]

This bringing out into the open through increased visibility was a key aspect of technoscience in the 1990s and 2000s, together with a potent mix of reverence for and suspicion of the scientific expertise underpinning it. Federal investment in NIH research remained relatively strong, despite moves by the George W. Bush administration to streamline the institutes. The NIH director in the early 2000s, Elias Zerhouni, saw the institute's research as "the engine for the biomedical future," but medical and political leaders repeated the need to improve communication between researchers, practitioners, and the public. Even Zerhouni believed it was "time for a new vision" for translational and clinical science.[20]

By way of contrast, media coverage of the 1990s was usually positive about private-sector biotech breakthroughs, linked to the excitement of recent start-ups such as Amgen (est. 1983) and Gilead Sciences (est. 1987), which joined the more established companies Genentech and Biogen to make California the epicenter of biotechnological research. The rapid growth of Silicon Valley in the southern San Francisco Bay Area was at the core of this tech acceleration. A 2005 report argued that this "knowledge intensive" sector, supported by a porous relationship between universities and industry, was "yet to reach its anticipated potential," mainly because what has since become known as health tech was overshadowed by information technology in terms of scale and revenue, at least until the 2010s.[21]

Health tech research in Silicon Valley initially focused on medical devices. However, by the millennium, over five hundred bioscience companies in the Bay Area had begun to draw on collaboration between medical geneticists, molecular biologists, and computer scientists, stimulated by revenue growth of 250 percent.[22] The adventurism of Bay Area companies sometimes led to wild ideas, including entrepreneur Peter Thiel's backing of blood transfusion therapy trials as "a pathway to radical life extension" and the interest of Elon Musk's Neuralink in brain implants.[23] The arrest of Elizabeth Holmes in 2018 for fraudulent claims about microscale blood testing and her company's neglect for patient safety shook Silicon Valley adventurism that had seemed unstoppable in the "Age of Unicorns," as *Fortune* magazine dubbed the culture of start-ups worth more than $1 billion.[24] Neither the Holmes scandal of 2018 nor her jail sentence five years later marked the end of acceleration, but they offered cautionary lessons. Holmes's company Theranos proved not to be the "laboratory of the future" that Vice-President Biden had hailed in 2015, and her public exposure was a setback for women entrepreneurs seeking to break into a white male–dominated industry.[25]

Imaginative writers and filmmakers were quicker to spot the reckless and self-serving behavior that helped fuel the acceleration of marketplace biotechnology. Cultural critiques of technocapitalism emerged in the late 1980s and early 1990s, particularly via the cyberpunk subgenre of science fiction and its offshoot biopunk, and these critiques of the dystopian dangers of Big Tech broadened after the millennium. An illustration of this trend is Dave Eggers's *The Circle* (2013), a near-future novel that exposes the insidious mental health effects of a surveillance-oriented Silicon Valley tech world masquerading as an open frontier. In the novel, the promise of the Google-like tech company The Circle to reveal the "TruYou" is a cautionary example of the "co-option of the language of creativity by corporate capitalism," foreshadowing the mission statement of the Silicon Valley firm BetterUp, founded that same year with the belief that "well-being and peak performance go hand in hand."[26] In its critique of the socially regressive potential of disruptive technologies (which often arrive on the market before the behavioral changes they may trigger have been fully assessed), *The Circle* reveals how surveillance capitalism fails to address existential questions.[27] To preserve good mental health within this tech-saturated world, individuals must grapple with the complex logic and many lures of capitalism. In responding to Eggers's view that such disruptive technologies are a "fast-flowing river that can't be turned back," this book examines how these conflicts play out within what Susan

Squier calls the "biomedical imaginary" at the confluence of industry technoscience, state governance, and cultural mediations.[28]

Millennial Biomedical Horizons

In assessing the complex relationship between the biomedical industry and federal politics, this book takes the 1990s as the horizon for understanding the entanglement of technoscience and American culture in the first two decades of this century and its consequences for mental health. The brain sciences were especially influential in embedding the biomedical imaginary in everyday life. Notably, the American Psychiatric Association's third (1980) and fourth (1994) editions of the *Diagnostic and Statistical Manual of Mental Disorders* steered away from psychoanalytic language toward a more organic lexicon, a shift that chimed with the Clinton administration's view that mental illness could—and should, if it was to reach parity—be treated as a version of brain disease. If we add to this perspective the portrayal in science fiction and film of cyborgs as integrated systems of neuronal and physiological networks, it is clear that in the 1990s there was a major re-navigation of conventional notions of selfhood in an accelerating technological climate.[29] This move beyond Cartesianism became possible, according to Nikolas Rose and Joelle Abi-Rached, because "a number of key mutations—conceptual, technological, economic, and biopolitical—enabled the neurosciences to leave the enclosed space of the laboratory and gain traction in the world outside."[30]

Instead of being "a face drawn in sand at the edge of the sea" slowly erased by the tide, as Michel Foucault famously closed his 1966 book *The Order of Things*, in the 1990s scientific ambitions scaled up and tested the boundaries and stability of selfhood like never before in modern history.[31] Ethical debates were central to the renegotiation of life itself, to evoke the title of Rose's 2007 book *The Politics of Life Itself*, especially when it came to questions of an individual's health and well-being. At times, these prospects took on scary forms shadowed by the ghosts of Icarus, Prometheus, and Frankenstein, provoking fears that geneticists were dangerously tampering with nature, perhaps more insidiously than in the 1940s when humanity for the first time had the potential to destroy itself with the development of the atom bomb. If, as Joseph Masco argues, the bomb "inverted the definitions of health and security, remaking them from positive values into an incremental calculus of death," then the biotech revolution of the post–Cold War 1990s offered redemption in promising to repair and enhance human life, at least to its proponents.[32] Yet this beneficent promise was overshadowed by what sociologist Michael Mulkay calls the potentially "monstrous changes that would inevitably follow if scientists were permitted to step beyond the boundary of legitimate conduct and to use living human individuals as experimental subjects."[33] In September 2019, British prime minister Boris Johnson recalled these millennial fears in an otherwise pro-tech speech to the United Nations General Assembly. He attacked "anti-scientific pessimism" while evoking the myth of Prometheus, whom the gods punished for stealing fire. "What will synthetic biology stand for?" asked Johnson provocatively. "Restoring our lives and our eyes with miracle regeneration of the tissues . . . or will it bring terrifying limbless chickens to our table? Will nanotechnology help us to beat disease, or will it leave tiny robots to replicate in the crevices of our cells?"[34]

Nikolas Rose shows how this "age of marvellous yet troubling new medical possibilities" generated "hopes and fears, expectation and trepidation, celebration and condemnation" regarding the technologies of biopower.[35] Although the 1990s began with a bold federal plan to improve the nation's health and reduce health disparities, as embodied in the ambitious Healthy People 2000 initiative, the uneven relationship between federal governance and industry innovation left the door open for a normalized biotechnological future at odds with public repulsion "at the prospect of genetically modifying the human species."[36] The *New York Times* symbolized this bifurcation on the first day of the new millennium, calling the "genetic future" both "tantalizing and disturbing" because biotech developments were giving humanity new ways "to play God."[37] These quotations reveal a gulf between the technical language of molecular science and a more diffuse understanding among the general public, yet they also underline the historical impact of the biosciences when "big things" were being envisioned, to quote Clinton's speech at the California Institute of Technology of January 2001.

In its interrogation of this confluence of policy and science, *Transformed States* sees the 1990s as a key phase of a thirty-year period when thinkers, writers, researchers, and practitioners engaged widely with biotechnological ambitions, applications, and analyses. Yet this trend was often accompanied by fears that an overreliance on technological solutions would jeopardize the "kinder, gentler nation" George H. W. Bush wished to return to, as he nostalgically described in his presidential nomination speech of August 1988 as the Cold War began to thaw. Within this context, the accelerating phase of the biosciences takes us from the beginning of the Decade of the Brain to the early months of the COVID-19 pandemic. In the mid-2020s, many of the future prospects that were envisaged in the late twentieth century are already with us, even as the global health emergency of 2020–2022 suggests that capitalist medicine and pandemic preparedness fall significantly short of the bioscientific aspirations of the premillennial period.[38]

This stark reality contrasts with the mythical cast of biology as a "science of becoming," particularly for those who imagine an expansive horizon that in which health limitations have eventually been overcome.[39] We might glimpse here a positive realization of the Heideggerian concept of "unthought" as "a burst of energy which transforms the tranquil order." Alternatively, we might follow Italian philosopher Giorgio Agamben's Heideggerian reading of existential anxiety that stems from recognizing that in our subjection to technology we are, in fact, "nothing and nowhere," a view that echoes Paul Virilio's vision of a tech-saturated world in which reality tips over into "electronic nothingness."[40] Importantly, though, by holding the kinetic and melancholic sides of Heidegger's thought in creative tension, N. Kathryn Hayles reminds us that technological problems raise issues of value, meaning, and purpose that undergird the "coevolution of humans and technics."[41]

If biotechnology came out of the laboratory in the 1990s to infiltrate everyday life, then it did so within a tech nexus that pushed many Americans to become reliant on technology. Eugene Thacker argues that "in its current state, we can describe biotech not as an exclusively 'biological' field, but as an intersection between bio-science and computer science," spanning a range of technical specializations that are only broadly comprehensible to the public.[42] Perhaps for this reason, baby boomer Clinton embraced this interconnected sphere by emphasizing the imminent medical benefits of biotechnological innovation "[that] has produced life-saving drugs that dissolve blood clots in heart attack victims and treat anemia in patients suffering from chronic kidney failure. It has helped produce disease-resistant plants, more nutritious foods, effective waste treatment systems, and methods to clean and protect the environment."[43] In this November 1995 speech, Clinton was looking to protect the patents of biotech companies so that American innovation on "the leading edge of change" could avoid imitation by international competitors, to quote his successor George W. Bush, who proclaimed the first National Biotechnology Week in May 2001.[44] However, Clinton recognized the need to safeguard citizen well-being in clinical trials (an aspect of his effort to tackle mental illness) and worried that what medical historian Harriet Washington later called "life patents" could have a corrosive effect on health and personal privacy.[45] Given this rhetorical slippage between "patents" and "patients," it is clear that we need to view biomedical research and practice through a multifaceted prism in order to evaluate how physical, digital, and biological networks affect human health holistically, rather than through a narrower lens that focuses on the efficacy of particular biomedical devices and interventions.

More than this, as a facet of what World Economic Forum chair Klaus Schwab calls the fourth industrial revolution, a study of the biotech acceleration compels us to adopt a historical view of its disruptive and creative impact on the bioeconomy: "The mind-boggling innovations triggered by the fourth industrial revolution . . . are pushing the current thresholds of life span, health, cognition and capabilities in ways that were previously the preserve of science fiction. . . . As human beings and as social animals, we will have to think individually and collectively about how we respond to issues such as life extension, designer babies, memory extraction and many more."[46] Whether or not we are "standing at the precipice" of a radically transformed future is a topic *Transformed States* tackles by exploring the health implications of biotechnology at the confluence of science, culture, history, and politics.[47]

One of this book's chief arguments is that cultural mediations are of equal weight to science and politics for understanding the biomedical imaginary, offering a vantage point and a potential praxis for an age of biotech acceleration. There is a risk that imaginative writing and film exaggerates, distorts, or misrepresents technology, which Don DeLillo's 2016 novel *Zero K* pictures as an uncontrollable "force of nature" that "comes blowing over the planet" and leaves nowhere to hide.[48] In speculating about the near future, there is another risk that such texts may retreat from or overly moralize about complex challenges on the horizon rather than seeing them with clear eyes. These are serious risks, but it is important to remember that cultural accounts can offer correctives to adventurist uplift narratives by exploring what values red biotechnology put at stake and charting future paths that might deepen rather than erode democratic values.[49] In emulating this recognition, *Transformed States* seeks an intermedial space in which a bioethical path can emerge between the extremes of technophilia and technophobia. As such, my aim is to replace the caricature of bioethics as lifeless regulation that only appears "when generative action is over" by developing an emergent and rejuvenated mode of bioethics that can balance continuity and change.[50] On this level, rather than echo Foucault's apocalyptic image of a human face in the sand washed away by the tide we can turn to this book's cover image, depicting one among a hundred identical sculptures looking out to sea that comprise Antony Gormley's installation *Another Place* (1997), to suggest that a version of humanity will remain in the face of biotechnological transformation.

Biotechnology and Life Itself

One of the most famous sections of Heidegger's 1954 essay "The Question Concerning Technology" (first translated into English in the mid-1970s) differentiates modern science from its ancient prototype. Heidegger sees the former as an exact science, while he presents the latter as a more capacious, questioning, and even ambiguous sphere that he believes could take us a substantial way toward truth, or *aletheia*. In this model, ancient thought did not make a substantive distinction between theoretical and practical reasoning and poiesis, or the poetic arts. When the severing of these realms took place is open to debate. Bruno Latour argues that an interconnected world view fractured in Europe in the early modern period, accompanied by a turn toward technology that Latour views as "epistemology's poor relation," and that fragmentation was clearly visible by the mid-nineteenth century, when the professionalization of medicine, engineering, and applied sciences segmented epistemologies.[51] Taking a philosophical rather than a historical perspective, Heidegger calls these applied sciences a "challenging forth" in their disguising of truth with instrumental logic, in contrast to the "bringing forth" of imaginative poiesis.[52] From this Heideggerian perspective, technical subjects are distant from theoretical reasoning and aesthetic contemplation because they cannot account for existential questions that surface at times of social turmoil and personal distress.

Heidegger did not propose that we abandon modern science, although he was doubtful that on its own it could reveal what he called *Dasein*, a "being in the world with others" that sees a meaningful realm beyond the strictly empirical. He believed that if technology could open itself up to a broader horizon of truth, free itself from instrumentalism, and begin to regard itself as "in a lofty sense ambiguous," then it might allow us to approach "the mystery of all revealing."[53] Heidegger believed that by supplanting rational thinking with the plenum of human activity, "we shall be able to experience the technological within its own bounds."[54] This puts technology in its epistemological place by tempering its assumed mastery. In Kantian terms, it brings into creative dialogue pure reason, practical reason, and judgment, the latter of which enables cultural practitioners to document, assess, and critique the place and status of technoscience in everyday life.

This is not an easy balance to strike. As technological entanglements deepen, it is difficult for patients, citizens, and critics to find a secure vantage point from which to assess gains and losses without appearing to be Luddites. Yet, as Kevin Aho's collection *Existential Medicine* makes clear, phenomenological aspects of health and illness are always in danger of being outpaced by biomedical instrumentalism.[55] With this in mind, this book seeks a Heideggerian "stepping back" to chart what is revealed and what is hidden in the biotechnological sphere over a consequential thirty years that span the millennium. Heidegger explained stepping back in his 1946 "Letter on Humanism" as a resource that reorients thought away from proceduralism and toward a speculative realm that poses broad existential questions. This resource equips us to both think through health consequences, some of which may be too distant to discern with clarity in our historical moment, and demarcate a space for countering grand designs with grassroots tech practices.[56]

Heidegger did not believe that a turn to philosophy is the solution, but instead advocated "more attentiveness in thinking."[57] His stance prompts us to ask questions about life in its fullness, while emphasizing the importance of reflection, recollection, and deliberation (embodied by the noun *Besinnung*) as important correctives to means-ends practices.[58] What Heidegger did provide are tools that interlink the technological and cultural facets of health and medicine. These tools help us think through the transformation of the self during this phase of biotechnological acceleration, although we should be careful not to fall into the traditional humanist trap of conflating the experiences of differing demographics that have witnessed widening disparities in income levels and health care access since the 1990s. On this issue, it is perhaps surprising, but also heartening, that President George H. W. Bush ended his June 1991 speech at the NIH swearing-in ceremony with two lines of progressive thought. He praised "unsung workers" in laboratories, offices, and hospitals while evoking the twelfth-century physician-philosopher Maimonides, who "spoke of medical practice inspired with soul and filled with understanding."[59] In this speech, Bush coupled science as shared labor with a recognition that the mysteries of human existence are more important than technological solutions. Despite evoking Maimonides as a non-Western spiritual and medical thinker, Bush was not in a philosophical position to articulate the concept of "unconcealment" that Heidegger believed that science, if viewed expansively, reveals about being in the world.[60] British sociologist Anthony Giddens frames this view in plainer terms, arguing in *The Runaway*

World (1999) that modern science in a globalized world endeavors to "colonize the future" through instrumentalism while in the process creating new forms of uncertainty by increasing levels of risk and unpredictability.[61]

We can turn to philosopher Nikolas Rose to probe the "politics of life itself" within the fourth industrial revolution and to appraise "our growing capacities to control, manage, engineer, reshape, and modulate the very vital capacities of human beings as living creatures," before returning to Heidegger through the eyes of postfoundationalist philosopher Richard Rorty.[62] Rose argues that a historicized view of contemporary biotechnology can offer a more expansive vision than a sociological appraisal of health care infrastructures or an epidemiological account of disease and pathology taken in isolation. Set against the view of the human body as an assemblage to be refashioned through a combination of personal design and biomedical intervention, Rose describes this expanded vision as a "molecular vital politics" that uncovers "multiple histories" and "pathways" of "an emergent form of life."[63] Facing the "maximal turbulence" of the millennial years, Rose discerns an enlarged concept of life with respect to reproductive and genetic technologies and identifies two conflicting forces that undergird biopolitics: "On the one hand our very personhood is increasingly being defined by others, and by ourselves, in terms of our contemporary understandings of the possibilities and limits of our corporeality. On the other hand, our somatic individuality has become opened up to choice, prudence, and responsibility, to experimentation, to contestation."[64] Within this conflictual zone of risk and possibility, Rose attempts to spatially map a cartography rather than trace a genealogy.

I agree with Rose that there is "no single point of culmination," temporally speaking, and with his later view that posthumanist discourses tend to "foreclose cultural debates" about "diverse ways of being human persons in our global present," particularly with respect to health inequalities and barriers to health care access.[65] However, I differ from Roses's cartographical approach in my view that temporal transformation is an intrinsic quality of biotechnology as a process of becoming. Whereas a biotech intervention might reconfigure or temporarily halt aging, it does not replace transition with permanence, even though anti-aging surgery may offer the illusion of such. If the primary goal of industrial biotechnology is to devise marketable products that can repair or enhance life, then it is important to recognize that "life" is never a fixed state.[66]

This somatic emphasis of biotechnology raises profound questions about mental health, which might suffer due to biotech interventions just as often as it improves, given the difficulty of avoiding unintended consequences. Rose argues that when "biological life" enters "the domain of decision and choice," we need to understand what it means "to live in an age of biological citizenship, of 'somatic ethics,' and of vital politics."[67] Rose argues that the somatization of ethics in an age of biotechnology means that the "language of biomedicine" shapes the ways in which we "experience, articulate, judge, and act upon ourselves."[68] However, instead of leaving ourselves overexposed to technological forces, Rose shows how an emergent and bottom-up bioethics can help navigate the politics of industry, medicine, science, and government that typically regulate "voices, bodies, needs, and desires."[69]

I will return to Rose's concept of somatic ethics periodically through the book. However, *Transformed States* goes further than Rose's studies by exploring how cultural practitioners project these fantasies and fears onto health, quite often in speculative forms as a means of tackling distinctly American questions of inheritance, transformation, perfectibility, and futurity. In their portrayal of a future dominated by biotech, these speculations often take a pessimistic turn in the literature and film discussed here. Yet they also sometimes return us to an affirmative horizon of ancient science and ancestral medicine that is indistinct from the poetic arts.[70] Even though Rorty did not believe that the two paths of ancient and modern science will ever converge, I argue that biotechnology can raise imminent and emergent questions about identities, values, and rights.[71] Addressing these questions is crucial if we are to meet the responsibilities of government, protect the rights of marginalized groups, and guide the communal possibilities of biohacking, citizen science, and environmental activism as alternative modes of health citizenship. Before discussing the implications for biotechnology in these arenas across the book's eight chapters, it is important to probe deeper into millennial debates about its dangers and benefits.

Redesigning a Posthuman Future

As a forum for addressing these millennial concerns, the Academy of Ideas staged a roundtable event titled "A Posthuman Future?" at University College London's Institute of Education on May 30, 2002. Featuring popular science writer Brian Appleyard (whose book *Brave New Worlds: Genetics and the Human Experience* had just been published), hematologist and director of the Wellcome Institute Mike Dexter, and medical ethicist Raanan Gillon, the roundtable hinged on exchanges between biophysicist Gregory Stock and political theorist Francis Fukuyama. It is worth pausing on the public significance of these two figures. Stock promoted himself as a scientific advisor to the Clinton administration (although there is no evidence in Clinton's papers to support this claim) and he cofounded Signum Biosciences in 2003 (which specializes in small-molecule novel therapeutics and skincare products) and Ecoeos in 2010 (which offers DNA tests to gauge personal susceptibility to environmental toxins), whereas Fukuyama worked for the RAND Corporation in the 1980s and was a leading figure of the neoconservative think tank Project for a New American Century (est. 1997), which promoted "military strength and moral clarity" in shaping "a new century favourable to American principles and interests."[72] These orientations guide their positions on biotechnology: Stock's bright utopian vision of a posthuman future contrasts sharply with Fukuyama's cautious bioconservative approach to Big Tech and genetic engineering.

Stock developed his affirmative view of the transformative effects of technology, as outlined in his book *Metaman: The Merging of Humans and Machines into a Global Superorganism* (1993), with the publication in 2002 of *Redesigning Humans*, in which he argued that "we are on the cusp of profound biological changes, poised to transcend our current form and character on a journey to destinations of new imagination."[73] He saw great promise in the belief that genetic interventions and "human self-design" will transform the current biological order "into a highly selective social process that is far more rapid and effective at spreading successful genes than traditional sexual competition and mate selection."[74] Stock's posthumanist vision may raise the ontological aspirations of *Homo sapiens* by positing a "metaman" with enhanced powers of strength, mobility, and intelligence. But his view is open to parody. For example, in his short story "The Evolution of Human Science" (2000), sci-fi writer Ted Chiang imagines that the future research outcomes of metahumans are available only via "digital neural transfer," while humans are consigned to a second tier from which they will "never make an original contribution to science again."[75]

At a remove from Chiang's meditation on human redundancy, Stock envisions a muscular future human overseeing an era of biotechnological prominence. He emphasizes the potential of new reproductive technologies (while dodging their gender politics) and believes that couples can redesign their futures, arguing that germline engineering will reinforce human continuity, making us "more human" by increasing the chances of living a healthy life. In *Metaman*, he cites the benefits of in vitro fertilization, bone-marrow transplants for infants, and the enhanced chance of healthy survival for babies born three months premature.[76] Stock believes that such developments should never slow, even though President Clinton did not approve the recommendations of the Human Embryo Research Panel about the benefits of generating human embryos for scientifically legitimate research projects.

Taking a more functionalist approach than the National Bioethics Advisory Commission (which Clinton formed in 1995), Stock viewed the millennium as a phase of natality that offered the possibility of moving out of childhood "into a gawky stumbling adolescence," before reaching maturity once we have learned how to manage our new powers "wisely."[77] Bone marrow research on leukemia and immune deficiency disorders were NIH priorities at the millennium (despite difficulties with donor sourcing and patient matching), and Stock worried that a retreat from adventurism would "deaden the human spirit of exploration, taming and diminishing us" rather than fulfilling our ability to inhabit possible futures.[78] In addition to avoiding questions of inequity, Stock did not consider how AI-enhanced technoscience might become so sophisticated that frail human subjects could be redundant in the near future.

Following French theorist Jean Baudrillard, we might envisage a future where technological supremacy hastens the process of humans declining "towards a pure and simple disappearance."[79] It is this bleaker vision to which Francis Fukuyama turned. In contrast to Stock's technoliberal optimism, Fukuyama focused on the political implications of biotechnology. In *Our Posthuman Future* (2002), Fukuyama argued for moral and political control over technoscience, including transnational legislation to restrict or ban research into cloning, echoing the strong anti-cloning stance of Leon R. Kass, chair of the recently formed President's Council on Bioethics, whom Stock had debated heatedly on NPR the previous month.[80] Fukuyama detected in biotechnology similar threats to those that Aldous Huxley and George Orwell portrayed in their dystopian fictions of the 1930s and 1940s, arguing that the possibility of reshaping "what we are will have possibly malign consequences for liberal democracy."[81] This evocation of Huxley's *Brave New World* has many millennial resonances, including a congressional enquiry on human cloning, a George W. Bush speech on stem cell research (delivered shortly after Kass's essay "Preventing a Brave New World" appeared in the *New Republic*), and a manifesto penned by the Christian Wilberforce Forum that sought to preserve "the sanctity of life in a brave new world" by ensuring that "all medical and scientific research is firmly tethered to the moral truth."[82]

As a counter to these conservative opinions, the Huxley evocation highlighted the speculative and cautionary role of imaginative writing as a corrective to ideological positioning. In the combined words of Margaret Atwood and Donna Haraway, this role encourages authors and scriptwriters to let "mad scientists [to] do their worst within the boundaries of our fictions" in an effort to "keep the real ones sane" by following threads and "plucking out fibers in clotted and dense events and practices" to reveal the health effects of biotechnology.[83] Approaching speculative fiction as a narrative mode of bioart that questions technological mastery, the literary and cinematic examples of the following chapters illustrate how that genre can help readers, citizens, and activists develop lateral vision and resistant tactics by probing the geopolitical and health effects of the biotech acceleration.

Fukuyama envisioned three scenarios: pharmaceutical supremacy, a dramatic rise in life expectancy, and bioengineered embryos that shape a child's genetic profile. Detecting dangers in all three, he held to the precautionary principle, believing that governments and health care providers had not yet fully assessed the implications of extending life spans in terms of shifting demographics and economic and ethnic variances in aging populations.[84] He also worried about parents who could not afford to enhance their children's intelligence and socially advantageous characteristics, dividing what Lee Silver calls "Naturals" conceived through traditional sexual interaction from "GenRich" children possessing genetic enhancements that may lead to a new uber-class—a topic to which chapter 2 turns.[85]

Paying little attention to the differing public perceptions of biotechnology, Fukuyama maintained his faith that capitalism is the best available economic and political model, as expounded in his 1989 treatise *The End of History and the Last Man*.[86] His argument is predicated less on calculated risk and more on his belief that genetic determinism denies agency and free will because unfettered biotechnology will forever alter the parameters of human nature. In his 1999 book *The Great Disruption*, he blamed the "information era" for weakening "social bonds and common values holding people together in Western societies" by widening the schism between rich and poor.[87] Whereas Fukuyama is vigilant about protecting his normative view of human nature, driven by his belief that biotech tampering will have disastrous social and cultural consequences from which he envisions no way back. This stance is in sharp contrast to Stock, who reveals the libertarian aspect of his techno-optimism with statements such as "if biological manipulation is indeed a slippery slope, then we are already sliding down that slope now and we may as well enjoy the ride."[88]

Instead of a "free, equal, prosperous, caring, compassionate" posthuman world "with better health care, longer lives, and perhaps more intelligence," Fukuyama envisions a future that is "far more hierarchical and competitive" in which "any notion of 'shared humanity' is lost" as the marketplace disrupts social order in insidious and far-reaching ways.[89] For this reason, he recommended that the federal government develop a robust regulatory framework for biotechnological research "to separate legitimate from illegitimate uses." Although the Federal Trade Commission, the NIH, and presidential advisory committees seek to demarcate bioethical boundaries for scientific research, Fukuyama envisages a compliance framework that spans public and private sectors and requires nation-states to sign up to a far-reaching international accord in order to avoid "the potential moral chasm that such a future opens before us."[90] In contrast, Stock thinks that biotechnologies such as cloning are overregulated— if they do not "arrive through the front door, they will come through the back"— and that humans were irrevocably en route to inhabiting this transformed world.[91]

This notion of a "biological imperative" at a genetic or cellular level was not unique to Stock. It sometimes manifested itself in doctrinaire forms, most notably by a group of self-proclaimed transhumanists linked to the Extropy Institute, which was based in Los Angeles from 1991 to 2006. Via its publication *Extropy: A Journal of Transhumanist Solutions*, which advocates for new and emerging techno-progressive practices that accelerate us into a future world, the British-born philosopher Max More and his Extropy Institute collaborators emphasized rationality and embraced the future, but they also recognized that some technologies can do damage to humans.[92] For this reason, More formulated what he called the proactionary principle:

> People's freedom to innovate technologically is highly valuable, even critical, to humanity. This implies several imperatives when restrictive measures are proposed. Assess risks and opportunities according to available science, not population perception. Account for both the costs of the restrictions themselves, and those of opportunities foregone. Favor measures that are proportionate to the probability and magnitude of impacts, and that have a high expectation value. Protect people's freedom to experiment, innovate, and progress.[93]

Extropy Institute champions tend to downplay the dangers of genetic discrimination and power grabs in favor of an intoxicating mix of futurism, scientism, and risk seeking that privilege biotechnological progress over healing practices. Although other transhumanists like philosopher Nick Bostrom argue that technologies should reduce existential risks, this quest tallies with the transhumanist views that Richard Powers parodied in his 2009 novel *Generosity* through the audacious opinions of genetic adventurist Thomas Kurton: "Enhancement. Why shouldn't we make ourselves better than we are now? We're incomplete. Why leave something as fabulous as life up to chance?"[94] Stock's contribution to *The Transhumanist Reader* amplifies More's mission to defect "a collective wisdom in our action."[95] But in other ways, Extropy Institute dogma strains against Stock's search for next-generation alternatives to conventional health care via precision wellness and environmentalist projects.

In such an agonistic environment it is often difficult to locate the conceptual and ethical middle ground I discussed in the preface that might balance a biological imperative with altruistic conduct, community values, and civil and consumer rights. One reason is because this biological imperative is often caught up in fierce culture wars, in which conservatives such as Fukuyama warn against the risks of a technocratic future and Stock and transhumanists argue that societies have the know-how to use technology wisely and that only useful technologies will prevail. Such dialogues are important markers of how the public understands biotechnology. Yet the following chapters show that in order to move beyond disagreement and rancor, we often need to turn to imaginative reflections on biotechnology, spanning the thirty years from 1990, when Michael Crichton wrote *Jurassic Park*, to 2020, when the first series of the German techno-thriller *Biohackers* aired.

Acceleration and Authenticity

The 2002 debate between Stock and Fukuyama is notable for the universalist yet masculinized language that often accompanies biotech discussion. Donna Haraway is one thinker who adopts an alternative stance when addressing the power networks technology spreads along and the "social relations of domination built into [its] hardware and logics."[96] Haraway is critical of masculinized humanism— "humanity's face has been the face of man . . . legitimate sons with the access to language and the power to represent"—yet she does not see this realm as wholly controlled by scientific and political leaders who dupe the masses into believing that no alternatives to heteronormative technological solutions exist.[97] Instead, Haraway views biotechnology as a "heterogeneous practice that enlists its members in . . . ordinary and astonishing ways" and detects as many "origins, natures, and possibilities" as there are dangers of subjugation.[98] In her 1997 book *Modest_Witness@Second_Millennium*, Haraway seeks to challenge heroic myths of "masterful subjectivity" that often accompany claims about technological progress by attending to subjects who operate beyond hegemonic norms.[99] In a 1989 speech, Haraway boldly stated that "feminist humanity must, somehow, resist representation, resist literal figuration, and still erupt in powerful new tropes, new figures of speech, new turns of historical possibility."[100]

Haraway is neither a full-fledged detractor nor an outright celebrator of tech-noscience. She discerns fluid spaces in which individuals can enact different kinds of mobility that may have transformative health implications at personal and community levels. What Haraway calls the "self-activating body" allows for healthy balance and dynamic movement but also offers an emergent health citizenship that is both personal and relational.[101] Postcolonial scholar Julietta Singh terms this kind of emergence "dehumanism," by which she means "an unexpected practice of recuperation, of recovering those forms of life . . . where we might find other ways of generative living," including the practice of bio-hacking that features prominently in this book's second half.[102] Singh's idea of "radical dwelling" as "an act of learning to live otherwise" is one model of how authenticity—which is under twin assaults by discourses of mastery and information overload—can actively reemerge in ways that improve wellness.[103] From this perspective, we must resist overpredicting or renouncing biotechnology, looking instead to evaluate its moral, cultural, and medical relevance in the unfolding present without losing scale or proportion.[104]

Writing in 2016, Klaus Schwab stated that the biosciences are pushing us toward the "new ethical frontier of ethics" by forcing us to interrogate what it means to be "better": "Should we use the staggering advances in biology only to cure disease and repair injury, or should we also make ourselves better humans? If we accept the latter, we risk turning parenthood into an extension of the consumer society, in which case might our children become commoditized as made-to-order objects of our desire? And what does it mean to be 'better'? To be disease free? To live longer? To be smarter? To run faster? To have a certain appearance?"[105] One pressing concern of this biotech age is how to anchor authenticity in such a fluid environment. For industry experts Paul and Joyce Schoemaker, this involves balancing the entrepreneurial drive for innovation with "regulatory oversight and moral compass."[106] In contrast, for Canadian environmentalist Bill McKibben, the task is to remain connected to the natural world as a refuge from tech saturation that often seems to trigger anxieties as we try to keep up with information flow.[107] McKibben recognizes that speed counts in some instances, such as the need for government agencies to respond quickly to the threat of global warming, but he argues that often advanced biomedical technologies aim to "blot out unpleasantness, to dilute confusion, distress, unhappiness, loneliness" rather than recalibrate the moral compass.[108] His argument is not as conspiratorial as Virilio's dystopian vision of an "arrhythmic" technocapitalist world full of fear, division, and "stressful claustrophobia."[109] Instead, McKibben echoes Virilio's search for lateral vision and promotes biophilia as an aspect of authentic living, but without seeing humans as the core of nature. This view approximates to Virilio's "dispersed moral philosophy" that tilts his pessimism toward what anthropologist Anna Tsing later called the "arts of living on a damaged planet."[110] In doing so, McKibben evokes a renewed sense of community attuned to the rhythm of nature that offers a refuge from the deleterious health consequences of tech overload.

McKibben was just one figure among many in the millennial moment who addressed questions of relativism, knowledge, and citizenship. Postfoundationalist thinkers of the 1980s and 1990s also voiced these concerns, prompting Richard Rorty to argue that reliance on metaphysical notions of truth and knowledge is increasingly untenable, just as the search for sustainable values is ever more pressing. In Rorty's rekindling of civic engagement in his 1998 book *Achieving Our Country*, he distinguished an affirmative cultural left both from a beleaguered left that observes more than it acts and the more disruptive views of the French post-structuralists who ostensibly shared his project.[111] For this affirmative vision, Rorty returned to the pragmatism of John Dewey and William James to develop an active ethical perspective that can work through the democratic potential of scientific humanism while sidestepping the criticism that this is just utilitarianism in disguise.[112] Such a philosophical move casts bioscience and health politics in a broader frame of reference than congressional health care finance debates and technocratic policymaking typically do. We can see echoes of pragmatic humanism in Nikolas Rose's emergent theory of somatic ethics as a mode of reinvigorated agency, but it is still difficult to clear a philosophical space without either evading technological questions or permitting technology to control the discourse.

A partial response to the biotech acceleration is to be found in a rejuvenated sense of community. Political journalist Thomas Friedman, for example, resurrects the ghost of moral humanism in the face of anti-humanist theories, claiming that "the best solutions for helping people build resilience and propulsion in the age of accelerations are things you cannot download but have to upload the old-fashioned way—one human to another human at a time."[113] The return of humanism that we glimpse in Friedman's writing is less the radical dwelling of Singh (see chapter 6) or the planetary humanism of McKibben (see chapter 8) and more a belief that good health and meaningful connectivity are necessary for combating social isolation in the face of tech acceleration—a view that health leaders in the Biden administration agreed with (see the conclusion).[114] In his reengagement in public life and an open culture, Friedman echoes Rorty in some respects, although Friedman recognizes the need for a vantage point whereas Rorty places agency over spectatorship. This position not only justifies the possibility of reforging democratic communities but also revives liberal hope for the future that chimes with both the progressive priorities of the Clinton administration and sociologist Robert Bellah's concept of a "good society."[115]

This theme of future hope runs through the chapters of *Transformed States* as a counterpoint to the dystopian speculation of writers and critics who worry that a functional approach to biotechnology disguises a host of ethical problems. Rorty sees Heideggerian hope as embedded in a more expansive and less functional view of science, although he is suspicious of Heidegger's melancholic mode of thought.[116] I return to this subject in the conclusion through the filter of what Bellah calls a "politics of imagination" that enables us to think beyond subject positions and seemingly inevitable horizons. This theme also returns us to

Nikolas Rose's recognition that the multiple biotechnological emergences of the 1990s traveled across state and national boundaries, thereby complicating Bellah's vision of a good society to be achieved inwardly, not through an elusive quest for a "vital center" (to recall Arthur Schlesinger Jr.'s Cold War concept) but through a moral transformation of public institutions that have both a national and global responsibility.[117]

In tracing these biotech pathways, the book's first two chapters focus on the politics of diversity and sameness within the spheres of genomics and stem cell research, then turns in chapters three and four to equally dramatic advances in brain science and AI-enhanced robotics that contribute both to biotechnological innovation and an expansion of the biomedical imaginary. I move from the biotech building blocks of genetics and consciousness in these two parts to a cumulative reading of the health effects of red biotechnology in the book's second half in terms of life spans, identities, and ecologies. As such, chapters 5 and 6 switch the focus to gerontology and gender transitioning to explore tensions between personal agency and health care access, before closing in the seventh and eighth chapters with the most consequential crises of our time relating to pandemic culture and planetary health, topics that challenge the heroic rhetoric of 1990s biotechnology and at the same time valorize vaccine and bioremediation technologies. To advance my argument that both perspective and praxis are needed in an age of biotech acceleration, this second half navigates micro and macro scales in which interventions at cellular, chromosomal, and neuronal levels implicate questions of personal identity, group agency, and global debates about how best to protect democratic values and nurture ecosystems in the face of epistemological uncertainty.

Throughout the book, readings of imaginative texts produced during these three decades intersect with debates in public policy, scientific research, and health care from sources such as industry reports, longitudinal studies, government papers, congressional hearings, public speeches, and media accounts. Some texts will be familiar, like Margaret Atwood's *Oryx and Crake* and the high-profile films *Gattaca* and *Avatar*; others will be less so, such as the anti-ageism film *Advantageous* and Daniel Suarez's biopunk novel *Change Agent*. But all these texts reflect on the sway of the biomedical imaginary over everyday life and act as correctives to the typically heroic tenor of biotech. A focus on fiction and film allows me to explore how technology plays out in narrative form and in moments of dramatic confrontation that often expose conflicting realities.

This brings the discussion up to 2020, the millennial horizon for many national and transnational health aspirations, although some of these goals are unfulfilled given the personal, social, and economic devastation of the COVID-19 pandemic. In this climate, *Forbes* writer Bruce Booth describes 2020 as a paradoxical year of "agonizing tragedy" and "buoyant optimism," and even the techno-enthusiast magazine *Wired* (est. 1993) now offers more scrutiny of the political and cultural power Big Tech wields.[118] As the fourth part of this book shows, the early 2020s offer few consolations in the face of colliding domestic and global crises. However, if a somatic ethics is both achievable and enabling in guiding us toward and beyond 2030 (as my conclusion considers), then we should look to assemble it from elements of Heidegger's interconnected thinking, Dewey's developmental pragmatism, and an ecological attention to the codeterminants of health. Not only might such an emergent position avoid the polarizing politics of the Stock-Fukuyama debate about the merits of a posthuman future, it might also help us avoid premature judgments about whether things are getting better or worse and work through the possibility of an affirmative bioethics.

PART ONE

GENETIC STATES

1   *Genomics, Diversity, and the Millennial Imagination*

On May 18, 1997, President Clinton delivered a rousing speech to the graduating class of the historically Black Morgan State University in Baltimore, encouraging the new graduates to see themselves as prepared for "the rapidly unfolding new reality of the twenty-first century."[1] The president praised Morgan State for producing most of the Black professionals in Maryland and spoke of new federal investments in education, health care, and science research. "This is a magic moment" he declared, "but like all moments it will not last forever." In affirming the "rich diversity" of American society, Clinton asked the graduating class

> to imagine a new century, full of its promise, molded by science, shaped by technology, powered by knowledge. These potent transforming forces can give us lives fuller and richer than we have ever known. They can be used for good or ill, [so] we must work to master these forces with vision and wisdom and determination. . . . We are now embarking on our most daring explorations, unraveling the mysteries of our inner world and charting new routes in the conquest of disease. We have not and we must not shrink from exploring the frontiers of science. But as we consider how to use the fruits of discovery, we must also never retreat from our commitment to human values, the good of society, our basic sense of right and wrong.[2]

The speech was impassioned but poised. Its rhetoric balanced the excitement of "transforming forces" and the quest to unravel the "mysteries of our inner world" with, on the one hand, wisdom and moral value and, on the other, the recognition that graduates of a historically Black public university are vital in ensuring that the future is shaped by a variety of modalities and accents, not by a white power elite. That President Clinton spoke about this millennial topic to Morgan State University graduates—instead of the more obvious audience at Johns Hopkins University, the premier place for medical and health research just two miles to the west—was part of his strategy "to inspire dialogue and conversation both about the issue of race itself . . . and the issues and values that bring us together."[3]

    The president's commencement address embodied three priorities that are national in character but that have broader transnational implications, mirroring the White House Office of Science and Technology Policy report, *Science and Technology Shaping the Twenty-First Century*, which went to Congress a month before his Morgan State University speech.[4] The first priority was the Clinton administration's commitment to creating new educational, social, and economic opportunities for Black Americans in an effort to eradicate racial discrim-

ination, as embodied in the president's initiative on race, titled One America in
the 21st Century.[5] Clinton was keen to stress Black health as a national priority.
To combat economic and racial disparities, he emphasized technological innovation, social opportunity, and community dialogues on race, themes he rhetorically united in an October 1996 campaign speech in Portland, Oregon, where
he asked "If we build a bridge to the future, is it going to be wide enough and
strong enough for every American to walk across?"[6] It also, more specifically,
linked to the fact that the Clinton administration named Baltimore an Empowerment Zone in 1994 and awarded the city a ten-year grant to stimulate jobs and
build community capacity during the tenure of the city's first Black mayor, Kurt
Schmoke.

The second source of the speech balances the twin emphases on opportunity
and equality by means of the president's interest in fostering what University of
California sociologist Robert Bellah called the "good society." In his 1991 book
of that name, Bellah and his collaborators argued that the economic boom that
followed World War II was predicated on rapid technological expansion that set
in motion "long-term processes affecting work, economic life, and the nation's
institutional structure as a whole" that continue to shape American aspirations.[7]
Bellah and Clinton wished to ensure that technological acceleration did not cast
off moral anchors, prompted by their beliefs that a good society relies on an ecosystem of intersecting communities that link "concerns for social justice, economic vitality, and environmental integrity" and enable meaningful public
debate.[8] This is a more inclusive social model than the one George H. W. Bush
described that year based on "common decency and commitment," although it is
important to note an exceptionalist quality to Bellah's concept of "good" that
emerges at times as a form of "civil religion."[9] Such exceptionalism (linked to Bellah's Episcopalian beliefs) contrasts with the secular approach of economist John
Kenneth Galbraith in The Good Society: The Humane Agenda, written five years
later, which posits achievable over utopian goals. Heeding Bellah's advice of 1991
that institutional reform is more important than the search for an elusive vital
center, Clinton contemplated giving a "good society" speech in early 1997, which
he noted in correspondence is "after all, what we are trying to establish."[10]
Although he did not deliver such a speech, Clinton recognized that rising inequalities jeopardize democratic values and that, in the words of Galbraith, "the good
society fails when democracy fails."[11]

Neither Bellah nor Clinton were anti-scientific. In fact, Clinton's credentials
as a technocrat can be glimpsed in his establishment of the National Science and
Technology Council in 1993, his emphasis in the Morgan State speech on a technological bridge to the future, his efforts to "raise scientific and technological literacy of all Americans" by creating a Technology Literacy Challenge Fund, and
his belief that economic growth was in large part "because of the ability of science and technology to rifle through our ordinary lives," as he described in a
January 2000 speech at California Institute of Technology.[12] Clinton's interests were strengthened by his vice president, Al Gore, who had published on

biotechnology as a senator, arguing that the pace of biotechnological development contrasts sharply with "the lethargy of the policy debate" and that robust
public conversations are needed to address "questions of how best to distribute
information, to empower others to use it."[13] Clinton's and Gore's opinions chimed
with the view of the Office of Science and Technology Policy that science is an
"endless resource" (recalling Vannevar Bush's 1945 report *Science: The Endless
Frontier*) and with Bellah's call for public debate—although Bellah was not always
in favor of Clinton's centrist and at times populist approach.[14]

However, Bellah, Clinton, and Gore were each concerned about the sustainable health of the nation (in his Cal Tech speech, Clinton spoke about caring for
those with disabilities and for the environment) and worried that unrestrained
technology might have "irreversible and dangerous impacts on communities," in
Gore's words.[15] Clinton foreshadowed what Gore later called the "complex ethical calculus" of responsible biotechnology when he warned that "being in the
grip of a big idea that is wrong can be absolutely disastrous."[16] This strong stance
opened Clinton and Gore to charges of bias toward *good* government-sanctioned
biotech that serves the public interest over *bad* commercial technologies, even
though biotech corporations such as Genentech had devoted significant spending
to research and development (compared to the spending of pharmaceutical companies) without extracting the excessive profits of Big Pharma.[17] I will return to
tensions between market forces and public interest periodically through the
book, illustrating that even within a single presidential term, biotechnology was
paradoxically seen as the equivalent of "putting a man on the moon" and the
opening up of a Pandora's box of unpredictable forces, especially without robust
government regulations that Galbraith argued were the social foundation of a
good society.[18]

If the first two sources of the Morgan State speech derived from Clinton's
commitment to balance opportunity and equality, the third source coupled pressing questions of bioethics and genetics. A trigger for these questions was the
leaked news in February 1997—three months before Clinton's graduation
address—that scientists at the University of Edinburgh's hub for molecular biology, the Roslin Institute, had cloned a domestic sheep. News of Dolly, the first
cloned mammal from an adult somatic cell, broke seven months after she was
born, causing media shock waves across the Atlantic. While embryologist Ian
Wilmut, who led the Roslin Institute cloning experiment, claimed that this
successful experiment in somatic cell nuclear transfer "will enable us to study
genetic diseases for which there is presently no cure," *Time* magazine jumped on
the sensationalist bandwagon by responding with the headline "Will There Ever
Be Another You?," while the *New York Times* warned that "Fiction Becomes True
and Dreaded Possibilities Are Raised."[19]

The Dolly case posed the issue of the accuracy of media reporting on genetic
breakthroughs and how media "genohype" shapes public attitudes.[20] The fear in
some quarters was that if scientists could clone Dolly, the door was open to
cloning humans—a scenario that might lead to unregulated experiments with

far-reaching bioethical and sociocultural consequences with respect to genetic discrimination and biomedical consumerism.[21] In defending the breakthrough, Wilmut asserted that the sheep cloning experiment "doesn't have anything to do with creating copies of human beings" and that he was "not haunted by what I do."[22] Nonetheless, there was so much clamor in the media and among government officials and religious leaders that Wilmut coauthored an article titled "Don't Clone Humans!," while the House of Representatives passed a bill seeking to criminalize the practice of somatic cell nuclear transfer to clone human embryos.[23] When the Democrats regained control of the Senate after a brief Republican majority, the Human Cloning Prohibition Act of 2001 marked a phase of intense federal anxiety (including a January 2002 warning by the National Academy of Sciences) about where lines should be drawn in the ethics and science of embryonic research (although the bill did not pass).[24]

Sensing these mounting congressional anxieties, President Clinton was sympathetic to genetic advancements but was mindful of existential and ethical concerns about cloning. As soon as the Dolly story broke, Clinton formed a commission with the aim of devising a policy within ninety days. He continued to highlight cloning over the next three years (although he was careful to distinguish human cloning from therapeutic cloning at the cellular level) and it remained a priority of the executive branch into the new century.[25] Cloning also featured in George W. Bush's early addresses and was the initial focus of the President's Council on Bioethics that Bush formed in November 2001. The council, which was led by University of Chicago ethicist Leon Kass, produced a report in 2002, *Human Cloning and Human Dignity*, that summed up ten months of debate as to whether there should be tighter regulations or a national moratorium on cloning research. Echoing George W. Bush's brand of conservatism, which led him to be more skeptical of scientific authority than his father, Kass framed the council's report squarely in moral terms: Bush referred to it in a 2002 speech as the "fresh breeze of sensible moral judgment, clearing away the fog of unthinking and easygoing relativism."[26] In its focus on "fundamental aspects of our humanity," the report posited that "legislative debates over human cloning raise large questions about the relationship between science and society, especially about whether society should exercise ethical and prudential control over biomedical technology and the conduct of medical genetic research."[27]

Set against this context, this first chapter analyzes the confluence of ideas in Clinton's Morgan State address with respect to scientific advancement, community identity, the politics of genetic engineering, the specter of techno-eugenics, and the role of government regulation in order to identify a vantage point between the extremes of technophilia and technophobia that can foster a bioethics that is both responsible and imaginative. Although we can criticize Clinton for not doing more to highlight technological inequalities along race and class lines, I argue that in tracing interconnections between these domains of knowledge, rhetoric, and practice we gain a more detailed picture of the medical applications and cultural implications of biotechnology at the forefront of debates about national health and democratic values.[28] My discussion of genetics in this first part of the book is a central aspect of thirty years of biotech acceleration, but this chapter focuses especially on the six years that bridged the millennium, 1997 to 2003, as an intense phase in which ethical concerns about human cloning offset the quest to read the genetic "book of human inheritance." In this contested terrain, congressional politicians often took an anti-cloning stance in contrast to the likes of biophysicist Gregory Stock, who touted the social benefits of responsible human cloning.[29]

The topic of cloning dominates the middle section of this chapter, flanked by two pivotal discussions. The first section focuses on the scope and achievements of the Human Genome Project, dubbed "the first great technological triumph of the twenty-first century," and the final section turns to the controversial science of gene editing in which DNA can be modified and then reinserted to create protective mutations, bringing the scientific and ethical debates up to the late 2010s.[30] By bookending debates about animal and human cloning with two faces of bioengineering—the first beneficent, the second riskier—we can broaden the mental and physical health implications of medical biotechnology. It is also important to reflect on how debates reverberated in the cultural sphere as potential correctives to partisan projections about genetic science via analysis of two speculative fictions: Michael Marshall Smith's *Spares* (1996) and Margaret Atwood's *Oryx and Crake* (2003). These scientific and literary intersections establish the epistemological and ontological horizon of chapter 2, which frames questions of life and nature with sharp disagreements about reproductive technologies and fetal personhood.

The Promises of the Human Genome Project

On March 23, 1990, four months before his proclamation of the Decade of the Brain, George H. W. Bush sent to congressional leaders his Annual Report on International Activities in Science and Technology in which he reflected on fiscal year 1989. Bush reminded Congress of the unprecedented pace of change of both science and foreign affairs. The fates of the two were interlinked, he thought, because with the fall of the Berlin Wall the United States would be able to cooperate fully with countries like Hungary, following the establishment in 1990 of the independent Regional Environmental Center for Central and Eastern European in Budapest. For Bush, the ideological spirit of "independence, democratization, and economic growth" undergirded these new collaborations, together with a more nebulous "desire to preserve and improve humanity's common heritage" that he associated with "the Revolution of '89."[31] This open spirit was underlined by the efforts to make the membership of the Council of Advisors on Science and Technology as "wide-ranging as possible" in terms of expertise, led by physicist D. Allan Bromley, who was keen to prioritize science education and translational research.[32]

Speaking in a year in which Congress spent $3.5 billion on biotechnology, Bush stressed the "global resource" of the science community, especially for a megaproject on the human genome for which he had signed appropriations in 1989 to support the ambitions of the National Institutes of Health (NIH) to understand how gene combinations create a unique set of human DNA.[33] However, the president warned Congress that the post–Cold War global marketplace was increasingly competitive and that he was wary of technological research in Japan and the expanded European community. To ensure that the United States remained a "world leader" on this "new frontier," he offset these challenges by encouraging "greater cross-fertilization" between private biotechnology companies and federally sponsored research to enlarge the country's scientific footprint and to ensure industrial growth.[34] Building on the Technology Transfer Act of 1986 and President Reagan's 1987 executive order that encouraged "exchange of research personnel between government laboratories and industrial firms," Bush's combination of cooperation and competition shaped the Human Genome Project from its inception.[35]

This grand publicly funded project stemmed from a May 1985 meeting at the University of California, Santa Cruz, chaired by its chancellor, Robert Sinsheimer. A biologist trained at the Massachusetts Institute of Technology in the 1940s, Sinsheimer was keen to establish a sequencing institute to propel Santa Cruz to the forefront of biotechnological research and development. Sinsheimer was captivated by the collective search for scientific control over "processes that have known only the mindless discipline of natural selection for two billion years," as he had stated twenty years earlier at the dawn of what he called an "age of transition."[36] Delegates at that 1985 meeting thought the complete sequencing of the human genome was achievable, although it would require effort on a huge scale to complete. Sinsheimer was ultimately frustrated in his effort to found a Santa Cruz sequencing institute, but the 1985 meeting took the international scientific community stem cell research to "the edge of knowing."[37] The Human Genome Project launched on October 1, 1990, across research teams in Britain, France, and Japan (joined later by teams in Germany and China), following five years of profile raising by prominent scientists such as NIH director James Wyngaarden and media reports that proclaimed that the United States was "on the brink of ushering in a golden age of gene therapy."[38]

The medical geneticist Robert Cook-Deegan claims in his 1995 book *The Gene Wars* that the "upper reaches of the Reagan administration, even more than most, were almost oblivious to biomedical research." However, congressional leaders and the George H. W. Bush administration were generally favorable to genomic initiatives and Wyngaarden successfully secured enough of a rolling budget to launch the project.[39] Before the launch, the Office of Technology Assessment weighed up the optimum size and speed of genome projects, but the scale of the transnational endeavor and projected fifteen-year timeline remained daunting, especially because genetics was still in its maturation phase.[40]

Coordination was achieved via a Genome Database held at Johns Hopkins University's School of Medicine that housed the gene map. This was initially funded by the U.S. Department of Energy and the NIH and plans were to make it publicly accessible as soon as practicable. Cook-Deegan argues that the project was less a holistic endeavor across its lifespan and more "the actions of many people, often working without knowledge of others treading on convergent paths," as symbolized by the movement of the Genome Database to Toronto in 1999 and then to North Carolina in 2003, circling back to Johns Hopkins in 2008.[41] He notes, though, that the global project linking the operations of sixteen international technology centers was vital to ensuring that genetic diversity was treated panoramically and to staving off criticisms that the project disguised vested interests that benefited the United States.[42]

Founded in 1988, the Human Genome Organization, located in Geneva, Switzerland, offered a global governance framework, with the Department of Energy and the NIH providing oversight of the American wing.[43] From 1993 through the early 2000s, the NIH side of the project was led by the first two directors of the National Human Genome Research Institute, molecular biologist James D. Watson (a co-discoverer of the DNA double helix in 1953) and geneticist Francis Collins, while David Galas initially oversaw the project for the Department of Energy. Their common goal was to address fundamental questions in pure science. The expectation was that the sequencing would lead geneticists and molecular biologists to a better understanding of hereditary disease that would enable them to develop forms of evidence-based medicine. In an early study, *Perilous Knowledge* (1993), Tom Wilkie saw this project goal as the "new hope of liberation from the shadows of cancer, heart disease, autoimmune diseases such as rheumatoid arthritis, and some psychiatric illnesses," in addition to identifying the genetic causes of muscular dystrophy, cystic fibrosis (the faulty gene for which had been identified in 1989), and Alzheimer's disease (this remained an elusive but pressing quest, given the disclosure of Reagan's condition in 1993).[44] Genetic research also had the potential to alleviate mental illness, as a *Science* editorial remarked in 1989: "The costs of mental illness, the difficult civil liberties problems they cause, the pain to the individual, all cry out for an early solution that involves prevention, not caretaking."[45] Even though it was unclear how gene therapy might eliminate deleterious psychological states that stem from complex codeterminants, not all of which are hereditary in origin, it is significant that mental health became a federal priority later in the decade, marked by the first surgeon general's report on the subject and an inaugural White House Conference on Mental Health in the summer of 1999, which recognized mental illness as a variety of physical disease that required early treatment to rectify what some physicians were calling a "system in crisis."[46]

Geneticist J. Craig Venter shared this "hope of liberation" by challenging the speed of the publicly funded Human Genome Project following his departure from the NIH in 1992 to work on automatic gene sequencing in the private sector. Initially via the Institute for Genomic Research and then from 1998 under the auspices of the new California company Celera Genomics, Venter's bioinformatics team pitted itself against the publicly funded project by practicing a shotgun technique (involving the shredding and reconstituting of gene sequences) and promising to speed up the public release of genomic data. Venter called this surge in research the "great gene gold rush" that was linked to his audacious decision to offer himself up as a human subject for full DNA sequencing, making him "the first person in history to be able to gaze upon his own genetic legacy," in his words.[47] This declaration was a significant reason why the federal project accelerated to ensure that its commercial rival did not outpace it and to prevent a monopoly on genomic data that might limit public access.

Tensions between public funding and private interests ran through the Human Genome Project, despite a joint public-private declaration from Collins and Venter that the genome had been fully sequenced in June 2000 (the pair appeared on the front cover of *Time* at the beginning of July) and the dual commitment of President Clinton and British prime minister Tony Blair to make genetic data openly accessible to the public.[48] A conflict of interest about the commercial patenting of genes and a dispute with NIH director Bernadine Healy were reasons why James Watson resigned in 1992 as director of the NIH genome program (Healy herself resigned the following year at Clinton's request). As Watson's successor, Collins thought that private investment actually aided the project and defended the public-private alliance at a congressional hearing, declaring it "both necessary and desirable," although he warned against the federal project being overrun by commercial interests and emphasized that cross-sector rivalries were tricky to navigate.[49]

In his 2005 book *Encoding Capital*, Leo Loeppky gives two reasons why the project received $3 billion of federal investment: first, its potential medical payoffs and, second, its "technological imperative" that fed "through the sinews of political and economic structures, relying, along the way, on the advocacy of specific individuals and organizations."[50] This second reason chimed with the broader biotechnological turn of the early 1990s and was why it was so important that Bush and Clinton (together with congressional leaders such as Senators Pete Dominici and Lawton Chiles) were champions of the project, even if they did not always grasp its technical elements. Yet according to Loeppky, the project's leaders did not fully consider the potential downsides, even though earlier grand initiatives such as the Manhattan Project offered instructive examples of how black box technology can release pernicious forces.[51] Federal backing also irked geneticists working on smaller projects who feared that funding would be otherwise scarce, while researchers in other NIH divisions worried that their endeavors would suffer, despite Watson's reassurances at an early stage.[52]

It is true that the Human Genome Project was predicated on an emerging digital technology that made possible the mapping of gene sequences "at increasing levels of resolution," as Department of Energy geneticist Charles Cantor described it, of "six or seven orders of magnitude."[53] The desire to make visible the complete gene sequence of humanity seemed promethean, yet technology made it feasible for the first time to map complete genetic data using computer imaging "as a large yet finite information database, a spatial, graphic ordering which acts as a digital archive."[54] Not only would the project enhance scientific knowledge and user access, it also indexed the human body, laying it open like a genetic book. Advances in computer and information technologies galvanized the project, but critics such as Catherine Waldby, evoking Heidegger's critique of modern science, worried about its instrumentality in transforming human subjects into searchable objects.[55]

If the science of the project could be questioned, then so too could its scale and ambition. From a distance, the Human Genome Project looks like a model of supreme organization in its spanning of government agencies, scientific teams, and international communities. It officially ended after thirteen years, two years before its aspirational date of 2005 (due partly to pressure from Celera Genomics), and it came in under budget. However, Charles Cantor and Robert Cook-Deegan argue that viewed close up, the project was actually "chaotic, marked by significant redundancy and disorganization" involving eclectic mapping methods from an early stage. These perspectives veer away from Clinton's official rhetoric "that investments in science are leading to a revolution in our ability to detect, treat, and prevent disease," as outlined in his final State of the Union Address.[56] Although it became cheaper and faster to identify base pairs of genes as the project matured and as sequencing moved from manual to robotic, it is worth pausing on these critiques because they pose searching ethical questions about conceptualizations of knowledge, diversity, and health.

Cook-Deegan identifies a combative tension between the technological and human aspects of the overall project and the emphasis of its two directors on "medically and economically useful applications."[57] However, it would be wrong to say that Watson and Collins did not recognize its ethical, legal, and social implications, especially as Watson established a working group at an early stage to ensure that a portion of federal funding (between 3 and 5 percent) was dedicated to these broader issues. Tensions remained, though. David Galas identifies issues of privacy, confidentiality, and discrimination—topics that featured in Clinton's speeches throughout the 1990s and prompted contributors of the 1996 collection *The Human Genome Project and the Future of Health Care* to ask "Who shall benefit from these new genetic technologies" and "Will genetic prediction of risk of disease be used to exclude from health care coverage those most likely to need it"?[58] Galas thought that the ignorance about genetics of those most concerned with ethical, legal, and social issues often led to a mindset of "naïve genetic determinism" and a belief "that there are good genes and bad genes or [that] genes alone control behavior."[59] He offered a warning about collapsing a complex science into simple moral categories, but this position also smacks of scientific protectionism and reveals a fault line within this ambitious international project.

In fact, ethical implications featured in debates even before the project officially started at two workshops in Valencia, Spain, in 1988 and 1990, overseen by the Banco Bilbao-Vizcaya Foundation. The ethics discussed at the Valencia workshop were not confined to those that Galas recognized as potential stumbling blocks, but rather revealed a fundamental "conflict among individual interests and those of society."[60] The Valencia Declaration on the Human Genome Project, drafted at the first workshop, was intended to ensure that "genetic information be used only to enhance the dignity of the individual," and it called for more vigorous public debate about the international project's "ethical, social, legal, and commercial implications" and for close collaboration between UNESCO and the Human Genome Organization.[61] This debate pushed the knotty concept of dignity to the forefront of genomic discussion and arguably played into the hands of conservative skeptics eager to alert the public to the dangers of genetic science. Delegates revised the Valencia Declaration's initial seven articles following the second workshop. This revised declaration acknowledged that the project "will have great benefit for human health and wellbeing" in minimizing deleterious inherited conditions and improving life expectancy, but the authors recognized the need to educate the public and offer genetic training for health professionals.[62]

Participants at the Valencia workshops were receptive to the project's international scope, yet it is surprising they did not debate racial politics at length given the atrocities that had been committed in the name of eugenics a half century earlier.[63] Others in the scientific community acknowledged that the question of race was a wake-up call. For example, the recognition that diversity should be considered more fully was embodied by the cover image of the February 2001 issue of *Science*, which featured six faces organized into a vertical DNA strand representing different stages of life and different world ethnicities. This striking image validated Clinton's view that science and technology could affirm "our common humanity" across countries and regions in the face of the upsurge in "ethnic and tribal and religious hatred and conflict" that the atrocities of 9/11 brought home later that year.[64]

The Human Genome Organization also emphasized the global scale of the project by hosting three workshops in 1992–1993 with the aim of launching a Human Genome Diversity Project that aligned with the NIH's new emphasis (via the NIH Revitalization Act of 1993) on ensuring that genetic sampling was more inclusive of minority groups. Although *Nature* proclaimed that the human genome was "everyone's genome," this 1994 project recognized the need to better account for diversity at the levels of cells and populations.[65] However, the Human Genome Diversity Project faced many pitfalls. The plan to collect blood samples from five hundred global ethnic populations met with a sharp backlash from indigenous groups, alongside the critique that the diversity project was little more than "21st-century technology applied to 19th-century biology."[66] These charges pivoted on the collision of scientific questions "about how to order and classify an aspect of nature" and political questions "about how to organize human differences for the purposes of creating credible and legitimate systems of governance." In seeking a middle ground, sociologist Jenny Reardon's 2005 book *Race to the Finish* steered between promoting Clinton's claim that science will triumph over racism and critiquing the project for being colonialism in disguise, although she argued that "questions about how to make authoritative claims about human diversity" will always be contestable.[67]

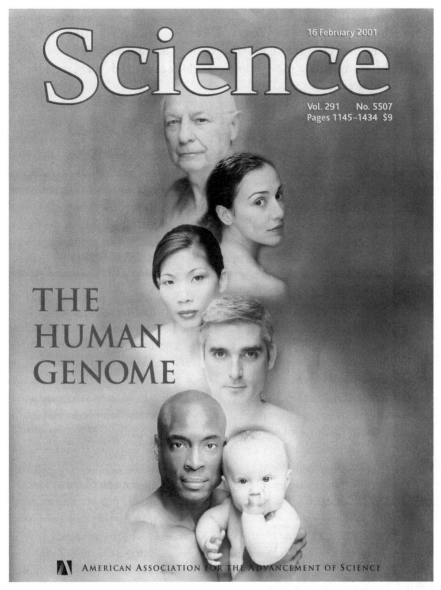

Figure 1.1. "The Human Genome," cover of *Science*, February 16, 2001. Photography by Ann Elliott Cutting/American Association for the Advancement of Science.

That the Diversity Project departed from its initial objectives did not lessen the fact that these "tensions and paradoxes" surrounding public-private relations, race, science, and statehood cast eugenic shadows over the Human Genome Project, as did aligned initiatives such as the 1000 Genomes Project of 2008 that added South America and North Africa to the regional spread of international partners.[68] This entanglement not only evokes one of Reardon's key questions, "Who can speak for humanness in this genomic age?," but also reveals how contested

humanism was in the 1990s, in that its universalism often masked power interests, as the NIH recognized when in 2010 it cofounded (with the UK's Wellcome
Trust) the Human Heredity and Health in Africa Initiative (H3Africa) to redress
the fact that many parts of the developing world had been "left out of the boom in
genomic science."[69]

This attempt to shift emphasis away from what sociologist Alondra Nelson
calls the "social power" of genetic science toward a focus on "social life" in the
genomic age is perhaps one reason why Clinton ensured that his public messages to
Black and Indigenous Americans addressed economic opportunities and how
advances in genetic research would be of medical benefit to not just all Americans
but to peoples across the globe.[70] However, the Clinton-era anti-discrimination
agenda was slow to move. What a 2003 Institute of Medicine report later confirmed
as racial disparities in health care access and mortality rates was earlier evident in
the view of George H. W. Bush's secretary of health and human services Louis W.
Sullivan (the second Black American in the role) that "deeply ingrained prejudices"
exist across the health sector and are "largely unrecognized and exceptionally difficult to eliminate."[71] Legal scholar Dorothy Roberts goes further by arguing that
the biological claims of the Human Genome Project that we are one race did not
usher a new democratic dawn; instead, assumptions about race-based genetic variation hardened in the early years of the twenty-first century.[72]

Reardon was not alone in revealing how occluded questions of race inflected
genetic initiatives. For example, Debra Harry of the Nevada-based Indigenous
Peoples Council on Biocolonialism (which was formed in order to safeguard genetic resources of indigenous groups) and the sociologist Jonathan Marks of the University of North Carolina asked in their criticisms of the Diversity Project, "Who
decides which genetic problems are important?"[73] The response from the scientific community aligns with Charles Cantor's view that the genetic factors behind
colon cancer, coronary disease, diabetes, schizophrenia, and bipolar disorder are
triggered by environmental factors. "These diseases are not purely genetic," Cantor contends, but probably everyone "is at risk for at least one of them because of
his or her genes."[74] The underlying question here is who is "everyone"? With
indigenous communities ever more marginalized, it is important to highlight the
cultural politics of these grand projects that tend to reinforce racial hierarchies
behind the rhetoric of togetherness.[75]

Part of the issue was that large population studies underpinned the Big Science agenda of the Human Genome and Human Diversity projects, while its participants tended to avoid questions of cultural identity and group politics in favor
of data mapping under the banner of scientific objectivity. Tempering this grand
scale, at least to a degree, were links between independent national research
teams and the bioethics of consent, ownership, and difference. Not only did the
health benefits of the Human Genome Project remain more latent than imminent, but the privileged status of the project's key players (mainly white men)
underscores inherent tensions around race and gender that parallel the culture
wars of the 1990s.[76] I will return to diversity toward the end of chapter with

respect to gene editing, but first it is important to address human cloning as the major fear of the genetic revolution at the millennium.

Faces of Human Cloning

Among the ethical issues posed by the Human Genome Project was the troubling question "Who owns the human genome?"[77] In partial answer, Tom Wilkie focused on the tension between the commitment of the international science community to make genomic data freely available and the private-industry drive to patent gene sequences. In *Perilous Knowledge*, Wilkie quoted James Watson's fear that this tension might lead to a competitively "nationalistic approach to science," an anxiety that prompted Watson to resign his NIH office in 1993 and return to Cold Spring Harbor Laboratory on Long Island.[78] In a 1990 article in *Science* on the "past, present, and future" of genomic research, Watson expressed his belief that the completion of this international project would inform a deeper understanding of "how we function as healthy human beings."[79] He characterized this long-term endeavor as a grand humanist project that would enable the scientific community and individuals around the world to understand their genetic inheritance and lead ultimately to interventions to correct faulty or deleteriously mutated genes. Yet Watson's dual emphasis on genetic mapping and human health also raises profound questions of agency and ownership that this section of the chapter brings together via a focus on human cloning.

Copying at the molecular level was at the heart of the Human Genome Project, but so was experimentation conducted on animals in an effort to understand genetic commonalities and viral behavior. Classical humanist thought categorically divides humans from animals, but the process of sequencing revealed only subtle differences in the genetic makeup of humans, monkeys, and sheep—and even nematode worms. A University of Cambridge project concluded in 1998 that a nematode worm has 20,500 genes, but this was put in perspective when the Human Genome Project revealed that humans have only 34,000 genes, a number later scaled down to closer to that of the nematode. The key distinction is that these genes are only 3 percent of the human genome; the remainder is composed of noncoded DNA that interacts with nearby genes. Psychologist Steven Pinker uses this statistic to argue that although human beings have more agency than biologists often credit because genetic sequences shape rather than determine behavior, the possibility of mapping a human's and a worm's genes similarly also pushes humankind off a privileged pedestal.[80]

The news of Dolly the Sheep, which broke in February 1997, six months after her birth in Scotland, posed two pivotal questions: How proximate are human and animal genetic profiles? And if a cloned sheep could be born and survive in a healthy state, then could a human also be cloned? These provocative questions sparked interest among politicians and journalists, but they unhelpfully skewed the debate toward fears by evoking the mythic characters of Icarus and Frankenstein, when in actual fact Dolly's conception was much humbler. As one of 277 attempts at somatic cell nuclear transfer, Dolly resulted from applying electroshock treatment to an unfertilized egg of a Scottish Blackface sheep fused with an udder cell of a white-faced Finn Dorset sheep. The team then surgically implanted the embryo into another Scottish Blackface that carried Dolly through to birth 148 days later.

The news of Dolly was a landmark moment, but the core ambitions of the Roslin Institute in Edinburgh, home to genetic research over the previous two decades, were to find out "how cells work" and to refine genetic technology rather than cloning for its own sake.[81] Wilmut, who explained the science of genetic transformation in *After Dolly* (2006), took pains to outline his aim to create a healthy animal, not a resource for a drugs farm. He contrasted Dolly with an older sheep named Tracy that had undergone transgenic modification to add human protein to her milk so that a private biotech company, PPL Therapeutics, could research possible cures for cystic fibrosis and lung cancer. Although both sheep were part of a long-term project to make healthier breeds of farm animals, what set Dolly apart from animal pharming in Wilmut's mind was the fact that she was cloned from adult somatic cells rather than fetal cells.[82]

Wilmut thought that media attention on human cloning missed the point, but he also received letters from the British public asking him if were possible to clone deceased relatives.[83] His book *After Dolly* is wide ranging in its history of cloning across multiple species, but it does not directly address the symbolism of Dolly or speculation about human clones that followed in Dolly's wake. This speculation ranged from what Cynthia Fox calls "world cloning wars" on either side of the millennium, to the "valid" and "in-valid" characters of the 1997 film *Gattaca* (see chapter 2), to the "dittos" that populate physicist David Brin's near-future novel *Kiln People* (2002) as a form of people-xeroxing in which personality and soul are carbon copied, to Neil Astley's speculative fiction *The Sheep Who Changed the World* (2005) in which a cloned sheep is granted a human level of intelligence.[84]

For psychoanalyst Adam Phillips, the symbolism of Dolly was just as important as her actual birth in challenging the casual assumption that all sheep are alike.[85] Phillips argues that because the fascination with cloning is rooted in childhood fantasies, it is difficult to separate desire and fear from genomics, particularly because psychic cloning happens on an everyday level in an individual's search for others fashioned in their own image.[86] There is some consolation (though also some psychic discomfort) in realizing that genetic clones will always grow up with different histories. James Watson gestured toward this in an important 1971 essay in *The Atlantic* in which he contrasted multiple replicas of celebrities with the recognition that if cloning could happen on demand, then it is as likely that "highly different fantasies" would lead to diversity rather than uniformity.[87] Yet the attractions and fears of "absolute identity" were too powerful for scientists like Wilmut to quell, especially when the seductive model of perfection is open to exploitation by commercial organizations wishing to biofacture carbon-copy life-stock.[88] This more exploratory side of the debate highlights that the symbolic aspects of cloning were virtually inseparable from its science and policy.

Another critique of Wilmut's experiment came from an official source, the National Bioethics Advisory Commission, the fifth federal bioethics committee to form, that released its report *Cloning Human Beings* four months after the news of Dolly broke. Recognizing that cloning at the cellular level was crucial for medical research, the chair, Harold Shapiro, an economist who was president of Princeton University, argued that the logical downside of making life-stock heathier through the process of reproductive cloning would also reduce its genetic diversity and was likely to have adverse long-term health consequences. The committee members acknowledged the therapeutic benefits of using transgenic animals to test drugs and regenerative agents, and they tried to allay fears about the mass cloning of humans, given the complex science that would be involved and the number of false starts in the production of Dolly. Nonetheless, the report recommended human cloning should be prohibited, both to assuage fears on religious and social grounds and because commission members believed that "any attempt to clone human beings via somatic cell nuclear transfer techniques is uncertain in its prospects, is unacceptably dangerous to the fetus and, is therefore, morally unacceptable."[89]

This perspective was not an attack on Wilmut's methods but an effort to maintain an ontological horizon that echoed the stance of the World Health Organization about the unfathomable health implications of human cloning and its efforts to prevent private businesses from advancing their own agendas by bypassing ethical regulations.[90] Guided by the Belmont ethical principles of 1978 and citing "unacceptable risks," the report recommended federal funds should not support human cloning. These principles advised that private sector companies should "comply voluntarily with the intent of the federal moratorium" and that national interests should align with those of the international scientific community in order to prevent rogue states from opening a Pandora's box that more responsible nation states would find hard to close.[91] The commission did not seek to prematurely end the debate, though, and its members recognized the effort required to educate the public without being either alarmist or complacent. It left open the practice of cloning DNA sequences for potential medical benefits and set a moratorium at three to five years to allow scientific and political leaders to consider the implications of somatic cell nuclear transfer technology.

When George W. Bush replaced this Clinton administration commission with the President's Council on Bioethics, he appointed ethicist Leon Kass as chair of a committee that included political scientist Francis Fukuyama and philosopher Michael Sandell—in contrast to members of the Clinton commission, whose expertise was focused on medical law, ethics, and care. In 1998, in an effort to develop a long-term conservative response to the National Bioethics Advisory Commission, Kass published *The Ethics of Human Cloning* with fellow council member James Wilson, including essays that Kass and Wilson had published in conservative magazines in the weeks after news about Dolly broke.[92] It was no surprise, then, that the President's Council on Bioethics highlighted the dangers and risks of permitting the private sector to have free rein on cloning.

Despite its aim to deepen bioethics, in fact this Bush-era commission did not propel the cloning debate much further than the Clinton-era commission had, except
to reinforce moral negativity toward new stem cell technologies. This anti-
scientific bias was noted by the medical director of the American Psychiatric
Association, who wrote to Kass in May 2003 to criticize the council for "some
serious gaps" in its biomedical information, especially with respect to diagnosis
and prescription drug use.[93]

The objections to cloning hung on what Kass, in his 1997 *New Republic* essay
"The Wisdom of Repugnance," describes as the intense emotions it provokes:
"Almost no one finds any of the suggested reasons for human cloning compelling;
almost everyone anticipates its possible misuses and abuses."[94] Kass channeled
pro-life Republican sentiments in reaching these conclusions, and his rhetoric
shaped President Bush's public remarks on prohibiting human cloning.[95] For liberal thinkers, this represented a "new conservative crusade" in which Kass sought
to develop what he called in a leaked memo of March 8, 2005, "a bold and 'offensive' bioethics" for the second-term Bush administration that might morally balance the scientific and technological emphasis of Bush's American Competitiveness
Initiative.[96] The executive director of the bioethics council, Yuval Levin, developed this offensive strategy in a previously redacted document of April 6th that
recommended a "rifle-shot approach" in order to maximize the chances that pro-
life bills prohibiting human cloning, stem cell research, fetal farming, and interspecies research would get through Congress.[97] Levin realized that a coordinated
defensive strategy by the conservative press was also needed, whereas Kass
believed that a Republican-controlled Congress favored his vision of "human life
and human dignity" and shared his suspicion of "runaway scientism."[98] This
emphasis on dignity echoed the UN's recent Declaration on Human Cloning,
which sought "to prohibit all forms of human cloning inasmuch as they are
incompatible with human dignity and the protection of human life." However,
for Kass, this was also a belief premised on a repugnant response to certain technologies ("in crucial cases . . . repugnance is the emotional expression of deep
wisdom, beyond reason's power fully to articulate it") and he warned his country
against becoming a "society that has forgotten how to shudder."[99]

We may credit Kass for locating a moral compass in the face of tech acceleration or castigate him for not sidelining personal belief when assessing scientific
innovation. Ignoring the fact that disgust often stems from phobia, Kass's particular project was to lay ethical grounds for prohibiting human cloning. Yet he did
not want to throw out emotions by ceding the intellectual high ground to rational scientists, especially when science blurs moral boundaries and, in his view,
threatens to undermine the foundations of human nature.[100] Kass made clear
ideological moves. He unfavorably contrasted the pluralistic position that identity is socially constructed with a conservative view that recognized that genetics
partially determine identity, wedded to the belief that human life is underpinned
by value and faith. This might seem like a reasonable position, but Martha Nussbaum argues that a philosophical stance based on disgust often links to "thoughts

about contamination and purity that are ubiquitously mixed up with prejudice and stigmatization."[101] It is in the universalist rhetoric of Kass that we see the cultural politics of sameness and diversity playing out.

Philosopher Adam Briggle discusses how Kass's desire that the President's Council on Bioethics embody a "richer and deeper public bioethics" supported his aim to develop an "overall philosophical anthropology, studying biomedicine within the context of the human lifeworld."[102] Briggle analyzes this desire for a rich public bioethics as an informed effort to move beyond instrumentalism and to recognize that "bioethical dilemmas are intertwined with power and conflicts of value, interest, opinion, and world-view."[103] Critics thought the bioethics council was heavily partisan, but Briggle argues that the Kass council "was about recovering a more adequate picture of being human, a wider, more robust ethical vocabulary, and a more inclusive, explicit public debate."[104] This characterization would have likely met with the approval of Bill Clinton and Robert Bellah in its channeling of the "rich diversity" of American life (to recall Clinton's 1997 Morgan State University), but it also served to justify the conservative undercurrents of the conclusions of Kass's council.

The publication of Kass's 2002 monograph *Life, Liberty, and the Defense of Dignity* coincided with the council's first report, *Human Cloning and Human Dignity*, which embodied this richer version of public bioethics, envisioned not as "an ethics based on biology, but an ethics in the service of *bios*—of a life lived humanly, a course of life lived not merely physiologically, but also mentally, socially, culturally, politically, and spiritually."[105] Despite its moral perfectionism, the report locates a space that links life ("for its precariousness and its sanctity, whether adult or embryonic") to a humanist concern for dignity, freedom, and equality.[106] The commission detailed seven policy options and two proposals. The first of these proposals, which ten of the seventeen members of the committee favored, added a "moratorium on cloning-for-biomedical research," while the second, favored by seven, sought tighter regulation for the research uses of cloned embryos.

The fact that both the Clinton and Bush administrations took human cloning seriously did not mean that federal commissions had a monopoly on bioethics. Mindful of Evelyn Fox Keller's premise that "the term *gene*" is a hindrance both to biologists and to the public at large, "misleading as often as it informs" especially in the years surrounding the millennium, I turn now to two speculative fictions that broaden the scientific lens by testing the potential and fear of genetic engineering.[107] The first of these fictions, published a year before the Clinton commission report, is Michael Marshall Smith's *Spares*; the second, appearing a year after the Kass council report, is Margaret Atwood's *Oryx and Crake*. I am especially interested in how these two texts speculate about cloning experiments, seeing in them consequences not only for physical and mental health but also for human rights and dignity.

Spares is set in Richmond, Virginia, in the near future, a city where the British-born Michael Marshall Smith lived as a child and later as an adult, making him what he calls "both outsider and insider."[108] Architecturally, new Richmond is a rationalized but radically transformed space; it has straight roads running into a center like a "giant's spider web" and is overlooked by transcontinental transport systems called Megamalls. Although new Richmond is a metonym of a futuristic United States ("just a city like anywhere else"), the Megamalls contain "all of the good, clean, *buyable* things in life crammed into a multi-storey funhouse."[109] As an example of gothic science fiction (signaled by its epigraph of ambivalent morality drawn from the midcentury crime writer Jim Thompson), *Spares* is a very visual novel. This is just one reason it was optioned by DreamWorks in 1996. Although it was never filmed, the slave theme that *Spares* explores is echoed in the 2005 thriller *The Island*, while class-driven hacker aspects of the novel are reprised in the interplanetary dystopia *Elysium* (2013).

Spares is not primarily concerned with the genetics that could lead to a culture of expendability or the possible contamination of humans and machines, as Greg Bear explored in his 1985 futuristic novel *Blood Music*. Instead, Smith probes the absence of dignity among the "spares," whose domain of dimly lit clone farms near Roanoke contrasts sharply with the Megamalls. Perhaps reflecting on the rapid expansion and growing demand for organ and tissue transplants over the previous decade, the spares are portrayed as the chattel of rich Americans who request organs and limbs when their own become worn or damaged.[110] Described as "docile, brainless, without purpose of any kind," the spares are not inanimate or unconscious, although most cannot speak and have damaged bodies.[111] For example, one female body has one arm and a skin graft taken from the left side of her face. The clones live in a twilight world of servitude from which the novel's protagonist, the ex-policeman and now drug addict Jack Randall, is keen to save them, despite his blurred motives.

While the company that manufactures the spares, SafetyNet, does not exactly mirror Craig Venter's Celeria, it is shaped by similar neoliberal values, driven by a marketized technocapitalist logic that values wealthy consumers over the replicas that supply replacements for damaged and worn-out body parts. This is far from the heroic horizon of the Human Genome Project and the breakthrough experiment of Dolly the Sheep, but it is not far from a realization of consumer genomics that epitomizes "the entanglement of the market in the development of the life sciences" in terms of who owns the body parts.[112] In this premillennial context, the clones are kept alive and fed at a minimal level to supply their originals when required, but they live in an existentially impoverished world and hover halfway between subject and object. This state is described as "one endless twilight of blue heat" in which they are forced to listen to the "mindless noise of other spares, and the slow blur of meaningless movement that takes place around them"; they populate "a butcher's shop where the meat still moved occasionally, always and forever bathed in a dead blue light."[113] The slow violence enacted on victims of an imperious state is a stark example of modern slavery in a lawless place, raising bioethical questions about poor individuals selling their body parts to raise money without comprehending the health risks.[114] The novel frames this power differential in terms of expendability: the spares are used when their owner requires surgery and are otherwise shoved back into a tunnel until needed again.

Smith's point is that human clones are more likely to serve wealth and privilege than they are to be granted anything approximating to co-equal status—or, if they are part of a fantasy of self-renewal, they are likely to be banished to a dark closet until their organs are harvested. Spares exist below the bodily level as "dead code segments, cut off from the rest of the program and left alone in darkness" rather than enjoying ontological cohesion or a semblance of rights.[115] The novel replicates the architecturally divided and class-riven world of Fritz Lang's 1927 dystopian sci-fi film *Metropolis* split into upper and lower realms. It also presages the shadowy existence of clones consigned to the "dark byways of the country" in one of the best-known contemporary cloning novels, Kazuo Ishiguro's *Never Let Me Go* (2005), which tests the hypothesis that in the right environment clones can "grow to be as sensitive and intelligent as any human being."[116] However, in *Spares*, the possibility of escape from servitude prompts Jack Randall's efforts to liberate the spares from their imprisonment via an alarm system, granting them some freedom of movement and education classes to foster awareness and, with the help of a developed droid Ratchet, relative independence.

On literary evidence, Smith has only a rudimentary knowledge of the science of human cloning and pictures the spares as little more than a wardrobe of replaceable parts "waiting for the knife" rather than cohesive, thinking, feeling beings—a subject Alex Garland takes up in his 2014 film *Ex Machina* (see chapter 4).[117] The South does not play a significant role in the book, but the specter of eugenics hangs over Roanoke Farm, particularly given that Roanoke is only just over fifty miles from Lynchburg, the site of the formerly named Virginia State Colony for Epileptics and Feebleminded, which oversaw a series of involuntary sterilizations after it opened in 1910. These sterilizations peaked in 1924 following the Virginia Sterilization Act, which targeted "mentally deficient" inpatients and justified medical violence toward Black Americans and poor whites.[118] Race is an underdeveloped theme of *Spares*, which is surprising given that it was one focus of Smith's debut 1994 novel *Only Forward*. Because the clones in *Spares* are at the service of wealthy originals, the major dividing line rests on class, yet the mental health implications of their underground life imply a caste or racial hierarchy. Randall's better instincts are triggered by this combination of deprivation and subjugation: he attempts to liberate the spares by working in the shadows of a surveilled world, which tallies with Smith's later enthusiasm for Harvard social psychologist Shoshana Zuboff's 2018 study *The Age of Surveillance Capitalism*.[119]

Not only does *Spares* force the reader to think about the edges of human dignity, it also raises questions of diversity and power. On first glance, the spares are alike, but they reveal differences; many of them have missing parts that leave them in a permanent state of damage. Smith's novel poses further questions about consumerism and dispensability while offering a left-leaning warning in the year of Dolly's birth that in the wrong hands or driven by the market rather than by bioethics, cloning in its future form is likely to undermine human rights and compromise health. In doing so, *Spares* raises ethical questions about market-driven science that promises to "rewrite our futures," warning that it is not the endless resource that fueled President Clinton's hope for a more democratic future.[120] In the search for a vantage point and a praxis that can foster responsible and imaginative bioethics, the chapter's final section turns to the early twenty-first-century practice of gene splicing, as foreshadowed in Margaret Atwood's 2003 novel *Oryx and Crake*.

Gene Editing and Interspecies Research

In contrast to the recognizable yet transformed world of *Spares*, Atwood's *Oryx and Crake* is set in a post-apocalyptic mid-twenty-first century when a devastating flood has virtually wiped out human beings. Atwood takes pains not to label *Oryx and Crake* dystopian, arguing it does not depict a true apocalypse because some "thin battered-looking" humans remain, despite their usurpation by genetically produced humanoids.[121] Instead, she prefers the label "speculative fiction" or "scientific romance" for the novel's exploration of "the consequences of new and proposed technologies" and the "nature and limits of what it means to be human."[122] Atwood, who is well versed in sci-fi traditions and contemporary scientific and environmental debates, leading her to document the "deep background" of *Oryx and Crake* on her (currently unavailable) website for the novel.[123] She describes her cultural role as a "dabbler" and "guardian of the moral and ethical sense of community" in her exploration of fears about technologies that are used for unethical ends.[124] As such, Atwood claims to write from the view of the general public, although her Canadian sensibility leads her to critique the worst excesses of technocapitalism that she sees in threatening form south of the Canada–United States border.

The world of *Oryx and Crake* is riven both physically and metaphysically. The technophile Crake lives in ease within the RejoovenEsense Compound, where he creates "once-unimaginable things," while Jimmy (or Snowman, as he is often called) struggles to exist as the last human being, a state of being that aligns with what a 2003 *New Scientist* interview with Atwood called "life after man."[125] Atwood stresses that *Oryx and Crake*, which was published toward the end of George W. Bush's first term, portrays a world in which national governments have collapsed and "everything is being run by corporations," echoing her warning that the United States was abandoning the rule of law in its invasion of Iraq.[126] More specifically, Atwood sees science as a vital investigative tool but is critical of its technological applications and a neoliberal ideology that commercializes nature. *Oryx and Crake* shows how the genetic experiments this chapter has charted—the Human Genome Project and transgenic cloning experiments—are likely to be used errantly when they are not guided by responsible legislation or when they are in the wrong hands.

Atwood takes some cues on the looming climate crisis from environmentalist Bill McKibben, but her MaddAddam trilogy, of which *Oryx and Crake* is the first volume, explores how transgenic technologies promise control over the environment yet actually create a more chaotic biosphere. The Crakers have been bioengineered to remove the "destructive features" of human life that are "responsible for the world's current illnesses," but in this terrain the boundaries between humans and animal life blur.[127] Writing before the emergence of inter-species research in the 2010s, Donna Haraway claimed that chimeras in and of themselves should not be seen as aberrations; with a nod to classical mythology, she wrote in 1997 that they are "the obligatory passage points, the embodiments and articulations, through which travellers must pass to get much of anywhere in the world."[128] However, in the world of *Oryx and* Crake, pigoons—pigs with human stem cell implants, just one of a number of transgenically modified creatures that roam the novel—are a frightening prospect of unregulated synthetic biology and genetic science that threatens human existence. On this point, Atwood agrees with McKibben that because "wisdom cannot be cloned or manu-factured," "perhaps we should leave well enough alone."[129] Rather than retreating from bioscience, she offers an imaginative bioethics that retains the philosophical reach of science while critiquing its applications. As such, *Oryx and Crake* can be read as a form of narrative bioart that explores the politics of nature while posing epistemological and ontological questions of personal and shared identity in a deregulated techno-world.[130]

Atwood's understanding of reflective and questioning science is captured in Snowman's attempt to remember the world as it once was as he struggles with "the blank spaces in the stub of his brain" and to cling to an elusive and vanishing identity.[131] The novel is full of chaotic life, much of it genetically manufactured, in contrast to Snowman's existentially sparse lifeworld in which he exists at "zero hour" because "nobody nowhere knows what time it is" anymore.[132] Whereas Snowman struggles with his mental health, the narrative embodies heroic technoscience in the shape of the hybridized pigoon: "bigger and fatter than ordinary pigs" so they can contain extra organs, pigoons are more intelligent and empathic than biological pigs but also more hostile toward humans.[133] Crake presides over the gene-splicing experiments at the ironically named Watson-Crick Institute, spurred by his belief that humans are faulty "hormone robots" that need transcending.[134] When it comes to the humanoid Crakers, the gene splicing is so sophisticated that it not only pre-selects genetic characteristics and "edit[s] out the fear" that haunts Snowman, it can also eliminate hierarchies, territoriality, and complex sexuality in favor of a low-footprint lifestyle.[135]

Oryx and Crake satirizes gene splicing even before its science became a reality, suggesting, at least in theory, that transgenic post-humans will push "thin battered-looking" humans to the social margins. In contemplating what a 1992 article called the "future fall-out of the genetic revolution," *Oryx and Crake* propels the reader to think through the proper uses and potential misuses of genetic technologies.[136] For example, there are biomedical benefits for creating transgenic mice from embryonic stem cells that can glow in the dark to trace cell types that might be useful for understanding Parkinson's disease. Yet bioethical

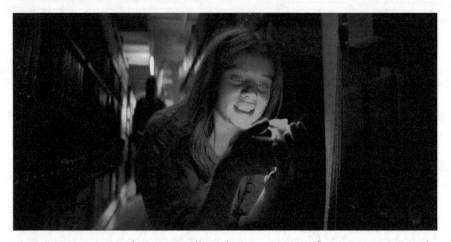

Figure 1.2. Emma Engels (Luna Wedler) admires a runaway fluorescent mouse at the University of Freiberg. *Biohackers*, series 1, episode 1, aired August 20, 2020, on Netflix. Everett Collection Inc./Alamy Photo.

questions should also be asked of such practices. Bioartist Eduardo Kac and French geneticist Louis-Marie Houdebine provoked such questions in 2000, when they created a genetic modification of Alba (an albino rabbit) so it would glow fluorescent green when exposed to blue light—a spectacle the *Biohackers* television series reprised in a seemingly innocuous encounter with a lumines-cent mouse running free in the University of Freiburg Library.

In its exploration of what Atwood calls the edge of the map, *Oryx and Crake* foreshadows bioart exhibitions, such as *Art's Work in the Age of Biotechnology*, held at North Carolina State University in 2019–2020, and transgenic practices, includ-ing a research program at the University of California, Davis, that aims to grow a human pancreas inside a pig embryo.[137] Made public in June 2016, the Davis experiment significantly advanced earlier trials such as one with rodents at the University of Tokyo, but the Davis scientists ensured that they terminated embry-onic development within the first month, mindful of the federal ban on human cloning and chimera research. NIH prohibited such research in September 2015, only to reconsider its prospects the following year in response to counterargu-ments by lobbyists. NIH officials continue to remain wary of interspecies research for its potential to "radically humanize the biology of laboratory animals," echo-ing Atwood's pigoons.[138]

By the mid-2010s, geneticists were using a new gene-editing tool called Crispr-Cas9 to intervene in faulty DNA by manipulating synthetic RNA strands in an effort to fix inherited mutations and to boost the immune systems of adults. Even though the Human Genome Project identified eight hundred genetic variants linked to common health conditions, NIH director Francis Collins acknowledged in 2010 that it had "not yet directly affected the healthcare of most individuals."[139] In contrast, Crispr promised a leap forward in the medical fight against cancer and cystic fibrosis, especially because it offered a relatively cheap gene editing tool with great potential applications for medicine and biodiversity.[140] The technique, which the transnational company Crispr Therapeutics pioneered, swiftly generated claims and counterclaims about its genetic efficacy and ethical dangers in newspapers and magazines. In 2016, an article in *Time* magazine claimed that Crispr had "the potential to change human lives forever," but scientific disagreements fed volatility in the stock prices of biotech companies such as Editas and Crispr Therapeutics.[141] These warnings tended to mask the huge medical potential of gene editing for helping to save endangered or extinct species. In fact, in 2019, the *New York Times* asked whether scientists should "toy with the secret to life," and that same year the *Japan Times* wondered whether edited human DNA might "destroy our humanity."[142]

The Crispr technique makes genetic manipulation for medical ends swifter and more effective but, as chapter 2 shows, it raises questions about the authenticity of a genetically modified being and what medical thriller writer Robin Cook calls the "dark side" of putting "the power of the creator in the hands of so many unregulated players."[143] The bioethical dangers of gene editing are illustrated by the birth of Lulu and Nana in Shenzhen, China, in November 2018. He Jiankui of the Southern University of Science and Technology used a germline intervention to make otherwise healthy embryos resistant to HIV by modifying the CCR5 gene. Yet in the process, he may have unwittingly left the babies more vulnerable to other infections. This provoked alarm from scientists, including former Food and Drug Administration commissioner Scott Gottlieb, who said it established a "terrible precedent."[144] Similarly, Francis Collins called for a "binding international consensus on setting limits for this kind of research," a plea that may have contributed to the suspension of He Jiankui's license, which was followed by a three-year prison sentence from a Chinese court for "illegal medical practice" as a deterrent to others. Although the World Health Organization has compiled a global registry of germline experiments, the rise of Crispr and DIY gene editing suggest that punishment and protocols might be insufficient to ease concerns that this may be the most dangerous Pandora's box to have ever been opened.[145]

In a more reactionary mode, this Pandora's box was conjured a decade earlier by the Republican Sam Brownback of Kansas and Democrat Mary Landrieu of Louisiana when they introduced to Congress the Human-Animal Hybrid Prohibition Act of 2009. Echoing Brownback's earlier opposition to human cloning ("the slippery slope that ultimately ends in a eugenic brave new world"), the two senators were concerned not only that chimera research undermines human dignity but also that the practice was "grossly unethical" because it blurs lines between individuals and species and is likely to give rise to radically humanized animals and new strains of disease.[146] Congress did not pursue the proposed bill. But such opposition suggests that lines between experimental and therapeutic biomedical practice are often hazy in policy debates and tricky to translate into what is required to sustain a good society, to return to the post–Cold War horizons of Bill Clinton and Robert Bellah with which the chapter began. These ideological tensions recall questions of diversity raised by the Human Genome

Diversity Project that cast a shadow over both genomic research and the historical arc of genetic intervention and eugenic practice, which was profiled in 2004–2005 by the *Deadly Medicine: Creating the Master Race* exhibition at the Holocaust Memorial Museum.[147]

Protocols that guide state-funded research in North America and Europe offer safeguards by ensuring that research funders and host organizations assess the consequences of such experimentation, including a 2005–2007 European Union–funded project called CHIMBRIDS that examined the scientific, ethical, philosophical, and legal aspects of chimera research. However, as chapter 2 discusses, looser regulations and black-market practices in some countries mean that on a global scale the door is already open.[148] Although it might be impossible to close this door, it is important to remember that interventions in genetic coding pose broader philosophical and health-related questions about humanness and postgenomic life. On this topic, Sarah Parry and John Dupré remind us that diversity is central to nature itself and that this should push scientific and political leaders to prevent biotechnology from simply becoming a capitalist tool.[149] This recognition should also ensure, as Jenny Reardon argues, that in order to respect human health we must keep to the fore the "dilemma of determining when and how to recognize and order human differences."[150]

Embryonic Entanglements

FETAL DESIGN AND LIFE CULTURES

On January 22, 1993, the newly elected President Clinton made a swift biopolitical intervention when he lifted the ban on federal research using fetal tissue. This was an effort to reverse Ronald Reagan's directive of five years earlier that instructed the NIH to temporarily cease all federal research activities using tissue derived from aborted fetuses, restrictions the Bush administration had extended indefinitely in November 1989. Clinton stated that the purpose of the memorandum lifting the ban was to "separate national health and medical policy from the divisive conflict over abortion" and to set forth "a new national reproductive health policy that aims to prevent unintended pregnancies."[1] Clinton's position that abortion is "safe, legal, and rare" pivoted away from his ambivalence toward abortion politics as Arkansas governor, although the term "rare" caused consternation among pro-abortion campaigners and, later, within the Democratic Party.[2] In signing this memorandum, Clinton sought to balance "individual freedom" and "responsible decision-making," to permit fetal experimentation up to the fourteenth day, and to redress restrictions on medical information, even though this emphasis on freeing biomedical science "from the grasp of politics" was not dissimilar to his predecessor George H. W. Bush's remarks as he sought reelection.[3] However, Clinton's stress on "unencumbered access" to biomedical research struck a very different chord, including in a March 2000 joint statement with British prime minister Tony Blair that lauded the capability of human genome research "to enhance the quality of life."[4]

Reproductive politics has long been a divisive public issue, especially in the half-century between the landmark *Roe v. Wade* legislation of January 1973 and the decision of the U.S. Supreme Court in June 2022 to overturn the ruling, which has led to a patchwork of states restricting abortion rights and a subsequent rise in self-managed abortions.[5] The topic of reproductive rights was a key plank in the women's movement and a prominent feature of the culture wars, marking a schism between Clinton's pro-choice politics (for example, increasing access to Medicaid funds for poor women who had been victims of rape and incest) and the strong pro-life emphasis of George W. Bush (who sought to placate the largely white party faithful).[6] These sharp reversals in federal policy depending on the power balance in Washington, DC, led Leon Kass to conclude in 2005, as he approached the end of a four-year term as chair of the President's Council for Bioethics, that "we are all living in embryoville."[7]

The polarization went far beyond abortion rights, making reproductive politics a flashpoint within broader scientific, medical, and ethical debates. Clinton began his eight years in the White House by stating that "we must let medicine and science proceed unencumbered by anti-abortion politics," including the establishment of a Human Embryo Research Panel and the lifting of a "near-total ban" on abortions in military facilities. In contrast, in his first month in office, January 2001, President Bush sent written remarks to pro-life activists at the March for Life on Washington's Mall. New Jersey representative Christopher Smith read aloud Bush's remarks, which pledged that the new administration would affirm the "infinite value of every life," build "a culture of life," and expand a "circle of inclusion and protection" for pregnant women and unborn children—even though First Lady Laura Bush had stated in an NBC *Today* interview that *Roe v. Wade* should be respected.[8] Newly elected Indiana representative Mike Pence, the next March for Life speaker, went further, calling for a "human rights amendment to the Constitution" (this proposed amendment had failed to reach to the Senate floor many times since an unsuccessful vote in 1983) and for Congress to prohibit federal resources to support abortion. The inaugural March for Life rally had taken place over a quarter-century earlier, on January 22, 1974, a year after *Roe v. Wade*, and Bush grasped the opportunity each year of his presidency to affirm this "culture of life," a term first used by Pope John Paul II in 1993.

A Republican majority in Congress for the first six months of 2001, and then throughout the 108th and 109th Congress, led to pro-life advances, buoyed by Bush's platform of compassionate conservatism (a message that anchored his 2000 presidential election bid) and the first lady's emphasis on children's health and literacy.[9] From 2001 onward, the Bush administration opposed public funding for abortion, especially partial-birth abortion in which the mother partially delivers the fetus. This stance was in part prompted by the inflammatory comments of Ohio representative Steve Chabot on reintroducing a bill in June 2002 that had twice failed to receive endorsement by Clinton, in which he described the physician puncturing "the back of the child's skull with a sharp instrument" and sucking "the child's brains out before completing delivery of the dead infant."[10] Chabot's opinion that this is simply "gruesome and inhuman" conflicted with Clinton's view that behind such caricatures was a "potentially life-saving— certainly health saving" procedure for mothers.[11] When Bush signed the Partial-Birth Abortion Ban Act in late 2003 (after delayed congressional approval) he imposed strict regulations on late-stage abortions, in line with the National Right to Life Committee, pro-life communities of faith, and secular conservatives such as Kass who argued that "the early embryo" is "protectable humanity" and "deserving of respect because of what it is, now and potentially."[12]

Whereas Clinton attempted to separate stem cell research and reproductive rights, Bush and congressional Republicans often conflated the two. In his 2002 March for Life speech, for example, Bush recognized that abortion "deeply divides the country," arguing that the nation "must overcome bitterness and rancor" and "seek common ground," especially as some Republicans were comparing partial-birth abortion to the death penalty.[13] Nevertheless, Bush was partisan in supporting the Born-Alive Infants Protection Act of 2002, which provided legal protection for an infant born alive after an induced abortion, and the Partial-Birth Abortion Ban Act of 2003, which prohibited the medical procedure necessary for late-term abortions.[14] He also mirrored his party's opposition to *Roe v. Wade* on the basis that the human embryo has at least coequal rights to the mother, a position the Supreme Court dodged in its landmark ruling when it proclaimed that "we need not resolve the difficult question of when life begins" in protecting women's right to have an abortion.[15]

On the recommendation of his National Bioethics Advisory Commission, Bill Clinton distinguished between reproductive cloning with "the intention of creating a child" (which he opposed) and cloning at the cellular level to advance medical research (which he believed was admissible).[16] Whereas Clinton likely established this commission to sidestep the controversy involved with approving the NIH-backed recommendations of the Human Embryo Research Panel, Bush walked a tightrope of a different kind.[17] To appease his Republican base and states opposed to funding genetic research, Bush officially declared his opposition to the destruction of embryos used for scientific research in order to ensure that "science serves the cause of humanity instead of the other way around." His compassionate conservatism softened hard-line pro-life views that condemned pro-choicers for promoting a "culture of death," which Pope John Paul II claimed was the fault of a "society excessively concerned with efficiency."[18] Bush's public speeches on dignity and family echoed the rhetoric of his Council on Bioethics, and on signing the Partial-Birth Abortion Ban Act, he spoke of protecting the "unborn" rather than using the more theologized term "pre-born" favored by March for Life president Nellie Gray.[19]

First Lady Laura Bush shared George Bush's compassionate message. She spoke about anxiety among children on *The Oprah Winfrey Show* following 9/11 and founded the National Book Festival, which linked advocacy for children's literacy to the passing of the No Child Left Behind Act.[20] But a softer Republican message was not always enough. In order to avoid disenfranchising the scientific community and states keen to provide funding for pioneering biomedical research, Bush conceded that scientists could continue to use existing stem cell lines while "respecting the sanctity of life," although this raised the ire of evangelical organizations such as the Family Research Council.[21]

When federal funds for expansive stem cell experiments were restricted, scientists became concerned about how much research this compromise would permit, especially given the weight of Bush's faith-based statements, which chimed with the likes of James Dobson, a radio personality and founder of the Christian ministry Focus on the Family, who liaised regularly with the White House.[22] Bush's public views were never as extreme as Dobson's belief that mental disorders and homosexuality were the result of inadequate parental discipline, yet the pair shared some spiritual beliefs and argued that the religious right should produce its own experts free of liberal bias.[23] Bush delivered all his annual March for

Life speeches remotely or by proxy, but he often gave his thoughts on unborn babies a spiritual twist, including at the January 2008 rally, when he envisioned "the glimmerings of a new America on a far shore" in which "the weak and innocent" are protected.[24] The pro-life emphasis on fetal rights and on giving "voice to the voiceless" is at the heart of philosophical, bioethical, religious, and legal debates surrounding fetal personhood and stem cell research that was often conflated with the controversial practice of reproductive cloning, not only in public opinion but also in the policy decisions of the Bush administration.

In this chapter, in order to locate an intermedial yet critical vantage point that avoids hardened ideologies, I want to unravel the health and rights implications of abortion from its medical and biotechnological practices, which, as political theorist Stefanie Fishel claims, are invariably entangled in the biosphere when it comes to reproductive technologies.[25] Not only were these entanglements evident in the wake of the Human Genome Project, but as early as the late 1970s, when the term "test tube baby" came into common parlance on both sides of the Atlantic. While John and Doris Del Zio of Florida were seeking to sue a Columbia Presbyterian Medical Center physician for terminating their laboratory-fertilized embryo of five years earlier in the name of procedural safety, the first test tube baby, Louise Brown, was born in Oldham in northwest England in July 1978 following successful in vitro fertilization.[26]

The political entanglement had spiked in the mid-1980s, when Ronald Reagan endorsed the anti-abortion propaganda film co-produced by the National Right to Life Committee *The Silent Scream*, which informed a 1985 Senate hearing on early-gestation fetal pain.[27] The Reagan administration struggled to take a consistent position on fetal transplants, mainly because of the tension between its free market ideology and Republican views about the sanctity of life. However, the trend toward recognizing fetal personhood has intensified since then, due in part to visual technologies that sharpened the crude ultrasound imagery of *The Silent Scream* to make the unborn fetus more familiar.[28] Lynn Morgan contends that during the George W. Bush administration, the human embryo moved from a potential human into an "icon of life."[29] Rather than taking us deeper into existential or health debates about fetal personhood, Morgan shows how Alexander Tsiaras's 2002 pro-life coffee-table book *From Conception to Birth* brought embryos viscerally to life, privileging the wonders of new life over the health experiences and rights of mothers.[30]

It is no surprise that entanglements in the biosphere are especially fraught when it comes to pro-life and pro-choice arguments. Given that every president since Reagan has tried to reverse the policies of the previous administration on embryonic rights, the language of reproductive freedom and fetal personhood has deep ideological implications. It is important to recognize that reproductive politics go far beyond abortion politics, where questions of rights, access, justice, privacy, and biomedical practice pose searching questions about national, gender, sexual, and racial identities.[31] Medical anthropologist Gay Becker argues that as "one of the primary frontiers in contemporary American society," the biomedical

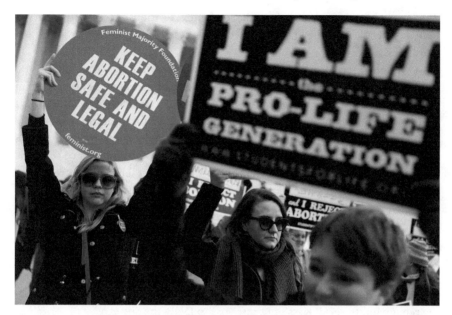

Figure 2.1. Pro-life and pro-choice activists gather at the Supreme Court for the January 2017 National March for Life rally in Washington, DC. Aaron Bernstein/Reuters Pictures.

sphere intersects with business and political interests that place the patient-consumer and the patient-citizen in tension, especially when it comes to deciding who owns health data.[32] This drama plays out on the national stage, for example in President Obama's almost immediate reversal of Bush's restrictions on reproductive rights. It also has global ramifications, particularly when reproductive technologies go offshore into less regulated territories.

By situating the eight years of George W. Bush's presidency at the heart of this chapter, I wrestle the science of reproductive technologies away from the viewpoint that "surgical interventions, microscopic examinations, and lab cultures" transform "the creation of a baby into a matter of technology rather than nature."[33] In the search for perspective and praxis, the chapter aims to rehabilitate the rich public bioethics proposed by Leon Kass as the first chair of the President's Council on Bioethics, yet without Kass's cultural conservatism or his blanket rejection of assisted reproductive technologies. The discussion of anxieties about genetic enhancement in Chapter 1 intensifies here, revealing that the clash between political, philosophical, scientific, and faith-based views on embryonics are more fraught in the United States than in many other countries. To this end, the chapter's second half draws upon two postgenomic literary texts that address the bioethical implications of assisted reproductive technologies from transnational perspectives. Daniel Suarez's biopunk novel *Change Agent* (2017) explores how revived Cold War fears play out globally in terms of access to and regulation of assisted reproductive technologies, and British crime writer Peter James's *Perfect People* (2012) contrasts a U.S.-based couple's plans to purchase a designer baby with the messier sides of family relationships to test what "is humanly at stake at the intersection of biology and biography," to adopt the words of Kass.[34]

Through these discussions, this chapter traces a lineage between cultural visions of reproductive technologies in the 1990s, represented by the 1997 film *Gattaca*, Nancy Kress's Sleepless trilogy (1993–1996), and Suarez's and James's more recent novels.[35] These texts are testing grounds for working through the health and social implications of genetic replication and exploring which regulations may be most effective without thwarting parental aspirations or scientific progress. These intensified debates hinge on tensions between unregulated technological practices and bioethical safeguards that raise fears about genetic disorders, the health of babies and mothers, the inequities of reproductive tourism, and what happens to filial relationships when technologies redefine the contours of identity and life.[36] Following Carlos Novas and Nikolas Rose's view that genetic risk can lead either to resignation in the "face of an implacable biological destiny" or to "new forms of genetic responsibility," I explore how responsible citizens can still "shudder" at human cloning without judging all forms of cloning repugnant, to recall Kass's gut response to Dolly the Sheep.[37]

These intertwined topics were particularly evident in the early years of the new century, following the birth in August 2000 of Adam Nash in Colorado with the assistance of in vitro fertilization (IVF). Adam was born with salient genetic traits that permitted a blood transplant for his six-year-old sister, Molly, who was suffering from a rare blood disease, although this specific donor trait was still far away from the concept of designer babies.[38] The complex subject of genetic surrogacy, both transnational and domestic, as explored in Jodi Picoult's 2014 novel *My Sister's Keeper*, for example, goes beyond the scope of this chapter. Nonetheless, here I explore philosophical and religious debates about the rights of unborn babies and fetal personhood that blur lines between biomedical interventions that aim to improve a baby's health and promethean practices that seek to gain future children a competitive advantage.[39] In this cultural crossfire we might conclude that there is "no outside to reproductive politics."[40] But this chapter contrasts transcendent pro-life notions of a "culture of life" with a pluralistic understanding of life cultures that demand a more granular and less ideological approach.

Bioentanglements: Politics, Science, Theology

In the *Roe v. Wade* ruling of January 1973, Supreme Court justice Harry A. Blackmun stated that in defending a woman's constitutional right to make her own reproductive decisions, it was not the role of the judiciary to speculate about when life begins. Blackmun based his wording on the understanding that "those trained in the respective disciplines of medicine, philosophy, and theology are unable to arrive at any consensus."[41] A lack of agreement about when personhood begins, plus a vagueness in public and legal discussions of embryonic rights, meant that opinion often rested on beliefs and fears rather than on reasoned arguments about the health of mothers and unborn children.[42] James Watson, a co-discoverer of the DNA double helix, epitomized the lack of consensus Justice Blackmun referred to. In May 1971, a few months after testifying to the House of Representatives on the potential consequences of experimentation of human eggs, he reflected on the potential and dangers of genetic engineering.[43] Watson spoke to Congress seven years before the first test-tube birth and ten years before the first successful in vitro case in the United States, but in his May 1971 *Atlantic* article "Moving toward the Clonal Man," he joined a debate about the proximity of successful in vitro fertilization and the more distant prospect of human cloning.[44]

Watson's immediate context, the "unexpectedly rapid progress" in test tube conception through to the blastocyst stage around five days after gestation, was coterminous with Minnesota senator Walter Mondale's efforts to introduce a Commission on Health Science and Society with the aim of establishing robust federal oversight. Mondale's endeavors helped shape the National Research Act of 1974, but the senator was frustrated by the "almost psychopathic objection to the public process" in Congress, epitomized by the reactionary attitude of the new neoconservative magazine *The Public Interest* that science was a threat to "liberal society."[45] In contrast to this renunciation of responsible science was the April 1971 issue of *Time*, with its heroic title "The New Genetics: Man into Superman," and Watson's cautionary "Moving toward the Clonal Man," which echoed his congressional testimony by pointing to the exploitation of surrogate mothers in countries that lack bioethical protocols.[46] Watson recognized that the benefits of IVF outweighed the risks of laparoscopic surgery to implant fertilized eggs in the mother, yet the reality of human cloning based on cell fusion techniques was, for him, a distant horizon.

Watson encouraged informed public debate about new reproductive technologies, even though he described scientists as often reluctant to take the discussion beyond the laboratory. Although he recognized the bioethical and geopolitical implications of commodifying artificially fertilized eggs, he failed to highlight the history of eugenics and the fact that the growing economic disparity between rich and poor Americans meant that such procedures were beyond the reach of many working couples. Watson ran into problems on the subject of diversity. His examples of white celebrities, musicians, artists, and "exceptional people" reveal culturally divisive notions of superiority and inferiority. Calling for an international protocol to prevent governments going rogue, Watson not only ignored diversity politics but did nothing in his essay to acknowledge the rights of mothers from differing demographics or embryos at an advanced stage in the gestation process.

Watson was just one voice in the "first phase of embryo politics" to navigate the contested topics of artificial insemination and human cloning. Those voices ranged from theological figures such as Paul Ramsey to ethicists such as Leon Kass, who both advocated caution, although the humanistic ethicist Joseph Fletcher saw many benefits of ending "reproductive roulette."[47] The subject shaped the founding in 1971 of the Joseph and Rose Kennedy Institute for the Study of Human Reproduction and Bioethics at Georgetown University, which aimed to bring together scholars from diverse disciplines. It also attracted feminist Shulamith Firestone, who believed that new reproductive technologies would enhance a woman's right to choose by replacing sexual reproduction with ectogenesis. This prospect excited Firestone because of its potential to release women from the burdens of pregnancy, but other feminists argued that this position was "non-nurturant" and Ramsey thought it would lead to "species-suicide."[48] Headlines often resorted to the Frankenstein myth, but the potential and the risks of artificial insemination and test tube babies were more culturally complex than simple position taking.[49] With the exception of Firestone's radically feminist tract, these discussions often sidelined specifics of gender and sexuality. Race was a largely absent category for Firestone, though, and even into the 1980s questions of race tended to be overshadowed by those of gender and sexuality, leading the authors of the 2004 publication *Undivided Rights: Women of Color Organize for Reproductive Justice* to decry the racial biases and silences of much reproductive health discourse.[50] That this first phase of public engagement occluded identity politics in favor of more universalistic views of biomedical research, population control, and government regulation meant there was little commentary about an emergent ethics at the cultural level that could propel questions of diversity, equity, and health to the fore.

Thomas Banchoff identifies the mid-1990s as the second phase of public interest in embryonic research, following successful IVF treatments and a hardening of pro-choice and pro-life positioning during the 1980s. At a time when Watson and NIH director Bernadine Healy were warning a members of Congress against the misuse of genetic data, IVF gave hope to many families who had difficulty in conceiving due to blocked or damaged fallopian tubes, although success rates remained variable and declined rapidly for older mothers.[51] IVF is a complex phenomenon, modifying existing technologies (such as egg fertilization and genetic testing) and giving rise to new ones relating to "animal research, pharmacology, fiber optics, advances in live culture media, instrumentation, microsurgery, ultra-sound technology and cryopreservation techniques."[52] As a matrix technology, IVF is much more than a procedure, in aligning ontological questions about the beginnings of life with what sociologist Sarah Franklin calls "biological relativity" that dissolves boundaries between (organic) biology and (manufactured) technology.[53] The fact that IVF creates more than one fertilized embryo to increase the chances of conception offended pro-life advocates, who felt that the practice compromised the sanctity of life (estimates were that only 4 percent of fertilized embryos led to IVF-assisted births in the late 1980s), at a time when Congress was considering consumer protection issues for parents choosing IVF. But, despite ongoing discussion in Congress, there has never been an overarching federal policy on IVF (aside from ensuring that Medicare or Medicaid only cover IVF costs for veterans), and the question of artificial wombs has not reached the level of serious national debate (as explored in the 2020 ectogenesis installation *Unbornox9* by the art collective Future Baby Production).[54]

IVF was markedly different from the big science of the Human Genome Project in that, as Franklin notes, it was prompted by the "narratives and hopes of couples seeking children" rather than by grand international designs.[55] Yet just as James Watson and Francis Collins believed that the Human Genome Project would eventually eliminate inherited genetic disorders, so, from the early 2000s onward, physicians used IVF to screen for genetic abnormalities before implanting the fertilized embryo into the mother's womb. The most obvious of these was Down syndrome, which is easier to detect than most other genetic disorders because of the presence of a third chromosome 21. Prenatal testing became more accessible and sophisticated after the millennium, but choices facing expecting parents differed markedly, depending on demographic pressures, how physicians present scales of risk, and attitudes toward disabilities.[56] This was the case even after the San Diego biotech company Sequenom released a new test, SEQureDX, in early 2009, claiming it was effective as early as ten weeks and was over 98 percent accurate in identifying the chromosome for Down syndrome. However, concerns about the precision of SEQureDX came to light a few months later amid queries about the company's data handling and sample size. Four years later, these questions led Sequenom to move away from invasive prenatal tests that involved removal and analysis of fetal tissue; instead, it launched the noninvasive test MaterniT21 PLUS.[57]

The absence of a federal mandate for prenatal screening has contributed to the influence of biotech companies on expecting parents who feel deeply connected to their evolving fetus but are often overreliant on medical professionals for prenatal direction. The combination of market-based pressures, the normalization of parental roles with respect to their unborn child, and variance in health care practices can prompt anxiety about screening results or even provoke fears about the hazy line between pre-implantation genetic diagnosis and eugenics.[58] Screening also has insurance implications for mothers who continue their pregnancy with knowledge of preexisting conditions like Down syndrome, such as former Alaska governor Sarah Palin, who pushed her baby Trig (born with Down syndrome) into the media spotlight when she ran as John McCain's vice-presidential pick in the 2008 election.[59]

In terms of regional variance, California is the most instructive case. George W. Bush's ruling that federal funds should not be used for stem cell research except for laboratory work on existing stem cell lines prompted the Union of Concerned Scientists to write publicly to the president in 2004 to protest the administration's tendency to distort scientific research.[60] Unhappiness with an anti-science White House led California legislators to pass a new state law, the California Stem Cell Research and Cures Act (or Proposition 71) to ensure that such research continues without reliance on federal funds.[61] This 2004 legislation, which led to the founding of the California Institute for Regenerative Medicine, made stem cell research a constitutional right in the state and was given bipartisan support, including from Governor Arnold Schwarzenegger and celebrities such as Michael J. Fox and Christopher Reeve, who had their own personal health battles. The fifteen-year mission (which was extended in 2020) was to provide oversight, encourage collaboration, and use funding from public bonds, including a $1.3 million project awarded to Stanford University in 2013 for the use of stem cells to explore chromosomal anomalies of Down syndrome.[62]

Despite the increasingly visible profile of disability rights groups and support networks such as the National Down Syndrome Society (est. 1979), overshadowing this variance of medical provision and scientific practice were heated debates among leaders who framed the "culture of life" in religious and moral terms. The belief that biotechnology threatened the sanctity of life had long roots, illustrated by a group of interfaith religious leaders who wrote to President Carter in June 1980 to warn of the "fundamental danger triggered by the rapid growth of genetic engineering."[63] However, reasoned religious and ethical cases competed with knee-jerk responses. It did not help the pro-life case that President Bush drew on the stigmatizing terms "weak" and "imperfect" in his 2002 March for Life remarks in outlining a vision of social responsibility toward vulnerable Americans, ignoring that some pregnancies might be deleterious to the mother's health.[64] This aligned with the views of pro-life Republicans and religious leaders who tended to blur different kinds of stem cell research in order to support their view that reproductive technologies disturbed the natural order.

Many pro-choicers and the scientific community believe that stem cells are vital for biomedical research because they give rise to other differentiated cells that can be used to study cancers (as was the case of the Stanford University grant) and to produce protein combinations. However, stem cell research was controversial because it seemed to involve the manipulation of life itself, especially when researchers at the University of Wisconsin created five immortalized stem cells lines in 1998 using human embryos left over from IVF treatment. Scientifically, this was a breakthrough moment, but its consequences could not be gauged until President Obama lifted the ban on embryonic stem cell research a decade later.[65] Obama, who wanted to return scientific integrity to federal policy, believed that his March 2009 ruling navigated between "a false choice between sound science and moral value," and he replaced the President's Council on Bioethics with a more pragmatic commission. He also championed disability advocates such as Christopher Reeve, who had died five years earlier and to whom he paid tribute.[66] However, a new backlash from faith and anti-abortion groups and Republican-leaning states revealed that the battle lines had not changed and that religious and moral arguments against stem cell research continued to influence policy.[67]

Contributors to *The Public Interest* believed that biotechnology debates were creating "a house divided," despite some bipartisan agreements such as the Stem Cell Therapeutic and Research Act of 2005, which supported a bone marrow and cord blood stem cell transplantation program. However, religious responses were not homogenous; they combined differing ethical and spiritual views that intensified public discussions, especially following Bush's announcement of 2001 that existing stem cells could be used for scientific research.[68] In reaction to the perceived triumph of the laboratory over the home, Christian groups such as the United States Conference of Catholic Bishops lobbied Congress to pass a permanent federal ban. For many conservative Christians, embryology redefined moral relationships and made the unborn baby "an object of knowledge, purpose, and will" rather than a wonder of creation.[69] Because of their concern that the manipulation of genetic material would mean that God's divine plan for normative procreation "vanishes into nothingness," some faith groups published their own resolutions in the early 2000s.[70]

In contrast to the vehement argument of the anti-abortion activist Nellie Gray that *Roe v. Wade* "is not settled law in America because it is evil," the South African theologian Jakobus Vorster, writing ten years later, presented a more reasoned case.[71] Vorster argued that the human embryo should be treated with dignity and rights as our "neighbor," based on the argument that an embryo even at five weeks (with a heartbeat and buds that will grow into arms and legs) represents the living breath of God as part of a covenant that requires protection like any other form of human life. Vorster's account made only passing reference to science, though, and in it the concepts of dignity and respect were underdeveloped.[72] From this deontological perspective, he gave little consideration to exceptions when abortion might be admissible or to the implications for the physical and mental health of the mother, either when she had experienced rape or incest or when the embryo has known chromosomal anomalies. Then and now, pro-life Republicans tended to weaponize mental health by arguing that mothers who choose abortion will experience "post-abortion depression and psychosis," even though Reagan's surgeon general, C. Everett Koop, thought there was insufficient evidence to substantiate this claim and neither the American Psychological Association nor the *Diagnostic and Statistical Manual of Mental Disorders* recognize post-abortion syndrome as a psychiatric condition.[73] In contrast to Vorster, Lee Silver argues that conceiving of genetic material as the "essence of human life" is a category mistake because "human life emerges only at a higher level, when the trillions of cells in the brain all function together."[74] Yet given the dual fears of pro-lifers about genetic engineering and rampant secularism, the religious response carried weight for many who envisioned the embryo as a transcendent life force instead of recognizing the more imminent cultural need to ensure access to health care for women from diverse communities.[75]

The President's Council on Bioethics, which was never entirely divorced from religious views of human nature, issued a report in 2002 that epitomized warnings about the moral dangers of embryonic research. Leon Kass, its chair between 2001 and 2005, claimed that media coverage of stem cell issues narrowed down what he wanted to be a far-sighted review of "deep human matters in order to articulate fully what is humanly at stake at the intersection of biology and biography, where life lived experientially encounters the results of life studied scientifically."[76] The *New York Times* claimed that in this re-privileging of sense over science, Kass delivered a "sharp dose of corrective medicine" and that his "special patient" was "no less than science itself."[77] Kass underlined his suspicion of scientists when he deselected three members of the Council on Bioethics, including molecular biologist and former president of the American Society for Cell Biology Elizabeth Blackburn, who went public in the spring of 2004 with accusations that the council had corralled its members in an ideological direction and misrepresented bioscience in its reports.[78]

Despite the resistance of pro-research council members like Blackburn, the 2002 report, *Human Cloning and Human Dignity*, addressed reproductive cloning. Even though this procedure was not yet a reality, the council shared the view of pro-life Republicans such as Pennsylvania representative Melissa Hart and Kansas senator Sam Brownback that the possibility of animal cloning meant that human cloning was a clear and present danger. However, unlike Hart's and Brownback's fervent speeches at the 2002 March for Life, the report tried to balance the benefits of stem cell research for treating diabetes, Parkinson's, and Alzheimer's with the dangers of cloning human embryos.[79] Nonetheless, its tone shifted when it moved from the issue of cell cloning to the thornier issue of assisted reproductive technologies. Recognizing that a cloned child might enhance the health of a family by giving infertile couples new hope, the report viewed the mass production of "superior people" as morally indefensible.[80] Closing off this eugenics prospect, the council critiqued the right to reproduce and arguments about well-being on two counts: first, parents should not impose their rights on an unborn child; and second, eliminating deleterious genetic conditions might unexpectedly lead to other conditions.

The *Human Cloning and Human Dignity* report concluded that genetic manipulation was "an enduring moral concern" and that it would always pose risks to physical health—and one assumes to mental health as well, although its authors did not address the psychological challenges a genetically engineered child might encounter. The main problem is that the report rapidly shifts from practical considerations to ontological ones, claiming that cloning would be an "experiment in human identity" and in "genetic choice and design," as well as being part of a broader social experiment that tests the conventional boundaries of family life and established social demarcations.[81] In taking a high perspective, the council did not consider the social and interpersonal challenges that genetic discrimination poses to individuals with disabilities and those assumed to have atypical genes—or even the possibility that a stigmatized genetic underclass might emerge.[82]

We might forgive the council, though only to a degree, for not developing this line of inquiry because it was six more years before the Genetic Information Nondiscrimination Act was signed in May 2008. Congress had received bills from lobbyists that sought to protect genetic data since 1995, fueled by concerns, including those of the Coalition for Genetic Fairness, that there were no federal standards for "the collection, storage, and use of identifiable DNA samples and genetic information obtained from those samples."[83] George W. Bush was in favor of such a bill under certain conditions and if it could ensure that electronic patient records were private and secure, an aspect of his drive to transform physical and mental health care through information technology.[84] When it was finally signed into law, when both chambers of Congress again had a Democratic majority, the act protected patients against the possibility that insurance providers would use genetic information in their assessment of coverage or that they would base premiums on DNA data. The legislation did not extend to long-term care or disability insurance, though, and it was ambiguous about what employers could do with health information about employees who participated in company-run wellness programs. Even then, as Bush prepared to depart the White House he issued the Provider Rule, which meant that the Department of Health and Human Services could cut federal aid to programs that discriminated against people who objected to abortion on the basis of religious or moral beliefs.[85]

While Obama rescinded the Provider Rule in February 2009, just a few weeks later, fierce disagreements about whether the Democrats or Republicans were the real champions of nondiscrimination against preexisting health conditions dominated debate in Washington, DC. This coincided with an intense phase in the culture wars stimulated by congressional Republicans and members of the Tea Party, who were keen to dismantle the insurance mandate of the 2010 Affordable Care Act. This chapter now turns to how these entanglements played out in the cultural realm, beginning with the 1997 film *Gattaca*, arguably the most cited cultural text about genetic manipulation, before considering two novels of the 2010s—Daniel Suarez's *Change Agent* and Peter James's *Perfect People*—that explore the health consequences of fetal design.

Design Fictions: From *Gattaca* to *Change Agent*

Gattaca is often approached as a design fiction that proposes a speculative model of our genetic future.[86] The film is based on an original screenplay by director Andrew Niccol and was released by Columbia Pictures in 1997, the year that Princeton biologist Lee Silver envisaged a future in which parents could enhance their offspring's innate talents by optimizing embryos. But *Gattaca* is also a meditation on what the President's Council on Bioethics six years later called "the human significance of procreation" and the "desire to protect what is valuable in it from erosion and degradation—not just from cloning but from other possible technological and nontechnological dangers."[87] This does not make it a reactionary film against the consumerist ideals that Silver describes. Michael Bérubé argues that in addition to affirming nonmanipulated human life and individual endeavor in the face of technocratic forces, genetic determinism, and a surveillance state, it is also a film about disability politics, identity passing, and employment discrimination.[88]

The design of *Gattaca* contrasts sharply with the world of Nancy Kress's Sleepless books. In her sci-fi trilogy, Kress treads a fine ethical line between valorizing the higher intelligence of "genemods" who do not need to sleep and recognizing the need for genemods to coexist with ordinary humans with lower IQs. In contrast, in *Gattaca* Vincent Freeman (played by Ethan Hawke) transitions from a genetically inferior being with a poor life prognosis to an elite position as he aspires to become an astronaut. Whereas Kress focuses on class conflict and minority status, *Gattaca* challenges the notion that genes determine destiny; Vincent adopts the identity of his lab-produced friend Jerome Morrow (played by Jude Law), who experiences a permanent lower-body disability following an accident. Released the year that biotech entrepreneur Martine Rothblatt was arguing for minimal state control over a family's reproductive decisions and open access to genomic data, *Gattaca* does not affirm individualism at all costs.[89] Instead, the film highlights the importance of empathetic relationships that can survive in a surveilled and atomizing environment.[90]

As a foundational biopunk text, *Gattaca* influenced other design fictions that test the role of biotechnology in what Andrew Solomon calls the "awkward interstitial territory" between genetic and experiential identities.[91] Dramatizing the intersection of these identities is a couple that gives birth to two boys: the first naturally conceived, the second engineered. Vincent, the firstborn, narrates his conception in the backseat of a car almost like a requiem, because a "child conceived in love" and with immediate needs is thought to be no longer suited to this future world. "The exact time and cause" of Vincent's death is known instantly at the moment of his birth. A nurse reels off a list of inherited conditions and mortality predictions, indicating that Vincent has a life expectancy of 30.2 years, a 60 percent chance of developing a neurological condition, a 42 percent chance of

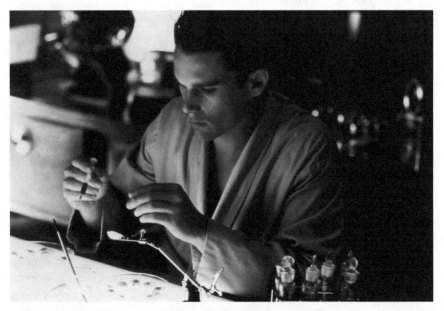

Figure 2.2. Vincent Freeman (Ethan Hawke) reassembles his identity in *Gattaca* (1997). Columbia Tristar. Pictorial Press Ltd/Alamy Photo.

manic depression, an 89 percent chance of attention deficit disorder, and a 99 percent chance of heart disorder, giving no indication that sociocultural factors might shape these predictions. On hearing this, Vincent's father veers from the plan to name his firstborn after him, branding his son less than legitimate, especially because the baby is not entitled to medical insurance because of his prognosis.

The conception of the second-born child, Anton, contrasts starkly with that of Vincent. In what is described as the "natural way," a genetic scientist displays four healthy embryos on a monitor and reassures the couple that there are "no critical predispositions to any of the major inheritable diseases." Vincent's voice does not control the narrative here. Instead, we see him as a toddler playing on the floor with a molecular model while his parents answer the geneticist's questions and choose his sibling's gender, skin tone, and eye and hair color. The geneticist even tells the couple that the pre-embryo screening process has removed any chance of "premature baldness, myopia, alcoholism and addictive susceptibility, propensity for violence, obesity, etc." The parents feel relief that these "prejudicial conditions have been eradicated" but want to leave a "few things to chance," although the geneticist states that he merely wants to ensure their child "has the best possible start." Exacerbating the stigma of genetic discrimination the young Vincent feels, his parents are gifted the "perfect" offspring in Anton, although they hold back from giving him enhanced mathematical and musical abilities in the film's extended cut, largely because they cannot cover the cost.[92] The two boys assume a genetic hierarchy: Anton (played by Loren Dean) is the taller and stronger of the pair, whereas Vincent realizes that his "real CV" is in his cells. The turning point comes when Vincent finally beats Anton in a swimming competition following a long series of predictable defeats. This victory destabilizes the assumed hierarchy, leading Vincent to aspire to greater heights while Anton suffers the shame of ignominy when he is unable to live up to his Olympian genetic code.

Everett Hamner describes *Gattaca* as a morality tale that "celebrates its hero's narrow escapes from genetic discrimination" because Vincent prevails despite facing the stigma of a natural conception and a predestined array of adverse health conditions.[93] Hamner questions its "biocultural plausibility," noting that the film exaggerates the medicalization of Vincent's health destiny, which is apparently sealed within seconds of his appearing in the world.[94] Although Vincent dodges his fate with his own ingenuity and a cool voice that offers an almost clinical perspective on this dystopian world of undisclosed violence, *Gattaca* does not readily allow for a more nuanced exploration of how environmental and cultural influences interact with genetic coding. Niccol explores these influences in his later films *In Time* (2011) and *Anon* (2018), whereas *Gattaca* opens up the black box of genetic determinism, with Anton's fate-changing swim triggering a different path to that supposedly predestined by his genes.[95]

Published twenty years later, Daniel Suarez's *Change Agent* can be read as a dynamic epilogue to *Gattaca*, developing the film's dystopian elements in a

futuristic design fiction that explores the global effects of the biotech acceleration on in vitro practices. *Change Agent* poses searching questions of power,
control, and care by projecting us into 2045, when rogue black markets have
replaced the regulatory role of the nation-state in a challenge not just to personal
privacy and data protection but also to the foundations of identity and health.
Suarez, who is best known for high-tech thrillers, shows in the novel's opening
pages how an average couple's desire to ensure that their future child is not
disadvantaged—just one among 1.5 million annual instances of assisted reproductive technologies—is the corporate veneer of a dangerous conspiratorial
world.[96] A self-professed science communicator and former IT consultant, Suarez
says that the aim of his design fiction is to provoke vigorous debate about synthetic biology so that we do not "stumble into the mid-twenty first century"
unaware.[97] This is not an outright rejection of gene editing, but Suarez believes
that synthetic biology poses serious safety and ethical questions that enterprise
often brushes over.[98] Appearing in spring 2017, when Crispr sequencing was featuring on television series such as *Westworld* (HBO, 2016–2022) and *Humans*
(Channel 4/AMC, 2015–2018), *Change Agent* pictures a world of unregulated technology in which the desire of average parents to eradicate inherited disease in
their offspring sits alongside illicit embryo harvesting and underground techniques that seek to alter the genetic architecture of adults.[99]

There are too many biotech elements in *Change Agent* to do it full justice here,
but I want to focus on two scenes—in the opening pages and halfway through
the book—that explore the health promises and dangers of unregulated assisted
reproductive technologies. The novel begins with a consumerist fantasy. Like
Vincent's parents in *Gattaca*, a middle-class Indian professional couple, the Cherians, are faced with a series of choices about determining the genetic fate of their
future child. It is ironic that an Indian couple travels to Singapore, given that
India was the primary destination for surrogacy in the early twenty-first-century
Global South, although legislative changes passed by the Indian Parliament in
2020–2021 sought to regulate both assisted reproductive technologies and exploitative outsourced labor.[100]

Instead of a team of medical personnel or a fertility therapist, the Cherians
meet only with a distracted genetic counselor at the unremarkable Trefoil Labs,
whose DNA-inspired logo consists of three interconnected circles (the logo later
unravels one of the novel's biotech mysteries).[101] Rather than relying on verbal
persuasion to convince the Cherians, the counselor beams an "in-eye" corporate
presentation onto their retinas, visually encoding what George Estreich calls
"images of what is 'natural'" by simplifying a complex genetic science into an
entrancing augmented reality.[102] Distinct from the underwhelming facility, the
luminous projection of an "utterly convincing" DNA double helix hovers in front
of the Cherians, accompanied by a female voiceover. Combining magic with reason, the voiceover presents gene editing as the only rational option for "ending a
legacy of suffering" and "putting humanity in control of its genetics." Yet despite
their allure, the projected images barely disguise global reproductive politics.

The DNA helix dissolves to present a despondent, naturally born blind African girl in contrast to a genetically edited, sighted child making cookies with her mother.[103] This fantasy is completed by a radiant image of a South Asian boy whose academic and athletic gifts seem to secure a patrilineal genetic future for the Cherians.

The scruples Mrs. Cherian voices that gene editing "seems against Nature" are countered by her husband's patriarchal hand on her knee and the counselor's reassurance that such choices are in line with natural selection, suggesting this is a reclamation of nature rather than a departure. However, before the couple can decide what gene edits are beneficial and affordable, the contrived tranquility of Trefoil Labs is disturbed by a security alert that dissolves the alternate reality into which the Cherians are being drawn. Despite reassurances that the police raid is a mix-up, the Cherians find themselves with other clients in a narrow corridor with no obvious escape. Before it is possible for the couple to assess the purpose of the raid, Mrs. Cherian is shot in the head, leaving her husband "shrieking in anguish," with both his wife and his genetic future extinguished in a flash.[104]

The patriarchal and natal fantasies of the novel's opening chapter are presented with subtle irony—the optical projection envisions the young boy as a healthy senior with his grandchild at the zoo. However, the slow build of this designer baby scene contrasts starkly with the police emergency and the ensuing chaos as other clients run pass the Cherians "in a panic toward an unseen rear exit."[105] The promise of enhanced natality ends in anxiety and sudden death, and the illusion that gene editing can make the future genetically secure by strengthening physical and mental health is shattered.

While the Trefoil Labs have no specific location, the second chapter portrays a deregulated global economy in which Singapore has become the "technology capital of the world" and the leading edge of the "Gene Revolution," revealing that Asia offers both more promise and increased danger for couples with the economic capital to design their progeny. It is likely that Suarez chose Singapore as the setting of *Change Agent* because of the opening of the futuristic biomedical research campus Biopolis there in 2006, following the establishment of the Genome Institute of Singapore in 2001. In this future world, the fact that genetic research in Southeast Asia is shown as less regulated has enabled that country to usurp the United States as a tech giant. In contrast, Americans are portrayed as anti-science individuals who mistake cell clusters as babies and resist vaccinations. Instead of exploring "extraterritorial trade" among poor American communities living close to "high technology corridors" such as Silicon Valley, unregulated bio-enterprises in *Change Agent* seek territories where national governments exert less control over marketable technologies.[106] *Change Agent* shares an anti-corporatist slant with Neal Stephenson's 1992 often-cited cyberpunk novel *Snow Crash* (1992), but it more squarely frames dysfunction within thorny bioethical debates about genetic regulation. In the novel, a news report underlines this a few pages later, indicating that these armed raids are in service of a UN treaty on genetic modification that is attempting to shut down illicit gene editing labs in order to preserve some semblance of world order.

The Cherians do not appear again after the opening scene, but their tragic story casts a shadow over Suarez's high-tech thriller. The main narrative follows the efforts of data analyst Kenneth Durand to break black market genomic cartels. Durand provides gene editing services via his work for the Genetic Crime Division of Interpol, a police agency that uses "advanced technologies in the fight against transnational crime," including human trafficking among vulnerable populations seeking to flee countries with extreme weather and fragile economies.[107] In its post-Crispr design, the world of *Change Agent* mirrors what biologist George Church and philosopher Ed Regis, collaborators on the 2012 book *Regenesis* (which is listed among Suarez's sources), describe as the exponential rate of technological change in which we can project "the consequences of taking two branches of the many forks in the road ahead . . . to its logical extreme."[108] The fact that Durand resorts to gene editing to modify the embryo of his young daughter Mia (and that he owns a neotenic pet "toyger") means that he is implicated in the deregulated world he seeks to clean up.[109] When his daughter asks about her genesis, Durand distinguishes between techniques that aim to eliminate genetic disorders (in Mia's case, Leber congenital amaurosis that causes severe visual impairment), as are permitted by the UN treaty, and unregulated practices geared toward enhancement, as is the case for the Cherians, who justify their choice to seek genetic modification with the claim that "weak memory [is] fatal to a future doctor or attorney."[110] Durand's explanation to his science-loving daughter steers a fine line between correcting genetic errors to prevent sickness and permitting "edits that don't fit the environment—even though we think they're cool."[111] The fact that Durand's mission focuses on the convergence of human trafficking and the rise of illegal embryo mills that could generate a "global genetic database" free from government regulation puts into context both the Cherians' meetings at Trefoil Labs and Durand's tender conversation with Mia.[112]

The second episode involves a visit by Durand and genetic engineer Bryan Frey (Frey has his own reasons for seeking genetic modification to correct his dwarfism) to infiltrate the Huli Jing cartel that has altered Durand's DNA, such that Durand now looks like his fugitive antagonist Marcus Wykes, including deep tattoos that intensify with strong emotions. Durand is relieved to later find only 0.006 percent of his DNA has been modified, but even with this small fraction, "he sensed how thin the cord was that tied him to himself."[113]

This facility Durand and Frey visit in Pattaya City, Thailand, contrasts sharply with the facility the Cherians encounter. It is presented as a cross between a fashion catwalk, a cabaret, a life-size diorama, and a showroom that is full of "lab counselors" and is hosted by "an adorable" and "effortlessly brilliant" six-year-old "Caucasian girl with blond hair and blue eyes."[114] With "flawless" pronunciation, the girl, Kimberly, presents to the guests other genetically edited children as embodiments of physical perfection with advanced linguistic, physical, and cognitive traits.[115] Whereas the projected natal imagery stimulates desire and attachment for the Cherians, the performance facing Durand and Frey, which includes a K-pop soundtrack, turns ethnic diversity and individual talent into genetic commodities that strip the innocence from childhood and colonize identity. In a parody of commodification, one young child is presented in "geisha-like makeup" and erupts "in a stunning operatic voice" to entertain the guests, as if the thread of her identity is destroyed in this consumerist marketplace.[116] In contrast to Durand's six-year-old daughter Mia's mix of childlike wonder and inquiring mind, this group of genetically upgraded children have unwittingly been granted a synthetic form of perfection at the expense of idiosyncratic traits and uneven health profiles that would distinguish them from an anodyne blueprint. Republicans might blame this dystopian world of genetically compromised childhood on pro-choicers or promethean scientists, but Suarez presents it in such a way that only the most aggressive technophile would think this is anything close to acceptable practice. After being asked to "favorite" the children on a tablet, Durand feels gut revulsion toward this display of medical tourism, recalling the visceral repugnance of Leon Kass in reaction to advanced reproductive technologies in general.[117]

Durand suffers physical, psychological, and ethical torment, at times verging on psychosis in his quest to regain his former identity and return to his family, but this "post-identity world," as the novel calls it, juxtaposes these two set-piece scenes to reveal just how easily parental desire and market commodification align.[118] Even at the end of the novel, when Durand makes a bedraggled homecoming, there is no sense that the "ethical quicksand" he navigates and the rogue genetic practices he witnesses will be easy to shut down.[119] It might seem, on this basis, that Suarez envisions less a reheated Cold War, in which the forces of civilization are pitted against genetic terrorists, and more global biotech anarchy premised on identity theft. Suraez's aim is not to renounce "technologically-empowered change" but to ensure that power does not become either too centralized or ceded to private-sector interests that privilege wealth over ethical or healthy practice.[120] In dramatizing the space between excessive governmentality and reckless enterprise, this shapeshifting novel is comparable to millennial sci-fi films such as *Face/Off* (1997) and *Minority Report* (2002) in its identity switches and web of conspiracies. At times, Suarez's voice as science journalist feels intrusive and at other times evasive, especially on the topic of reproductive labor. Yet at its heart is Durand's love for his daughter and wife, which helps stabilize his health, in sharp contrast to the alluring promises made to desirous parents by adventurists in a deregulated market, which the novel reveals to have profoundly adverse health consequences.

Designer Babies and the Family Romance

At first glance, the British crime writer Peter James is not an obvious contender for exploring the impact of embryonic interventions on family life. Best known for his Roy Grace series of crime thrillers, James has at times forayed into the

mysteries of science, religion, and the supernatural. Not a writer of science stories of the ilk of Michael Crichton's *State of Fear* (2004) and *Next* (2006), the latter
of which mixes "a catalogue of what could go wrong with biotechnology" with
policy recommendations on genomics, James has conducted sufficient research in
order to tackle big pharma and alternative medicine in *Alchemist* (1996) and *Faith*
(2000) and the clash between religion and science in *Absolute Proof* (2018).[121] The
concept of perfection recurs in James's crime fictions and coalesces in the exploration of genetically engineered children in *Perfect People*, a novel James shaped in
response to advice from geneticists and neurologists to give the story veracity.[122]
By taking us into the heart of "the family romance" (as Sigmund Freud coined it
in 1909), this chapter's final section further explores the bioethical entanglement
of embryonics, politics, and culture via a reading of James's *Perfect People* in order
to navigate concepts of design and perfectibility that inflect a quasi-eugenic
approach to procreation.[123]

The novel introduces us to John and Naomi Klaesson, an Anglo-Swedish
couple living in Los Angeles, where John works as an untenured research scientist at the University of Southern California. The couple have scraped together
enough money to afford an unorthodox offshore fertility procedure on a cruise
ship. This is a very different family dynamic from the one that conservative
thinker James Q. Wilson envisioned in the book he coauthored in 1998 with Leon
Kass, in which parents become largely dispensable because "getting a clone from
a laboratory would be like getting a puppy from a pet store."[124] *Perfect People* presents two committed parents who seek assisted reproductive technology to eradicate a faulty gene. The procedure, to be conducted by "maverick geneticist" Leo
Dettore, would help Naomi conceive without the risk of passing on the (invented)
genetic Dreyens-Schlemmer syndrome that killed their first child Halley at the
age of four a few years earlier.[125] The effort to compensate for the loss of a child
lends the novel a melancholic tone, although there is no mention that Naomi
received mental health support for the loss of her first child or fertility counseling
before she and John decided upon an experimental assisted reproductive technology. Nonetheless, the naturalism of its opening and the candor of Naomi's diary
entries set the novel apart from a high-tech film like *Replicas* (2018), in which a
grieving and remorse-stricken biomedical researcher (played by Keanu Reeves)
strives to resurrect his wife and children following a fatal car crash by cloning
replacement bodies with replicas of their neural maps.

Rather than the immortal cloning ambitions of *Replicas*, the narrative of *Perfect People* normalizes John and Naomi's parental desires. However, because they
also choose enhancements—in part because in Los Angeles you "found yourself
wanting things you'd never wanted before"—they rouse the attention of headline-
hungry media and the Disciples of the Third Millennium, a fanatical sect that
condemns "fooling around with human life itself" as a form of satanism and
tracks down the progeny of parents undergoing such procedures.[126] This a far cry
from pro-life activists taking their cause to Washington's Mall. However, when
Mike Pence (who used incendiary language in his support of the partial-birth

abortion ban) misquoted Billy Joel at the March of Life 2003, saying "it just may be a lunatic America is looking for," it legitimated the actions of extremist groups like the Army of God that used what they considered to be righteous violence against abortion centers and medical staff, as Joyce Carol Oates exposes in her 2017 novel *A Book of American Martyrs*.[127]

From the outset, the narrator of *Perfect People* stresses the Aryan features of the couple: John's "resolute Nordic features and a light Californian tan" are in sync with Naomi's Anglo-Saxon heritage.[128] John works on modeling replicas of primitive brains in order to deepen understanding of evolutionary processes. But he is as naïve as Naomi when he gauges the potential risks of an offshore artificial insemination procedure conducted by MIT- and Stanford-educated Detorre, whom scientists suspect of eugenic motives because he has patented an "efficient high-fidelity replication of genes" that uses a laboratory intervention to bypass the natural polymerase replication.[129] (The risks of stem cell research moving off-shore into unregulated waters was an issue NIH director Elias Zerhouni warned Congress about in 2004, following legislation that prohibited scientists from using all but existing stem cell lines.[130]) Detorre embodies this rogue culture on the fringes of orthodox science; he has been debarred from practicing medicine in the United States after he conducted genetic experiments on embryos that had "subsequently gone to term."[131]

The contrast between the Everyman couple and a potentially promethean scientist whom the Klaessons meet aboard a mysterious cruise ship carrying "a Panamanian flag of convenience" just off the New England coast provides the mise-en-scène for both an unregulated pre-Crispr procedure and an embryonic mystery that evolves slowly. The novel's domestic and global elements intersect subtly, presaged by Naomi's search on the first night on the cruise liner for an elusive point "where medical ethics, the acceptable boundaries of science, indi-vidual responsibility and plain common sense all meet."[132] Her diary entries give the reader access to her initial distrustful of Dettore, his "mediagenic" air of "great wealth," and his brazen defense of eugenic practices.[133] In their first con-versation, she recalls the *Time* depiction of him as a contemporary Dr. Franken-stein. His fingers and voice reassure her, but the fact that he presents the couple with a sixteen-page list titled "Klaesson, Naomi. Genetic defects. Disorders" adds to her consternation about the level of intervention. Faced with the dilemma of whether to agree to edits that would reduce the risk of inherited disease or could enhance their future child's health, the couple have no guidelines to fol-low. Naomi justifies their decision by noting in her diary that non-assisted repro-duction is too much of a lottery, given that her dead son Halley "got a shitty [genetic] deal."[134]

Perfect People does not present a world as extreme as Ken Macleod's futuristic 2012 novel *Intrusion* in which "nature kids" are close to illegal. Nonetheless, James's novel explores what Joan Rothschild calls the tendency in reproductive medical practice to conflate the words "healthy" and "perfect," which serves to amplify the "discourse of the perfect child [that] distorts the pregnant woman's hopes and plays on her fears."[135] James's literary interest in the supernatural is inflected by exploring how phenomena just out of focus dominate the lives of protagonists who are not wholly in control of their future despite their efforts to design it perfectly. It plays out in Naomi's anxious efforts to cope with her dream, although her anxiety remains undiagnosed in clinical terms and she receives no advice about a possible multifetal pregnancy. Naomi's hauntings intensify after a "ghost ship" sequence and the seemingly accidental death of Dettore in a helicopter accident. When she discovers that she is carrying a daughter and not a son, the couple has no one to contact about what they initially consider a mistake until Naomi realizes that she is about to have twins, followed by a very painful double birth procedure that foreshadows the discord and violence awaiting them.

The mutual dependency of non-identical twins Luke and Phoebe from an early age is not so developmentally surprising. However, when the Klaessons return to England to escape the threats of reporters and a fanatical sect, it is soon apparent that the twins have cognitive and linguistic skills far beyond their age, including command over a secret language in which they pronounce words backward with every fourth letter removed (perhaps a joke about genetic codes).[136] Despite John's expertise in experiential learning and simulation modeling, which he takes with him across the Atlantic to a new job at Sussex University, he is ill equipped to deal with the twins' advanced learning arc or to predict genetic modifications that might influence their emotional needs and self-concepts. The Klaessons are moderately concerned about genetic resemblance but cannot cope with the prospect of the twins outsmarting them. Seemingly unaware of the psychodynamics of this emerging family struggle, John dismisses their secret language as a form of invented speech, or idioglossia, before realizing that it is the sophisticated code of advanced intellects.[137] Instead of consulting reproductive health or twin concordance studies, James relies on correspondence with Caltech neurobiologist David Anderson, whose coauthored book *The Neuroscience of Emotion* (2018), explores how emotions are encoded into neural circuits and distinguishes between base emotions (joy, fear, anger, sadness, disgust) and social or moral emotions (shame, embarrassment, pride) that emerge after socialization.[138]

The maladaptation and behavioral problems the twins display seem to worry John and Naomi more than their mental health. Initially they think the twins are "backward" rather than intellectually advanced posthumans asserting their dominance in the family. After seeking professional opinions from a psychiatrist and behavioral psychologist who observes the twins in their home, John resorts to buying the three-year-olds a home computer, convinced that their brain development is already that of a typical teenager.[139] However, this only hastens their growth curve, leading them to dismember the family guinea pigs after reading about kidney dissection on *Gray's Anatomy* online, in one of the most gruesome moments of the novel.[140]

This scene is not a conduit for monstrous progeny or parents on a par with horror sci-fi films such as *Splice* (2010) and *I Am Mother* (2019), nor is it a portal to

the serious explorations of gender and race that we find in Octavia Butler's speculative fiction, including in her final novel, *Fledgling* (2005). Instead, *Perfect People*
exposes the Klaessons' naïveté in their failure to seek the opinion of a neurobiologist or to recognize the dangers of uncontrolled internet access. This neglect
reinforces their naïveté about technology in general, especially when John realizes that the twins are outsmarting him when they override his efforts to change
their computer password. More viscerally, the precocious puberty we see in the
Pattaya City scene in *Change Agent* materializes when Phoebe begins her period
very prematurely at age three (half the age when precocious puberty is likely to
occur in girls), and the twins' sharp experiential learning curve means that they
have no interest in interacting with children of their own age. That *Perfect People*
does not probe the mental health impact of these changes may be explained
either by the Klaessons' myopia or the generic limits of the crime thriller.

In the novel's final quarter, the distraught Klaessons seek to track down the
twins following their disappearance when a fanatic assassin bungles his attempt
to eliminate them. This search entails a chase south to Greece and then east to
Dubai. John and Naomi feel compelled to go alone without police protection
to unknown global locations when the twins contact them initially by encrypted
email (stating that their parents are "unable to provide [them] with the level of
stimulus and education [they] require") and then by videocast.[141] Eventually, the
Klaessons not only find Detorre alive but also realize that they have carelessly
signed a contract that means that the twins' custody defaults to Detorre if the
children freely choose this. The naturalistic tone of the novel's earlier parts is left
far behind when the twins reject "Mother Nature" as an imperfect system, a nod
to the eerie new species of children that emerges in British sci-fi writer John Wyn-
dham's 1957 novel *The Midwich Cuckoos*. Slowly, John and Naomi recognize that
through genetic modification they have given rise to a new species of "perfect
people" in which parents are unnecessary except as a vessel for gestation,
although this need is also likely to pass in time.[142] What the parents do not fully
realize, though, is that the voice of designed children comes with freight that
enables them to demand the right to independence at an earlier age than children
typically would.

However, the final irony of the novel is that the precocious puberty theme
that makes the twins so advanced in their childhood years quickly catches up
with them. In an epilogue to the novel, set eight years later, John and Naomi
excitedly await the twins' return after receiving an unexpected message from
them. At the airport, the couple are shocked to meet two figures in wheelchairs
who have physically aged into their eighties; only their piercing blue Nordic eyes
single them out as their twins in this startling scene of progeria.[143] Their perfection, then, is not only a category mistake but an unsustainable ideal that slips
away from both parents and children, their innocence and youth disappearing in
an instant.

While we may wish to dismiss Suarez's and James's novels as biodystopias
that will not, or at least are unlikely to, come true, Richard Storrow argues that

such fictional representations "can be transformative in addressing not only exist-ing bioethical dilemmas but also ones that yet remain in the realm of specula-tion."[144] In excavating the complex bioethical terrain of embryoville, both novels cut through the rancorous ideological positioning of Washington, DC, broaden-ing readers' perspectives on bioscientific entanglements in the hope that a good society (or a better society) is possible by combining responsible practice and international standards, such as the World Health Organization's Human Genome Editing Registry, introduced in 2019, a database of clinical trials that use human genome editing.

Mental health in these future worlds is an underdeveloped theme. But we can still read the two novels as testing grounds for what Carlos Novas and Nikolas Rose term genetic "life strategies" and what Leon Kass calls "a life lived humanly," while critiquing the moral perfectionism of Kass's world view by assessing it both within the family circle and against the standards of global health governance.[145] There are also absences in both novels with regard to diversity and engagement with the sociopolitical issues Alondra Nelson and Ruha Benjamin pose with respect to race and technology.[146] Nonetheless, Suarez and James ask us to think about cultures of life as pluralistic rather than in exceptionalist terms. Their shared theme of precocious puberty is relevant when assessing genetic proce-dures that are designed to protect and enhance yet may leave children vulnerable to forces that they and their parents are ill equipped to deal with. More than any-thing, these fictions revisit perfectibility less as the province of biotechnology and more, in the words of Joan Rothschild, "a transformed vision" that has the potential to replace "the dream of 'perfect babies' with the goal of health and well-being for all children . . . in all their differences and diversity."[147]

PART TWO

CONSCIOUS STATES

3   *Health in the Neuronal Workspace*

RETHINKING CONSCIOUSNESS
AND INTELLIGENCE

A short article published in *Nature* in October 1993 peaked professional and public interest in what in utero fetuses and young children can sense and learn. The lead author, Frances H. Rauscher, a postdoctoral researcher at the Center for the Neurobiology of Learning and Memory at the University of California, Irvine, assessed how music triggers differing modes of awareness, especially those that shape spatial reasoning skills.[1] Involving thirty-six students, the experiment conducted by Rauscher and colleagues concluded that listening to ten minutes of Mozart's Sonata for Two Pianos in D Major temporarily enhanced the subjects' spatial awareness. The researchers calculated that this enhanced level of activity temporarily increased IQ eight and nine points higher than listening to relaxation instructions and silence, respectively.

The experiment had many limitations. It did not test other Mozart sonatas or other forms of music. It did not consider whether similar effects might be detected in young children, even though Rauscher started with preschoolers in mind. And it did not test the relative effects on the verbal reasoning and memory of the student sample. In fact, Rauscher made no claims beyond the limits of the experiment. Yet the "Mozart effect," as the media termed it, stimulated further research into fetal auditory perception of both language and music. Just as important, it triggered cultural debates about what expecting and actual parents might do to improve the musical sensibility of their children and to maximize potential cognitive benefits, especially as research showed that the auditory capabilities of fetuses begin at twenty weeks of gestation.

In fact, the "Mozart effect" has taken on a life of its own in terms of its popularization and its possible effects on general intelligence. There are Mozart effect CDs for final-trimester fetuses and babies (a version of which was funded by Georgia governor Zell Miller in 1998 and distributed to new mothers), brands offering inflated claims about the educational qualities of their products (notably the Baby Einstein brand based in Atlanta), popular columns offering to separate fact from fiction regarding the special qualities of music for sentience, and therapeutic claims that verge on New Age speculation by the likes of the Colorado music educator Don Campbell, who popularized the term "Mozart effect."[2] In addition to fueling a culture of "neuroparenting" stoked by anxiety and what writer Jonathan Franzen calls "the wired paradigm" (see chapter 5), this potent mix of science and speculation also influenced Washington politics.[3] Michigan representative Vernon Ehlers cited research behind the Mozart effect in a 1997 debate on arts funding, and President Clinton profiled the positive influence of music education on academic performance in 2000, when he visited the public Joseph C. Lanzetta School in East Harlem, appearing with Billy Joel to encourage the public to donate musical instruments to schools.[4]

An experiment conducted at the University of Belfast that was published two years before Rauscher's piece in *Nature* showed that the rhythm and melody of music has the capacity to stimulate alertness in late-trimester babies. Studies since 2000 have broadened this focus, including those that tested the effects of music on fetal arm movements (2010), on memory four months after birth (2013), on fetal heart rate (2019), and on maternal well-being (2021).[5] There have also been counterclaims about whether the temporary benefits on IQ in Rauscher's paper withstand scrutiny, an issue to which Rauscher herself has returned, claiming that the "Mozart effect" label has "been grossly misapplied and over-exaggerated."[6] Others have commented favorably on how music enhances the neuroplasticity of young minds and manual dexterity without buying into the hype of the Mozart effect. In his plea for better music education, neurologist Oliver Sacks cites Canadian musicologist E. Glenn Schellenberg's view that music primarily affects mood rather than cognition, although it is important to distinguish between the benefits of playing or singing from the benefits of simply listening to music and between its long-term and instantaneous effects.[7] Physicist Philip Ball agrees, claiming that "we perform better if the music makes us feel good" and concluding that "Mozart has no intrinsic, mysterious power to make your child smarter."[8]

Debates about the Mozart effect illuminate the dangers of limited experiments that have a wildfire effect, but they also point in two other directions.[9] One direction is the explosion of research conducted during the 1990s about how the human brain generates consciousness and interfaces with the body. This intersection of neurological and biotechnological research poses questions about how music stimulates diverse neural networks in different areas of the brain and body; the relation between music and language; the transfer effects of music for cognition, dexterity, and emotional intelligence; and the extent to which music can have a sustained impact on well-being.[10] Such an approach to what Nikolas Rose and Joelle Abi-Rached term the "neuromolecular brain" falls squarely within the sphere of neurobiology instead of seeking to distance neurology from biotechnology.[11] The other direction is the commercialization of intelligence products since the 1990s that aim to capitalize on neuroplasticity, especially enhancement technologies that are marketized to give children a competitive advantage or special programs that promise to aid the education of those experiencing developmental disabilities. In the early twenty-first century, although some educational providers envisaged a child's growth holistically, questions of mental health rarely entered discussions of IQ as a measurement of cognitive ability unless the discussion is fueled by worries about how the neuroeconomy controls the "management of the mind."[12]

Taking debates about the Mozart effect as one of many paths through the neuropolitics and biopolitics of the 1990s, this chapter focuses on the mounting interest in consciousness during the Decade of the Brain, how this interest dovetails with rival progressive and conservative views of intelligence, and the implications for those experiencing neurological challenges, especially among younger and older Americans. At the time, the mid-1990s seemed like a breakthrough moment when researchers and practitioners were collaborating with computer scientists to expand the therapeutic possibilities of artificial intelligence and with molecular biologists to develop techniques of personalized neurology that have the bandwidth to respond to both "genetic and environmental factors that influence response to therapy."[13] This remained an open and expansive field into the 2000s, as neurosurgeon Kewal Jain illustrates. Jain tracked over twenty different "blood–brain" relationships that link biotechnology and neurology, echoing a 1990 memorandum that health secretary Louis Sullivan sent to President Bush in which he promoted Decade of the Brain initiatives on the basis that more than a third of "known genetic diseases affect the brain."[14] Amid excitement about the possibilities of neuroenhancement, philosophers and scientists raised questions about brain disorders that erode a sense of perspective and selfhood and often provoke anxieties about identity and belonging. Jain injects a tone of realism into his more heroic claims, noting that despite neurobiological advances, "there are serious deficiencies in our understanding of the pathomechanism of several neurological disorders as well as our ability to diagnose and treat these disorders."[15]

Accordingly, in opening the second part of this book, "Conscious States," this chapter addresses the nosological and operational dangers of reducing mental ill health to brain disorders and of pronouncing grand claims about breakthroughs, given that there were so many challenges to what Jain calls "biomarker identification in neurological disease."[16] As a prelude to discussing technological applications of neurobiology for addressing learning disabilities and degenerative disorders, the next section focuses on philosophical and neurological debates about consciousness that run from 1990s through the 2010s. This enables me to highlight the developmental and sociocultural implications of intelligence debates, before discussing in the final section Canadian educator Barbara Arrowsmith-Young's *The Woman Who Changed Her Brain* and the 2015 film adaptation of New England neuroscientist Lisa Genova's 2007 novel *Still Alice*, in which selfhood is both learned and unlearned in dialogue with cognition enhancement and pharmaceutical technologies. Despite the strains exerted on a stable sense of selfhood within narratives of neurological challenge or loss, I show how an emergent mode of bioethics helps thread the needle between philosophical and scientific approaches to consciousness and intelligence, revealing how discourses of advancement, transformation, and uplift typically overshadow those of emotional and psychological well-being. Just as the first part of *Transformed States* explored Jenny Reardon's question "Who can speak for humanness in a genomic age?," this chapter restates the question, "Who can speak for humanness in a neurological age?" with respect to individuals and families living with atypical neurological conditions, as a prelude to the focus on augmented biotechnologies in chapter 4.

Consciousness as a Neuronal Workspace

When George H. W. Bush proclaimed the 1990s as the Decade of the Brain, he aimed to stimulate biotechnological initiatives, strengthen medical understanding of experiences at each end of the life spectrum, enhance awareness of the neurosciences via public discussion, and decrease the social and economic burden of mental illness.[17] The proclamation followed a joint resolution of Congress the previous summer, championed by Massachusetts representative Silvio O. Conte, a veteran Republican who promoted the NIH's call to develop a national mental health plan. The joint resolution noted "a technological revolution occurring in the brain sciences" that combined "such diverse areas as physiology, biochemistry, psychology, psychiatry, molecular biology, anatomy, medicine, genetics, and many others working together toward the common goals of better understanding the structure of the brain and how it affects our development, health, and behavior."[18] Conte had long been an advocate of expanded health coverage and investment in biomedical research at state and national levels, and the joint resolution was his final congressional triumph before his death in February 1991. An Office of Science and Technology report, *Decade of the Brain, 1990–2000: Maximizing Human Potential*, that was released two months later acknowledged Conte's "foresight and leadership" and his influence on improving "the health and well-being of Americans."[19] The NIH also recognized Conte's crucial role in promoting the congressional mission to raise awareness of mental health issues by naming its network of centers for neuroscience research after him and by integrating neuroscience into its strategic plan as "the foundation for understanding mental disorders and/or transform the understanding and treatment of mental illnesses."[20]

Bush recognized the "daunting task of educating the public—as well as scientists themselves" about the fundamental importance of brain research, but he did not always strike the right tone.[21] For example, although he followed the American Psychiatric Association in declaring the week beginning October 7, 1990 as Mental Illness Awareness Week, instead of acknowledging vulnerability to mental ill health in certain demographics, such as among teenagers or in communities of color, he stressed the technological side of neuroscience in tracing "intricate pathways through which the brain's messages flow" in order to learn "more about normal and abnormal behavior, emotion, and thought."[22] Despite this emphasis on the "multidisciplinary efforts" of scientists and physicians to understand the neurological causes of mental illness, Bush was criticized for using stigmatizing language in a 1989 ABC interview and for referring to Alzheimer's patients as "victims" being ravaged by disease in a dedication ceremony that year.[23] In addition, there is no evidence to show he engaged with Decade of the Brain activities, aside from commenting on the reorganization of the Alcohol, Drug Abuse, and Mental Health Administration in July 1992 as an effort to pool expertise and bring mental health research "into the mainstream of biomedical and behavioral research at NIH."[24] The president's office received Decade of the Brain briefings in 1990–1991, but had Bush attended more events at the Library of Congress over the next nine years, he would have witnessed how interdisciplinary conversations were deepening an understanding of cognition, learning, memory, and adaptability, alongside topics aligned with White House priorities, such as the aging brain, the subject of a November 1993 symposium that was held a year before former president Ronald Reagan announced that he had an advanced form of Alzheimer's.[25]

The philosophical aspect of these debates ran alongside efforts to raise public awareness about brain capacity and disease. This was primarily via collaborations between the NIH and the Library of Congress and included the launch of an international Brain Awareness Week in May 1996. This initiative promoted new technological advances in medical imaging that increased the "capacity to map the biochemical circuitry of neurotransmitters and neuromodulators" in order to facilitate "the rational design of potent medications" that could strengthen an understanding of the neural causes of complex physical and psychological conditions. In this respect, philosophical and neurological investigations intersected with genetic mapping for understanding inherited and degenerative aspects of dementia, an increasingly prevalent condition that the World Health Organization believed posed "one of the greatest societal challenges for the 21st century."[26] Significantly, little federal regulation accompanied the neurological revolution, except for ethical protocols to safeguard human subjects in research environments. This trend contrasts with a dearth of congressional concern for potential misuses of data and violations of privacy, even though neuroscientific evidence was emerging increasingly often in courtrooms.[27]

At arm's length from clinical trials and congressional activity, philosophical debate in the 1990s stepped back from laboratory applications and returned to fundamental questions of mind and body, subjectivity and selfhood. These debates hinged on disagreements between, on the one hand, behaviorists such as Daniel Dennett and Paul and Patricia Churchland who saw the mind as the epiphenomena of brain activity and, on the other, thinkers drawn to the irreducible aspects of subjectivity. This second camp included analytic philosophers John Searle and Thomas Nagel and British molecular biologist Francis Crick, who had shifted away from his genetic research with James Watson in the 1950s to work on the neurobiological underpinnings of consciousness at the Salk Institute for Biological Studies in La Jolla, California. Paradoxically, although these debates had historically been shaped by federal initiatives and neuroscientific advances, they were also ahistorical in picturing selfhood as a nebulous abstraction instead of something that is embedded in sociocultural and biographical particularities. This did not mean that debates returned to essences, especially after "the linguistic turn" that Richard Rorty heralded in the late 1960s, which argued that we must acknowledge how words and discourse mediate questions of thought and action.

Daniel Dennett, an outspoken professor of cognitive science at Tufts University, echoed the linguistic turn in his provocative 1991 book *Consciousness*

Explained, in which he concurred with Rorty that metaphors are all we have when we approach truth.[28] Understanding that the power of language sets humans apart from animals, Dennett broadened his work from his training in cognitive science to tackle big philosophical issues. He tested the power of this approach in his 1987 book *The Intentional Stance*, then shifted gears in *Consciousness Explained* by seeking to resolve mind-body dualism and dispel mysteries about the mind for a popular readership. The secular humanism Dennett's philosophy rests on is often aligned with the work of British evolutionary biologist Richard Dawkins, whose reputation as a provocateur and hostility toward the arts is evidenced in his 1998 book *Unweaving the Rainbow*, which assaults what Dawkins considers to be the delusory wonderments that inspired John Keats and other Romantic figures and that circulate as folk beliefs through contemporary culture.[29] We can see a similar attack on ingrained beliefs in Dennett's critiques of the Cartesian idea of a "Central Meaner" as an engine of sense making and the polyzoic theory of "the pontifical neuron," which posits that certain master neurons are conscious.[30] Although Crick criticized Dennett for being "overpersuaded by his own eloquence," Dennett, undeterred, developed a philosophically serious "intentional stance" toward the subject of utterances on the premise that they are rational beings.[31]

Consciousness Explained, arguably more than any other book of the decade, delivered a sophisticated riposte to Cartesian mind-body dualism with "boldness, originality, and panache," in the words of Richard Rorty.[32] Harkening back to his former teacher Gilbert Ryle's famous attack on the "ghost in the machine" in *The Philosophy of Mind* (1949), Dennett presented a "multiple drafts" theory of consciousness that dispensed with the idea of a special center to consciousness, a place where "it all comes together; and consciousness happens."[33] Instead, Dennett predicated his multiple drafts theory of consciousness on the premise that when we observe a scene carefully there will always be perceptual gaps in our internal description of it. He saw consciousness as intrinsically "gappy," but argued that trained perception fills in these gaps to present the illusion of a plenum, brought about via "parallel, multitrack processes of interpretation and elaboration of sensory inputs."[34] Dennett framed this philosophical position in terms of the evolutionary development of a flexible mind that processes sense data rapidly and that we give names to. In his embrace of the human mind as a "complicated, evolved machine," Dennett was encouraged by the developmental interest in neuroplasticity to dispense with a single dominant narrative of self—"the 'final' or 'published' draft"—based on the premise that we continually revise sense impressions in light of new data.[35] This model does not deny agency, but neither does it surrender it to an essence that is anterior to consciousness.[36]

Dennett used a broad palette in explaining his multiple drafts theory of consciousness, including a discussion of patients encountering neuronal disconnections between their left and right hemispheres due to brain damage. However, in cases of the neurological disruption that split-brain patients experience, Dennett denied the "narrative gravity" he affords to a fully functioning individual.[37] We might feel repelled by this denial of agency for patients with neurological damage or consider Dennett too vociferous in his challenge to rival models that he deems incompatible with his own. Francis Crick, for example, argued that Dennett's dismissal of the Cartesian theater overlooks the idea that there might be multiple such theaters in a distributed model of the mind—a theory that might preserve a degree of agency for all conscious individuals no matter what their neurological condition.[38]

Among other disagreements, Dennett publicly locked horns with John Searle of the University of California, mainly because Searle's theory of mind was too phenomenological for his liking. In his 1992 book *Rediscovery of Mind*, Searle agreed with Dennett that consciousness is an emergent concept "caused by neurophysiological processes in the brain," but argued against Dennett's version of functionalism in an effort to retain private subjective experiences as a "special feature" of the brain.[39] Aside from his specific critique of the computational model of the brain (as he elaborated in a Decade of the Brain speech at the Library of Congress), Searle claimed that consciousness is a biological feature of the brain but in its "first-person ontology" is also a higher-level mental phenomenon that stands apart from neuronal processes.[40] This view was shaped by the biological research of Gerald M. Edelman, director of the multidisciplinary Neurosciences Institute in New York City, particularly Edelman's quest to put "the mind back in nature" without resorting to an outmoded dualism, which he elaborated in his pioneering books *The Remembered Present* (1990) and *Bright Air, Brilliant Fire* (1992).[41] Edelman's theory of a "dynamic core" of consciousness—as presented in the Decade of the Brain symposium series and developed in his coauthored 2000 book *A Universe of Consciousness*—was based upon reentrant neuronal activity in the thalamocortical system that forms feedback loops within the cortex, some of which are drawn into a state of conscious awareness.[42] Evoking William James's interest in the flow of consciousness a century earlier, Edelman asserted that "matter itself may be regarded as arising from processes of energy exchange" and that "mind is a special kind of process depending on special arrangements of matter." To Searle's mind, Edelman's neuronal theory lent biological justification to the argument that consciousness emerges as a "special feature" of the brain—a feature that is not entirely reducible to background neuronal activity because it produces intentional states toward which the self is motivated.[43]

In a heated exchange in 1995 between Searle and Dennett in the *New York Review of Books*, Searle claimed that Dennett's eliminative account failed to do justice to the brain's "special features" and to ontological questions of being. In response, Dennett accused Searle of circling around paradoxes of subjectivity.[44] In rejecting selfhood as a magical notion that is unavailable for scrutiny, Dennett later called his distributed model of self a "heterophenomenology" that takes a "third-person approach to consciousness" by focusing on what consciousness reports instead of attempting to know much about who is doing the reporting.[45]

This exchange is less about solving consciousness and more about the ways the biosciences and cognitive sciences reanimated old philosophical debates about whether selfhood is monistic or dualistic. The differences between Dennett and Searle are those of temperament and approach: Dennett believes that consciousness can be explained by dispelling folk beliefs, whereas Searle recognizes that there "is no simple or single path" in either philosophical or scientific terms.[46] Each used neuroscience to underpin their ideas, but whereas Searle believed that these pathways lead us inward to the "rediscovery of the mind" and outward to forms of human sociability, Dennett warned against "interdisciplinary miscommunication" and remained skeptical about whether problems that neuroscience and philosophy tackle are exactly the same. Regardless of the validity of Dennett's criticism that Searle's biological monism hides a vestigial dualism and seeks comforts in an unknowable knower, ultimately Searle rescues the category of the human, in all its multiplicity, whereas Dennett's materialistic behaviorism replaces this baggy concept with a systems model that redescribes human behavior computationally.

I will return to the Dennett-Searle disagreement in the next chapter with respect to artificial intelligence, but in their divergent approaches to consciousness neither fully considered the question of how we ascribe meaning to certain types of experience over others or how a mode of living is pieced together from the fragments of sense perception that create an impression of flow. If, as Thomas Nagel argued, we see ourselves only "from outside," then we might lose conviction and "find it difficult to take our lives seriously," whereas seeing ourselves from inside gives sense to life, even though it may lead us to retreat from ever-changing flux beyond the self.[47] For Nagel, who wrote before the rise in diagnosed anxiety disorders, the solution is to recognize that we are "simultaneously engaged and detached" in the lives we lead.[48] Rejecting the centerless view that he tacitly associates with Dennett, Nagel goes beyond epistemological concerns in his 1986 book *The View from Nowhere* (and more explicitly in a 2017 review of Dennett's *From Bacteria to Bach and Back*), pinpointing morality as a form of "objective reengagement" that accounts for the views and lives of others, although he notes that this does not dissolve the sense of life's absurdity.[49] Although this ethical turn is absent in many accounts of consciousness, Nagel's view is similar to Searle's position in its alignment of science with common sense yet without collapsing one into the other.[50] The implications of a life led both as observer and participant poses problems when one of these perspectives becomes dominant— out of personal choice or shaped by a health condition or compelled by a distorted sense of reality, as the 2001 movie *Donnie Darko* explores for a Virginia teenager. Nonetheless, Nagel sees the alternative view as one of denial, repression, and a repudiation of "full awareness."[51]

While Nagel's model allows for ethics to sit alongside epistemology, what it lacks—and, arguably, what Dennett's Darwinian model possesses—is a conception of selfhood as a dynamic and unfolding process rather than a static thing to be known and oriented toward a goal. Illuminating this process-oriented perspective, developments in narrative medicine have, since the early 1980s, considered how the self is partly a construct of language that unfolds in narrative terms and in dialogue with others. This approach was epitomized by the launch of the journal *Literature and Medicine* in 1982, in which practitioners of narrative medicine critiqued the format of the medical chart (which downplayed the subjective experiences of the patient) and instead promoted what Larry Churchill called "the moral primacy of stories over stages" in narratives of health and illness.[52] This conceptual and institutional shift away from charts to stories raises a number of operational, epistemological, and ethical questions, especially about who owns the narrative voice for patients experiencing profound neurological impairment.[53]

Writing three decades later, the British neuroscientist Anil Seth argued that the mapping of first-person (phenomenological) and third-person (neuronal) descriptions of consciousness is still a work in progress but that it is in the textual realm that Nagel's idea that we are both detached and participatory comes to life, leading us back toward a biomedical entry point.[54] Oliver Sacks, arguably the best clinical exponent of this double view, explored how individuals experience pain on the inside but can also be observed empirically. He developed his ideas through case studies on right-hemisphere damage to the brain affecting speech, writing, and memory in *The Man Who Mistook His Wife for a Hat* (1984) and *An Anthropologist on Mars* (1995). Importantly, Sacks's notion of a "clinical tale" moved beyond the behaviorist approach of Dennett and the defectology orientation of neuroscience.[55] Because many of his patients had lost the capacity to construct their own narrative, the physician had to assist in extrapolating the "elemental form" as a patient tried to give words to experience in order to produce a layered "history of illness from its first intimations, through all its subsequent effects and evolutions."[56] In his writing style, Sacks favored an organic language of effect and affect over a more procedural rhetoric of stages. He saw stories as elemental and therapeutic, in which a patient who cannot fully recover from illness or brain damage can, in some instances, accommodate themselves to a new reality, facilitated by the physician as healer-scientist.

There is a danger in privileging narrative over medicine here, by granting it magical rehabilitative properties that rarely exist in degenerative conditions or those in which there is a complex interplay between soma and psyche, as Angela Woods reminds us.[57] Nevertheless, the epistemic and ontological shifts that narrative medicine explored in the 1980s and 1990s were consequential not only for the doctor-patient relationship but also for thinking about broader practices beyond the clinic. While Sacks enjoyed the relative luxury of private practice, which enabled him to observe his patients with a more considered eye than would a typically hurried physician in a public hospital, he only occasionally resorted to narratives of overcoming and more often focused on an individual's efforts to adapt to neurobiological flux.

Dennett's functionalism is at odds with Sacks's radically empirical perspective that thoughts have an owner that lends them a personal quality no matter what the extent of brain's capacity to form words and meaningful phrases is.[58] However, there are some resonances between Dennett and Sacks. For example, Dennett notes in *Consciousness Explained* that brain damage often forces a patient to invent "new paths," to find "new ways of doing old tricks" and to seek rehabilitation through "active exploration," especially when drug therapies only go so far in alleviating the disruption of brain function.[59] Sacks would frame these quests in person-centered terms, but his interest in evolutionary versatility led him to detect in many of his patients a capacity to compensate for neurological loss even in instances when the coherence of their world is in jeopardy. Sacks was more attentive than Dennett to the sounds and words—as well as to the language of music—that gives style its individuality. Dennett recognized this when he credited Sacks for recognizing the "riches language brings to a mind," but Sacks went further by viewing language ability as anterior to the capacity to meaningfully arrange spoken and written words.[60]

The challenge for physicians and psychologists is how to bridge the subjective experience of patients and the health realities they face. Underlying this tension between experience and reality is what cognitive psychologist Jerome Bruner calls a "classic human plight" that structures all stories. Bruner detected that the structural unity of the story rests on the relationship between "plight, characters, and consciousness" that manifests itself variously as "steady state, breach, crisis, redress" along an extended timeline.[61] Bruner saw the mythic structure of storytelling as having therapeutic benefits in its capacity to place different kinds of frames around experience, even though his universalist template may lead us toward grand archetypes and away from recognizing particularities of cultural and gender difference.[62]

Taking a more neuroscientific approach to Bruner, Antonio Damasio adhered to the emergent theory of consciousness as a feature of neuronal brain activity but also saw consciousness as "the feeling of knowing" in which a wordless core is extended through mental images that are given shape in thoughts and expression through words and stories. In his 1999 book *The Feeling of What Happens*, Damasio recognized the danger of impairments that affect the whole of consciousness, but Damasio's model of an extended consciousness with a neurobiological core is persuasive.[63] He refined this model in *Self Comes to Mind* (2010) by describing three layers of consciousness: a "protoself" arising out of "primordial feelings" is given initial shape by a "core self" that is intentionally oriented and is then given more recognizable shape via a third-level "autobiographical self" that generates pulses that interlink past and future.[64]

This understanding of the primacy of elemental stories and how they are given shape at a higher level of consciousness would satisfy neither a hard-core realist who would point to disruptions in brain functioning as an explanatory framework nor a poststructuralist focusing on textual fissures, ambiguities, and detours in which a linear story dissolves into a series of often-contradictory iterations of a messy, human life. Narrative medicine steered between the poles of realism and relativism, allowing enough free play to account for variations of consciousness while retaining story structures by which we make some (if never complete) sense of otherwise inchoate sense impressions.

It is notable that questions of expression and narrative were often missing in the largely consensual neuroscientific understanding that consciousness is the "global neuronal workspace" that Bernard Baars of San Diego's Neuroscience Institute postulated in 1997.[65] Dennett embraced the concept of a global workspace, in which conscious states are broadcast, as one that explains how consciousness works through "sideways influences, from competitive, cooperative, collateral activities" that can often be mistaken as a top-down process.[66] This ensemble model resonated with Edelman's idea of open-ended maps with a dynamic core that integrates different types, bundles, and levels of neuronal activity, some of which are drawn into higher-level consciousness. The crucial difference is that Dennett sees consciousness as a "postlanguage phenomenon," whereas Damasio and Edelman argue that language begins at the wordless core of a primordial brain map and becomes more sophisticated at higher levels of consciousness.[67]

This view of language is compatible with the workspace model in that it can be assembled in different ways to produce meaningful utterances but is where conscious information sits alongside unconscious intentions and meanings. However, the workspace model strains against the noncomputational argument about the plasticity of the human brain and the essentially "nonmechanical" quality of human consciousness, which logician Robin Gandy asserts cannot be replicated by computers, "however complex their programs."[68] There are also questions to ask about what happens when Edelman's dynamic core fractures in cases of schizophrenia and for those experiencing right-hemisphere damage, but it is important to note that Dennett does not give up entirely on human agency, even if he tries to dispel its metaphysical implications. In 2003, he argued that "partially coherent agency" is compatible with this view of sorting through the plenum of consciousness, admitting that what we call selfhood is a construct of both language and evolution.[69] In one provocative line, Dennett described the mind as "the control system of a chameleonic transformer," suggesting there is still some shaping agency in the open-ended neuronal workspace.[70]

It is notable that Bush's Decade of the Brain proclamation of 1990 focused on brain diseases that affect both memory and language ability and that directly influence the ability to tell a coherent story from a first-person perspective. Edelman considers language and consciousness to be of equal importance, particularly because "possession of true language with syntax in humans gives rise to higher-order consciousness[,] allowing its possessor to be conscious of being conscious."[71] In this view, higher-order consciousness is predicated on the capacity to configure experience through feedback loops and contextual awareness of environment. This raises the question about whether Edelman is just reframing computer organization in organic terms. But it also nudges us away from needing to decide whether subjectivity is a construction or a delusion and toward the recognition that in most cases, language is intertwined with thoughts and emotions.[72] The next section turns to these topics of human intelligence and emotion.

Intellect versus Affect

At a May 1998 symposium at the Library of Congress on the neurobiology of emotion, Second Lady Tipper Gore opened day two of proceedings with a short, impassioned keynote. Librarian of Congress James H. Billington and NIH director Steven E. Hyman described the theme of the symposium, titled "Discovering Our Selves: The Science of Emotion," as "critical to our individual and societal health" in helping us understand not only the mysteries of emotion but also "serious mental illness—the common and debilitating scourges of depression and anxiety disorders, the lack of motivation and emotional abnormalities in schizophrenia, the devastating problems of autism."[73] Lewis Judd, the director of the National Institute of Mental Health, was confident at the end of the 1980s that biomedical research was starting to make "major advances in understanding the biological and genetic underpinnings of affective disorders," and a decade later, as mental health advisor to President Clinton, Tipper Gore joined the NIH's effort to elevate emotion from the "dark basement" of neurobiology by giving it a human face and an executive branch profile.[74] In addition to arguing that the neuroscientific "almanac is being written as we speak," Gore stressed the importance of "total health." By this, Gore meant both basic research and its biomedical applications, highlighting the vital role of health care workers in "translating this virtual explosion of knowledge into ways to improve the lives of millions of Americans who suffer the symptoms of various mental illnesses."[75]

Tipper Gore highlighted the historical importance of this moment in giving a "voice to the voiceless" during the early planning stage of the inaugural White House Conference on Mental Health the following June. This compassionate commitment was of a piece with her founding of the Tennessee Voices for Children coalition in the early 1990s, which promoted health and education services at the state level, and the touring Homeless in America photography exhibition she curated with the National Mental Health Association in the late 1980s.[76] Gore stressed technological solutions and contributed to a growing emphasis on identifying organic biomarkers for mental health. But she also believed that tackling stigma regarding mental illness and nurturing the emotional landscape of lives and communities deserved equal priority with questions of intelligence, until "the chink in the walls of suspicion and fear and ignorance about mental illness gets larger."[77]

Debates about the Mozart effect in the 1990s often blurred the intellectual benefits and emotional affects of music—understandably, given that music stimulates both sides of the brain. Although Tipper Gore did not contribute to this debate (she instead tackled perceived misogyny in heavy-metal music), she was keen to mark this historic moment. The fact that the Library of Congress symposium focused on children's health and everyday emotions indicates a broad view of intelligence and a more nuanced understanding of the supportive and creative structures needed to foster it in young children. Child psychiatrist Stanley Greenspan touched on this in his presentation at the 1998 Decade of the Brain symposium, noting that "societal patterns are eroding rather than strengthening these critical emotional building blocks. Impersonal group-oriented infant and child care (the case in many day care centers), decreased human interaction in play and education, growing family problems, and decreased adult-to-adult interactions: all erode the emotional interactions necessary to abstract thinking, moral judgment, and intimacy with others."[78] We may see this as a culture wars statement in its criticism of prevailing social values and the direction of national educational policy, but this view is central to Greenspan's work on pediatric health and emotional intelligence.[79] A believer in the benefits of music, Greenspan focused on how infants and children use language as a tool of emotional organization and metabolic activity, especially at six to twelve months, when typically a developing brain displays a high degree of plasticity. Thinking of language as "emotional interaction" that has both generative and reflective aspects, Greenspan believed that through careful observation, a parent or educator could guide a child showing signs of "apathy, self-absorption, impulsivity, concrete and disorganized thinking, and/or language and learning problems" toward more emotional affirmative interactions.[80]

This returns us to the roles of language and narrative structure and highlights the need to conduct psychodynamic work with children instead of simply resorting to drug treatments for autism and attention deficit disorder, to take two examples. We might see Greenspan's perspective as an idealistic approach to tackling the challenges children with learning needs face. Conversely, we may read this view as a criticism of educational models that privilege cognitive intelligence over emotional intelligence. Either way, it places the creative solution to developmental disabilities (and their implications for mental health) in human hands instead of relying on technological solutions. Greenspan's twin goals were to unlock a child's potential and reduce the stigma associated with lack of sociability or language and numeracy challenges.

Greenspan's research marked a sharp contrast to the most prominent intelligence theory of the time, as postulated by Harvard University psychologist Richard Hernstein and political scientist Charles Murray in *The Bell Curve* (1994).[81] Focusing explicitly on how IQ often correlates with income, education, and employment, Hernstein and Murray proposed the bell curve theory to explain how higher levels of intelligence index to social advantage.[82] Classifying the population with one of five intelligence labels from left to right on the curve— Very Dull, Dull, Normal (the median category), Bright, and Very Bright—they pointed out that individuals labeled with the first two terms are those that are most socially disadvantaged and less able to compete for well-paying jobs. Hernstein and Murray's theory of economic stratification and their biodeterminist view of a cognitive underclass relied on a narrow statistical conception of intelligence measured as IQ. They saw "musical abilities, kinesthetic abilities, or personal skills" as falling into the realm of talents rather than intelligence and sidelined "intrapersonal and interpersonal skills," although they at least admitted that measures of intelligence are "a limited tool for deciding what to make of any given individual."[83] Using IQ to plot social trends meant that Hernstein and Murray's classifications relied on stigmatizing labels. In addition, their conclusions about race and heredity offended Black communities, especially their efforts to turn a statistical view of intelligence into public policy, as Henry Louis Gates Jr. noted.[84]

The Bell Curve does not present a coherent model of the mind or consciousness. Instead, the analysis relies on a statistical method shaped by a Social Darwinist belief in the genetic composition of intelligence and the social advantages that certain forms of intelligence are granted within a capitalist system, producing both a "cognitive elite" and an underclass. Hernstein and Murray did not attend to the rich life-worlds that Oliver Sacks discerned in his patients or to an increasing number of autobiographical accounts. For example, Cole Cohen shows in her compelling memoir Head Case (2015) how her diagnosis of Gerstmann's syndrome in her mid-twenties, caused by "a partial atrophy of the right parietal lobe" that profoundly affected her handwriting, numerical skills, and spatial awareness, was not a measure of her intrinsic intelligence, especially with regard to language development.[85]

The Bell Curve received much criticism for its correlation of educational levels and racial stratification, but questions were also asked of the authors' statistical methodology and their suggestion that poor parenting and behavioral problems are more likely to arise among families with lower IQs. Paleontologist Stephen Jay Gould was especially concerned about Hernstein and Murray's reductionism, stating that "intelligence, in their formulation, must be depictable as a single number, capable of ranking people in linear order, genetically based, and effectively immutable."[86] As an aspect of his broader critique of biological determinism, Gould argued that not only were Hernstein and Murray's correlations weak, but they also failed to note that the causal patterns they posit are at best speculative. Gould did not deny that genetics play a role in intelligence, but he highlighted the ecological role the environment plays in shaping consciousness and rejected the fact that general intelligence could be represented by a formula because this suggests that intelligence might be cloned or bought.[87] The argument for cloning intelligence was a step beyond what Gould calls The Bell Curve's "manifesto of conservative ideology."[88] Hernstein and Murray did not argue that intelligence could be enhanced by a pill, as fantasized in Alan Glynn's 2001 novel The Dark Fields and its 2011 film adaptation Limitless, in which the performance-enhancing drug MDT-48 (loosely based on Modafinil, which is used to treat sleeping disorders) turns an unfocused writer into a genius, helping him identify hidden connections between data while boosting his language skills and musical talents.[89] Yet there is a pharmacological urge here (at least figuratively speaking) that enables certain demographics to attain normative forms of intelligence while simultaneously denying it to others.

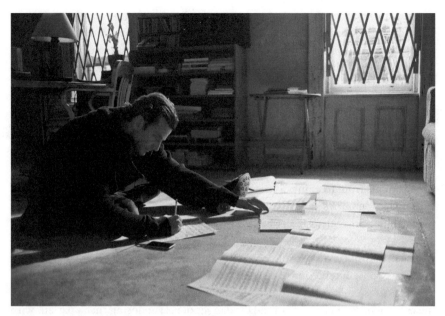

Figure 3.1. Eddie Morra (Bradley Cooper) experiences a boost in cognitive powers after taking MDT-48. *Limitless* (2011). Moviestore Collection Ltd/Alamy Photo.

I will return to the topic of smart drugs, but it is important to note here that Gould's critique did not explore the extent to which Hernstein and Murray's position is predicated on theories of social and racial superiority.[90] Especially alarming was James Watson's adherence to the racial implications of Hernstein and Murray's thesis, a position that led the former director of the Human Genome Project to make disparaging remarks about Africans in his 2007 memoir.[91] However, while *The Bell Curve* dominated scientific and cultural debates about intelligence in the mid-1990s, it ran alongside discussion of the Mozart effect, which veered away from IQ and toward other spatial and emotional forms of intelligence. Hernstein and Murray's biodeterminist model allowed no room for this broader view or for the different educational routes that interested Stanley Greenspan. They also did not discuss the links between intelligence and language or what happens when neurological impairment or mental ill health prevents an individual from expressing themselves coherently. In fact, Hernstein and Murray were uninterested in variations to the bell curve norm that may account for alternative modes of intelligence.[92] Their social scientific perspective veered away from a neurobiological anchoring of consciousness that might have pushed them to address more nuanced accounts of intelligence—both natural and artificial—beyond their cognitive-elite model. The next chapter returns to such AI questions, but it is important first to consider implications of these accounts of intelligence when faced with neuronal disruptions in expressive meaning making.

In Oliver Sacks's theoretical writings and clinical tales, he was critical of the scientific reductionism epitomized by *The Bell Curve* and advocated for a holistic approach to neuroscience to account for the neuronal substructure of the brain and the higher realms of consciousness with which his patients voiced often profoundly disruptive conditions. Sacks was fascinated by language in its broadest sense—not just the speech acts that interested John Searle or patients with savant traits but also the deeper rhythms of language that reveal themselves through the body or alternative forms of expression. Sacks saw cognitive intelligence as continuous with more affective forms of consciousness and creative expression that have a "binding power."[93] This includes the power of music to help Parkinson's patients from freezing, as Sacks explored in his 1973 book *Awakenings*, or that can trigger memories and "depths of feeling and meaning to which [patients with frontal lobe damage] normally had no access," as described in his 1992 clinical tale "The Last Hippie."[94]

Sacks did not overlook patients who fall in the margins of a statistical bell curve or whose interactions between what Gerald Edelman calls "core systems, nonconscious memory systems, and signals from value systems" defy easy measurement.[95] There is an attendant danger of presupposing that a patient with dementia or aphasia retains an intuitive grasp of their world even if it is beyond their ability to mobilize language. However, Sacks offers enough of a human bond between himself and his interlocutors to give the reader faith that meaning making continues in all circumstances, except for coma or brain death, although brainwave research shows that even those in minimally conscious states can respond to commands and word repetition.[96] This emphasis on meaning making aligns with the clinical work of Damasio, who sees in the "improvised vocabulary of nonlinguistic signs" of aphasic patients the possibility of communicating richly and "humanly."[97] Damasio and Sacks believe that empirical study reveals how consciousness emerges from complex neuronal activity, even in cases in which consciousness is profoundly disrupted. This is not categorically different from the global neuronal workspace model, but Sacks sought to give a voice to patients living with the kind of "gappy consciousness" that Dennett discerned. Sacks's immanent approach to language and rhythm revealed that just because a patient loses the capacity to fill gaps between sense impressions, it does not mean they lack intelligence or the ability to interact meaningfully.[98] It was precisely the individuals living with a gap between expectation and experience—to use Searle's phrase—who interested Sacks, prompting questions of expression, being, and knowledge.

The romantic aspect of Sacks's work and his emphasis on the natural world are not only diametrically opposite to the behaviorist reductionism of Dennett on the one side and the statistical reductionism of Hernstein and Murray on the other, it also reveals continuities within profoundly disrupted states without elevating intellect above affect. As Sacks stated in the mid-1980s, a patient who might seem profoundly withdrawn or who requires institutionalized care may still be "truly and creatively intelligence, and not just have a mechanical 'knack,' in the

specific realms—musical, numerical, visual, whatever—in which they excel. . . .
It is this intelligence which must be recognized and nurtured."[99] The forging of
new paths is a capacity a patient may need assistance with via interpersonal care,
augmented speech technologies, or neurologic music therapy. The latter is effective for poststroke patients experiencing aphasia or those with other forms of
brain damage, such as former Arizona representative Gabrielle Giffords, who
found singing therapy effective after being shot in her left hemisphere in 2012.[100]

Sacks veered away from drug treatments (even though *Awakenings* recounted
an experimental drug therapy for Parkinson's symptoms) because he was wary
about quietening the primitive rhythms of an individual as an aspect of their core
consciousness. To his mind, drug interventions might mute inherent creativity
that has its own "connections and synchronizations" that cannot easily be captured on brain imaging devices.[101] The semiotics we use to give meaning to sense
impressions push Sack's neuroscientific account away from the "coldness and cal-
culation" of cognitive philosophy toward an imaginative realm shot "through
with passion, longing, and romance" that seeks emotional and imaginative connections between physician and patient.[102] Sacks recognized that language,
including the rhythmic structures of music and nature, is woven into the varied
fabric of life itself. To this end, the final section of this chapter returns to the
affective emotional realm that fascinated both Sacks and Damasio, posing mutually informing questions on epistemological, ontological, and bioethical levels.

Learning and Unlearning the Self

Debates about the layering and scope of consciousness in the 1990s were not
always attentive to how disruptions to basic and advanced functioning often have
a profound impact not just on individuals but also on their support networks.
When Daniel Dennett playfully asked the question "Where Am I?" in 1978, it was
an abstract thought experiment rather than a profound existential question about
perception, embodiment, and memory, issues that are especially acute for conditions that affect speech and cognition. This final section applies debates about
consciousness, intelligence, and selfhood to two conditions that George H. W.
Bush identified in his Decade of the Brain proclamation that were of particular
concern in the 1990s: developmental disabilities and dementia. These conditions
have complex health biomarkers relating to genetics, epigenetics, and environment, and they continue to evoke the question "Where Am I?" despite two further decades of research into and a federal emphasis on the revolutionary
potential of the neurosciences. The final section of this chapter illustrates how
the relationship between the neurosciences and narratives is not unidirectional.[103]
I want, first, to briefly return to Stanley Greenspan and Oliver Sacks for thinking
about alternative forms of intelligence and modes of neuronal connectivity
before testing neuroscientific models with reference to Barbara Arrowsmith-
Young's *The Woman Who Changed Her Brain* and the 2015 film adaptation of neuroscientist Lisa Genova's novel *Still Alice*, both of which, from different ends of the
life spectrum, explore processes of learning and unlearning.

We have seen how Greenspan's developmental model illuminates the cognitive and affective aspects of young lives. Because children's brains have plasticity, their neurons make new connections when "activated by experience," but in cases of intellectual and developmental disabilities, neurotropic pathways cannot be unblocked by nurturing environments alone.[104] The explosion of memoirs published in the 1990s and 2000s that explore the thin line between mental health and mental illness coincided with the growth of popular scientific accounts of neurological deficits and excesses, to cite the titles of the first two sections of Sacks's *The Man Who Mistook His Wife for a Hat*, arguably the most recognizable of this group. Disability rights advocates argued against this deficit neurological model because it can easily be equated with a damaged identity instead of simply describing a neurotropic reality. Still, growing clinical and popular interest in savantism and superintelligence ran alongside research on language disruption, in early lives, in midlife and among older Americans experiencing dementia.

We can find an embedded version of Greenspan's developmental model in Barbara Arrowsmith-Young's 2012 book *The Woman Who Changed Her Brain*, which charts her journey from the severe learning difficulties she experienced at school in the late 1950s and 1960s (including dyslexia, dyscalculia, and what she calls a "kinesthetic speech disorder") through to the establishment of an educational system she began to develop in the late 1970s that sought to unlock the hidden potential of a new generation of schoolchildren by forging neuronal pathways that seem to be blocked or inhibited.[105] Arrowsmith-Young chose not to address the topic of learning difficulties from a state perspective, which—in the United States—included the White House endorsement of the First National Congress on Adults with Special Learning Needs in 1987, President George H. W. Bush's America 2000 education strategy for addressing the over 40 million recorded cases of American adults with reading difficulties, and the efforts of First Ladies Barbara Bush and Laura Bush to destigmatize the labels "remedial" and "slow learners" by promoting literacy. Instead of reflecting on policy initiatives, Arrowsmith-Young documents how her personal encounters and the stigma she felt as a girl who was identified as a slow learner inspired her to develop pedagogical techniques that focus on the visual and auditory stimulation that strengthened her cognitive capacities, aligning with Nikolas Rose and Joelle Abi-Rached's recognition that neurobiology is often approached "not as destiny but *opportunity*."[106]

Arrowsmith-Young recalls the breakthrough moment in her mid-twenties (in the late 1970s) when she read the writings of Russian neurologist Alexander Luria, whose *Man with a Shattered World* (1972) focused on what traumatic brain injury teaches us about cognitive capacity and how brain processes adapt around damage to core functions. Primarily, Luria helped Arrowsmith-Young reconceptualize brain activity as a form of neuronal networking.[107] Focusing less on the repetitive tasks championed by Barry Kaufman in his controversial Son-Rise Program, which he believed could enhance the IQ of children with autism, Arrowsmith-Young focuses on actualizing brain potentiality. She does so by drawing on Toronto psychiatrist Norman Doidge's 2007 book *The Brain that Changes Itself* and University of California psychologist Mark Rosenzweig's experiments of the early 1960s that showed how rats in an "enriched environment" perform better on maze tests than those in "impoverished environments."[108]

This notion of an "enriched environment" is a leitmotif for the Arrowsmith program, which was instituted at a private school in Toronto in 1980 and has since grown globally, including a research network spanning North America, Europe, and China. Although Arrowsmith-Young is Canadian, *The Woman Who Changed Her Brain* reveals a transformational perspective that seems distinctly American, tapping into what Julie Passanante Elman calls a "rehabilitative journey" that promises to "culminate in 'stable' adulthood and ensure national health" by acknowledging learning differences as a step before reinforcing normativity.[109] Arrowsmith-Young's personal success story is interwoven with her educational entrepreneurship, but it also echoes President Clinton's belief that educators should do more to create stimulating and supportive environments (linked to the 1997 White House Conference on Early Childhood Development and Learning) and the George W. Bush administration's emphasis on early-stage diagnostics to ensure that children are not "left behind" on reading and comprehension.[110]

The Woman Who Changed Her Brain complements Arrowsmith-Young's biography. In contrast to IQ-based diagnostics, the book presents stories of children who have benefited from the program, focusing always on how the unlocking of neuroplasticity can overcome just about any cognitive deficit. This view is predicated on the potential for such a release, which is why the uplift stories veer away from brain trauma and atrophy or cases where disadvantageous socioeconomic conditions would prohibit a child from entering the program. Part of the problem with Arrowsmith-Young's account is that it places supreme belief in transformation and neuroplasticity over and above children who do not respond to these exercises or whose stories do not help advance the Arrowsmith program. The book is heavy with references, yet it lacks extended neuroscientific research into classroom techniques and meaningful sample sizes. Instead, it relies on uplifting stories and the increased feeling of well-being and sense of self that educational success can bring, as Arrowsmith-Young herself experienced in her mid-twenties. The intertwining of autobiography and educational potential is illustrated by the book's formal design: it jumps around historically to ensure that the author's "joy and excitement of being able to really communicate" for the first time chimes with stories of children who have positively responded to the Arrowsmith program.[111]

The objective of the program is to clear brain fog by improving the connectivity and functionality of the prefrontal cortex in problem solving and self-direction. *The Woman Who Changed Her Brain* outlines techniques to clear and stimulate the brain on differing cognitive and affective levels but, surprisingly, does not focus on the potential benefits of music therapy. However, since 2017, the Arrowsmith Program has promoted a complementary educational program, Soundsory, which aims to develop neuroplasticity and improve sensory processing through cognition-enhancement technologies that combine rhythm and movement to support "the integration of the brain and body through a developmental progression."[112] Echoing the emphasis that Australian neuromedia researcher Jill Scott places on sensory, haptic, and immersive experiences in sentient learning, Soundsory is technologically sharper than Arrowsmith's paper-and-pencil and computer exercises in its aim to stimulate bones in the ear and sound contrasts via electronically manipulated pulses through a headphone.[113]

The manufacturer of Soundsory is Sound for Life Ltd (est. 2014), a Hong Kong–based neurotech company that has also developed a Forbrain product to improve attention, speech, memory, and learning for autistic children. While the educational benefits of music therapy have been established for children diagnosed with autism, the science behind Forbrain and Soundsory lacks evidence of rigorous peer-reviewed trials.[114] This trend highlights both the recognition of the affective sphere when it comes to special needs education and the extent to which claims around sentience are open to exploitation. Two commercial examples of this trend are the education tech company Mindvalley (est. 2002), which promises to unlock extraordinary levels of cognition, and Neuralink (est. 2016), which aims to restore neurological functioning and autonomy for Americans with quadriplegia by transforming the brain-computer interface.[115] Despite the heroic promise of the Mindvalley and Neuralink promotional materials, commercially oriented tech routinely ignores instances in which uplift narratives grant only limited or temporary agency, especially in cases of degenerative disease—a topic to which I now turn to conclude the chapter.

Two of the most poignant moments in the 2015 film adaptation of *Still Alice* are when Alice Howland, played by Julianne Moore, barely recognizes herself in a mirror due to early onset Alzheimer's. These two moments are part of a haunting sequence, corresponding to the three-quarter point in a two-year narrative cycle (2003–2005) that structures the episodes of Lisa Genova's novel and makes visible the diminishment of neuroplasticity in Alice's brain. By focusing on questions of personhood, Genova's prologue melodramatically frames neurological diminishment as the silent strangulation of neurons: "Whether it was molecular murder orcellular suicide, [the neurons] were unable to warn her of what was happening before they died."[116] The filmed sequence takes a phenomenological approach to the fragmentation of Alice's consciousness and self-awareness. Following a bright childhood memory flashback featuring her dead father and sister (her father has passed familial dementia on to Alice), we see Alice's dim reflection in the screen of her laptop, which, alongside her cell phone, has been a lifeline, enabling her to retain contact with her daughters and her neuronal connections to memory via tasks and games. For five long seconds the camera focuses on the dark screen that frames the blurred outline of Alice's hair, face, and dressing gown before cutting to a side shot from the far side of the room. We see her sitting passively on the sofa in the background as a cleaner works industriously in the foreground, emphasizing that Alice can no longer perform basic tasks.

Following another memory flashback of the child Alice with her father on a sunny beach, the second existential moment (fifteen seconds later) shows her disheveled hair and face in close-up as she stares at herself in a bathroom mirror. Alice looks down momentarily, half blankly, half quizzically, to find that she is brushing toothpaste into her open palm. She lifts her hand and then seemingly absentmindedly daubs toothpaste on the mirror to entirely obliterate the image of her face as the scene shifts to another childhood memory flashback. The scene recalls a number of mirror shots in one of Julianne Moore's earlier films, the 1995 movie *Safe*, in which a largely inarticulate Californian homemaker suffers from an unnamed disease that affects her both physically and psychologically. The silence of the *Still Alice* sequence is telling, with just a melancholic refrain linking the two scenes. In Genova's novel, the equivalent scene prompts Alice to pose two unspoken questions, "What's wrong with my face? . . . What's wrong with these mirrors?," before she covers the mirror with toothpaste in a confused state of mind.[117] The film uses a blurred lens to signify how the previously articulate Alice only dimly experiences a turning point in which her consciousness is gappy (what a *New York Times* review called Moore's ability to convey the "pathos of emptiness"), accompanied by a loss of basic capability as we see her struggling to tie the laces of her trainers a minute earlier.[118]

Alice's inherent intelligence, which has helped her gain elite status as a professor of cognitive psychology at Columbia University (Harvard in the novel), is increasingly compromised by her degenerative condition. That she is "fascinated by communication," linguistics, and phonology makes early onset Alzheimer's more marked than it might otherwise be when her professional and domestic lives begin to unravel. The film implies that her career has been a singular pursuit for Alice, whereas references to William James in the novel suggest a personal meditation on brain health rather than a critique of the work stresses of higher education or the consumerist emphasis of marketized health care.[119] In fact, because Alice's privileged social status has enabled her to enjoy a healthy lifestyle in terms of exercise, diet, and self-care, there is little room in either version to explore environmental or social factors, including the growing burden of Alzheimer's in communities of color where resources are often scarcer, as the NIH recognized in the early 1990s.[120] We might criticize *Still Alice* for not being sociological enough or for not engaging with the public side of Alzheimer's, including an exploration of the "biomarkers of prediction and prevention."[121] Nonetheless, in its emphasis on the inner and outer lives of Alzheimer's, *Still Alice* asks the twin questions "Where am I?," by focusing on the embodied effects of memory loss on cognition and consciousness, and "Who am I?," which haunts the disassembling experience of dementia.

The occasional memory lapse at the start of the film increases in frequency (most poignantly when Alice searches for the word "lexicon" during a public lecture at UCLA), and we also see the shift in the ever-simpler language she uses when playing Words for Friends on her phone: Alice plays "hadj" on a triple word

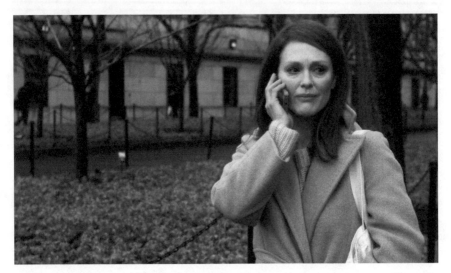

Figure 3.2. Alice Howland (Julianne Moore) begins to experience memory lapses in *Still Alice* (2015). Artificial Eye/Alamy Photo.

score early in the film (for 66 points) but struggles to think of "tone" only 45 minutes later (for only 5 points when she could have made either a double-word or a triple-letter score). This shift is also marked by more symbolic moments, such as when she texts her husband "where r u?" on returning from Los Angeles before forgetting her location during a familiar run on campus. The phrase echoes that more abstract question "Where am I?" that Dennett poses when he imagines that his brain, his body, and his consciousness are separated from each other geographically and biotechnologically, leading to dizzying confusion as he tries to locate a sense of self. Alice's research on past-tense irregular verb forms in infants eighteen to thirty months old initially gives her confidence that we can learn much more about "the relationship between memory and computation that is the very essence of communication."[122] However, her own life arc contrasts starkly with this cognitive view of intelligence and spatial awareness, leading not only to short-term memory loss but also to category mistakes, spatial disorientation, and loss of self, as is apparent when she watches a home movie titled "Alice Howland," which she can "only stomach" watching once. Her surname "Howland" suggests a modern-day Alice in Wonderland, bewildered and lost in the transformed world of Alzheimer's: what Alice in the novel describes as feeling "neither here nor there, like some crazy Dr. Seuss character in a bizarre land."[123]

Genova notes that the catalyst for the novel was her grandmother's Alzheimer's, which became apparent in her eighties but "systematically disassemble[d] her" when she became increasingly childlike.[124] Using the novelistic form as a mode of science education, Genova contrasts her inarticulate grandmother to the initial articulacy of Alice. This gives phenomenological insight to the typical experience of Alzheimer's, even as Alice is portrayed as an exceptionally talented person who is deeply conventional in her family life, leading her to deter her younger daughter, Lydia, from pursuing an acting career. The epistemological gap between Alice's own experience and the narrative is shortened in the novel because she is given a voice, albeit a diminishing one, in contrast to a dementia narratives like Michael Ignatieff's *Scar Tissue* (1993), in which the narrator tries to imagine the life world of his aging mother "at the dark edge where everything is crumbling" or Jonathan Franzen's interwoven autobiographical and imaginative reflections on brain disease and memory loss (see chapter 5).[125]

Alice's self-care and memory retention in the early stages of dementia are important, but so too are relationships with her daughters. Anna (Kate Bosworth), who discovers that she has the familial Alzheimer's gene, has the economic means to use genetic screening to ensure that the twins she conceives do not carry the gene. Her sister Lydia (Kristen Stewart) refuses to take the genetic test so as not to cast a determinist shadow over her life. In fact, despite some initial conflicts, Lydia offers the strongest lifeline to Alice when her husband (Alec Baldwin) puts his career ahead of his responsibility as caregiver. It is Lydia's role—especially when she plays Irina in a performance of Anton Chekhov's *Three Sisters* in the film—that provides emotional connectivity for Alice once medical science has reached its limit.[126] Alice empathizes with Lydia's ability to convey Chekhovian despair and joy, although she forgets that Lydia is her daughter. This empathic bond seems to stem from what anthropologist Janelle Taylor terms the "moral laboratory" of new modes of interaction as a "site for experimentation, creating conditions for the emergence of new virtues."[127] In this instance, at least, Alice retains intersubjectivity, even as subject-object distinctions and maternal feelings are eroding in her neuronal workspace.[128]

The film's ending is overly sentimental, especially as Alice retains the capacity to identify love as the primary theme of Tony Kushner's AIDS-era play *Angels in America* (as read to her by Lydia), even when she is in the process of disassembling, losing basic facets of cognitive functioning and control over her voice.[129] The power of dramatic theater takes the place of music in stimulating an affective emotional response in Alice. However, it is surprising that her family does not try different modes of therapy (beyond her husband bringing her DVDs to watch when she can no longer read novels), especially as clinical trials in the mid-2000s were showing that music and art can reduce anxiety and agitation in moderate to severe forms of Alzheimer's, together with evidence that suggests that the nootropic supplement choline can assist in nerve repair and cognitive functioning.[130] Although creative approaches that might retain narrative continuity for Alice are extremely limited, technology is a lifeline as her cell phone and laptop function as portals of prosthetic memory until a late stage of her disease. Nevertheless, the film—more than Genova's novel—contrasts the diminishing existential aspects of Alice's health experiences with her professional world, represented by her role as an Ivy League scientist and the neurological experts she consults. However, medical science has marked limitations: physicians are unable to treat or slow down her Alzheimer's, especially once the early diagnostics have indicated that it is a familial genetic strain inherited from her father.

Alice is prescribed two drugs in combination that are thought to increase the intensity of neurotransmitters: Aricept (or donepezil, which has been available for medical use since 1996 and can have mild cognitive benefits) and Namenda (or memantine, a new drug at the time that was thought to slow down the progression of dementia).[131] The story does not focus on the side effects or the efficacy of the combined prescription on receptor uptake, aside from Alice's sense that the drugs might be futile (it "felt like aiming a couple of leaky squirt guns in the face of a blazing fire"), her difficulties with managing her pill regime, and flashbacks to her childhood in the film that might be stimulated by the hallucinogenic side effects of Namenda.[132] Although there are no critiques of medical paternalism or profit-seeking physicians, *Still Alice* illustrates Genova's belief that neither Aricept nor Namenda "gets at the heart of the matter. They don't stop the disease from progressing. They just make the most of what is still functioning."[133] There is a further pharmaceutical layer in the novel as Alice is also prescribed the experimental drug Amylix, which, as the penultimate chapter states, is thought to have failed in its initial promise as an amyloid beta–lowering agent.[134] Such pharmaceutical limitations are cruelly emphasized when early in her illness, Alice leaves a message to a future Alice to consume a full bottle of Rohypnol (prescribed for chronic insomnia), only for the future Alice to lack the capacity to execute the detailed instructions to commit suicide by prescription drug overdose.

Yet the novel and film might have dealt with the messier side of Alice's decline more starkly (what the novel describes as "layers of disturbing filth") and might have looked beyond the fact that as an Ivy League professor Alice does not experience socioeconomic pressures that might otherwise have deepened her struggle or led to diagnosis at a much later stage. Questions of stigma and fear are not analyzed in sociological terms. Instead, the novel focuses on the sense of loss that Alice feels when she is forced to step away from her professorial duties and her fleeting recognition that she is no longer in the "ninety-ninth percentile" for "abstract reasoning, spatial skills, and language fluency," as her neuropsychologist describes it.[135] Nevertheless, both versions of *Still Alice* are successful in showing Alice's transitions as key elements of what Damasio would call the stripping away of her autobiographical self and core self. This leads to a form of "social death" for Alice in her experience of what Dragana Lukić calls the "multiple ontologies" of dementia as she loses a grip on where she is and who she is.[136]

Although Genova's novel probes Alice's incremental memory loss in more granularity than the film, in contrast to writer David Foster Wallace's neuropessimism that leads him to muse about the impossibility of getting close to someone else's pain, both versions of *Still Alice* strive for a balanced perspective on different levels of consciousness, seeking to show how Alice's emotional intelligence survives, albeit in fragmented and diminished form, even after she loses her capacity for cognition and speech.[137] The film's humanistic emphasis is most acutely apparent when, suffering from moderate memory loss, Alice prepares a lecture for the Alzheimer's association, only for Lydia to suggest that her mother focus on the personal side of the illness rather than technical descriptions of amyloid plaques and neurofibrillary tangles. This exchange is absent in the book, which arguably overemphasizes Alice's ability to still perform as a public speaker, only for the euphoria she feels after the event to contrast sharply with the cognitive and physical decline of her final six months.

The emphasis in *Still Alice* on what poet Elizabeth Bishop called the "art of losing" as an embrace of unlearning offers a leitmotif for Genova's career as a neuroscientist-turned-writer. It stresses the need to think through strategies of survival that go beyond the aims of the federal government to "prevent and effectively treat" Alzheimer's by 2025 to think through what intelligence means beyond typically measurable limits and to recognize the psychological burden on individuals and carers.[138] *Still Alice* is not a radical literary experiment that seeks to capture the "syntax of gaps and silences" that characterizes, for example, the late work of poet George Oppen as he started to experience dementia in the late 1970s that eventually made him incapable of writing.[139] Yet in a health environment in which perspective and praxis are put under increasing strain, Genova tries to account for lapses, pauses, repetitions, and silences in the novel's diaristic form. Rather than portraying Alice's diminished life-world as a form of zombification, she remains humanized. Straining against the idea that biotech "happiness pills" are the best option for alleviating low-level depression, Alice experiences (seemingly nonpharmacological) moments of "pure happiness and joy," even in late-stage dementia, and retains some emotional intelligence even when her self-consciousness and awareness of others' feelings weaken.[140] Moments of love between daughter and mother are not only reconciliatory but also a form of person-centered care that does not require Alice to cognitively perform, offering a "temporal solution" of "interpersonal possibility" to offset the stripping of personhood.[141]

Bishop's idea of the art of losing loops back to the question "Who can speak for humanness in a neurological age"? It also illustrates the bioethical balance between art and science that Sacks sought in his clinical tales of patients inhabiting worlds that are simultaneously familiar and unfamiliar, conditions that led him to identify alternative routes for communication when habitual channels are blocked. This is not to summon a magical Mozart effect—even though music therapy can be beneficial for autism and dementia—but to call for work in a more embodied and less prescriptive field than scientific accounts often allow. Such an expansive field can address existential questions of being, hope, and longing that complement scientific research and medical care. As chapter 5 discusses, there is a long road ahead for Alzheimer's research, despite the FDA's approval of Leqembi in 2023 following clinical trials by Biogen and the Japanese biotech company Eisai—which, in cases of mild dementia, may slow the Alzheimer's arc by reducing the buildup of amyloid plaque.[142] Nonetheless, this expanded field can revive the richer public bioethics that Leon Kass called for, but without Kass's conservative ideology that tends to push diverse and idiosyncratic experiences into a generalized category of human nature.

Augmented Lives

ARTIFICIAL INTELLIGENCE AND
ROBOTICS IN A TIME OF CONFLICT

In October 2016, late in his presidency, President Obama spoke inspiringly at a White House Frontiers Conference at Carnegie Mellon University in Pittsburgh about what his Democratic predecessor in the White House had called the "endless resource" of science.[1] Two decades before Obama's speech about the "pretty cool" devices on display at the conference, President Clinton and Vice President Gore had envisaged a convergence of exciting frontier technologies with "dramatically valuable results for humanity."[2] Inspired by a National Academy of Sciences forum titled "Science in the National Interest," Clinton and Gore recognized the need for long-term investment to ensure that "scientific enterprise" would develop "at a rate commensurate with its growing importance to society" in order to enhance education, health care, national security, productivity, and quality of life.[3] Obama echoed this vision as he praised Pittsburgh's entrepreneurial spirit as a city bouncing back from recession through investment in artificial intelligence, robotics, and regenerative medicine.[4]

All three of these Democratic leaders gave equal weight to the nation's health and the nation's economy. They did so to ensure the federal government's aim of maintaining the "competitive advantage" of the United States "as the world's most innovative economy" but ensuring that this goal did not overshadow "the chance to cure cancer or Parkinson's or other diseases that steal our loved ones from us way too soon," in the words of Obama, who underscored this balanced agenda by recalling his inaugural address of 2009. Back then, after eight years of Republican rule in the White House (Republicans controlled Congress for four and a half of these years), the newly elected president promised to "restore science to its rightful place and wield technology's wonders to raise health care's quality and lower its cost."[5] At the 2016 Frontiers conference, Obama reiterated his belief that "reason and science" are not "inimical to faith and feelings and human values and passions," even though the "Republican war on science," as political journalist Chris Mooney called it, was fueled by this dichotomy.[6]

This balanced agenda was given a human face when Obama met Nathan Copeland, one of the delegates at the October 2016 conference. As a science student in 2004, the eighteen-year-old Copeland had injured his neck and spinal cord in a car accident, leaving him paralyzed from the chest down, although he retained some shoulder movement and sensation in his wrist and fingers. A robotic limb study at the University of Pittsburgh's Medical Center gave Copeland hope he might regain some of his former abilities. The study was supported by the Revolutionizing Prosthetics program of the Defense Advanced Research Projects Agency (DARPA), an arm of the U.S. Department of Defense that invests in breakthrough technologies. The pioneering project involved a surgeon implanting four microelectrodes in Nathan's brain that enabled him to manipulate his arm, hand, and fingers "by just thinking about it." This halved the time it took to grasp an object (compared to earlier limb prototypes that relied on vision) and restored his ability to feel through his prosthetic fingertips despite his damaged nervous system (although he still could not sense hot and cold).

Not only did Copeland experience the restoration of a previously intuitive set of physical actions through a brain-computer interface, but his increased manual dexterity was married to the "ability to hold a loved one's hand and feel that emotional connection," as the Johns Hopkins mechanical engineer Jeremy Brown later described.[7] This breakthrough technology was a major step beyond the myoelectric prosthetic limbs of ten years earlier. In 2006, war journalist and amputee Michael Weisskopf, who had a myoelectric prosthetic, described his "fake" arm as moving like a "dumbbell—fat, clunky, and heavy"; in his memoir *Blood Brothers*, Weisskopf recounted his feelings of clumsiness and loss of control before he slowly adapted to his prosthesis. [8] In contrast, in Copeland's case there was a much stronger potential to reintegrate mind and body via a cortical modem that had the potential to restore his dexterity and sense of connectedness. The Pittsburgh conference gave Nathan the opportunity to shake hands and fist bump with the president and to hear Obama speak about what might be possible in the future "if we keep on pushing the boundaries."

This boundary-pushing agenda set the stage for the first Senate hearing on AI in November 2016, titled *The Dawn of Artificial Intelligence*, following a House hearing two months earlier on advanced robotics.[9] In the Senate hearing, Gary Peters of Michigan pictured a technologically driven nation as an "ever-evolving innovation ecosystem that's rooted in robotics, machine learning, and . . . artificial intelligence."[10] The two hearings investigated the "opportunities and potential threats" of convergent technologies. But neither touched on the mental health implications of this convergence, even though Obama made efforts to invest in neurological research in his second term, notably in April 2013 when he launched the BRAIN (Brain Research through Advancing Innovative Neurotechnologies) initiative to ensure that innovative neuroscientific research received an injection of federal funding.[11]

This did not mean that mental health was neglected in Washington, DC. Obama spoke passionately about ensuring that Americans with mental health challenges did not suffer in silence when he opened the National Mental Health Conference in June 2013, and a House hearing in April 2014 addressed the barriers veterans with brain trauma faced.[12] Nonetheless, Obama missed an opportunity to respond to the human side of Copeland's story. What was not emphasized at the conference Copeland appeared at were the facts that technological performance was only a small part of the story and that DARPA requires industrial investment to move a trial technology to the marketplace.[13] Rachel Mabe highlighted these aspects in a 2017 article in the *Atlantic*, where she noted the view of Copeland's surgeon that an initially withdrawn young man became more gregarious as the project advanced. However, Mabe's interview with Copeland undercut a simple narrative of overcoming. He expressed his wish that the breakthrough technology could become embedded in his everyday life, but he also recognized that feelings of depression were likely to return once the DARPA funding expired at the end of five years. In contrast to the heroic tenor of the Frontiers conference, Mabe concluded that Copeland was only borrowing the prosthetic arm in the name of bioscience instead of having permanent access to a technology that would fully augment his identity.[14]

If Obama had publicly recognized the broader consequences for Copeland's mental health, he might have deepened this public relations opportunity. A more nuanced statement would also have helped frame the heroic rhetoric that Obama, following Clinton and Gore, used for disruptive technologies, especially those at the confluence of artificial intelligence and advanced robotics that accelerated biotech innovation in health tech during the 2010s. In 2016, Eric Horvitz, director of Microsoft Research Labs in Washington state, reminded a Senate hearing that "the acceleration of AI competencies" had great potential to transform health care, but also that "AI is a constellation of disciplines . . . all aimed at a shared aspiration, the scientific understanding of thought and intelligent behavior, and developing computer systems based on these understandings."[15]

The emphasis of the hearing was on tool-based (or weak) AI, but the subcommittee chair, Texas senator Ted Cruz, asked Horvitz and Greg Brockman, cofounder of the San Francisco research laboratory OpenAI, for their thoughts on general (or strong) AI. He prefaced the question by quoting tech entrepreneur Elon Musk's 2014 comment that the realization of strong AI would be like "summoning the demon."[16] Instead of addressing Musk's comment (perhaps because Musk was a cofounder of OpenAI) or the views of other public figures such as Stephen Hawking, who had warned against the approaching dangers of singularity (when technology will be uncontrollable having surpassed human powers), Brockman stated that general AI capability was between ten and one hundred years away. Horvitz agreed with Brockman's view that the nation should instead be focusing on "concrete safety problems." General AI was too far off for serious discussion, whereas tool-based AI could more immanently address short- and medium-term technical and social problems and still grapple with "known unknowns."[17] He blamed the hyperbole surrounding the AI focus of Hollywood films such as *The Matrix* (1999) and *Lucy* (2014) that imagined singularity, although he admitted that these were "great themes" that "keep us enamoured with interesting possibilities."

Arguably, the possibilities of biotechnology at the interface of robotics and AI were both more immense and more concerning than the Senate hearing admitted. Cognitive robotics expert Murray Shanahan had argued three years before the hearing that they "demand serious debate," even though the most outspoken advocate of singularity, inventor Ray Kurzweil, flirted with what Shanahan called "ideas that seem so speculative as to border on the absurd."[18] Nonetheless, instead of abstract ruminations on futurity, Robert Carlson, the author of *Biology is Technology* (2010), argued that market demand was already fueling augmented technologies, "rooted in the desire to augment inherited human and physical potential with technology."[19] Given that three congressional terms have passed (at the time of writing) since the *Dawn of Artificial Intelligence* hearing—and that the House called AI a "game changer" in 2018—it is significant that congressional leaders did not probe the ethical implications of AI until 2019 and a full discussion of ethics did not take place until October 2021 by the newly launched bipartisan congressional Task Force on Artificial Intelligence. Titled *Beyond I, Robot: Ethics, Artificial Intelligence, and the Digital Age*, this 2021 hearing placed higher standards on AI than on humans, as outlined by the task force chair Bill Foster, in order to avoid discrimination by race, gender, class, or age. (Protecting children was a key theme, but it was not explicitly linked to mental health.)[20]

These Washington discussions raise crucial questions about social inequality and exploitation that Neda Atanasoski and Kalindi Vora argue "underlie the contemporary conditions of capitalist production."[21] Taking this view of technoliberalism seriously does not mean we need to "summon the demon," to recall Elon Musk's view, by projecting ourselves into doomsday scenarios of robot invasions and human extinction—although Musk's words are ironic in the rearview mirror, given the launch in 2022 of the humanoid robot prototype Optimus by Musk's Tesla company, named after the leader of the heroic Autobots from the *Transformers* franchise. Instead, we should reflect on what the acceleration of disruptive technologies means for embodied consciousness and whether it will drive "struggles for cultural prestige" instead of offering an endless resource by creating job opportunities via automated manual work practices, as Musk claimed the perfected Optimus would do.[22] Atanasoski and Vora argue that such a vision of big-box technology liberates human potential only by degrading and devaluing others as robots become "surrogate humans" that "take over the dull, dirty, repetitive, and even reproductive labor performed by racialized, gendered, and colonized workers in the past."[23] This mode of "digital eugenics" is not wholly apocalyptic, but it nonetheless threatens the basic building blocks of a good society by creating a "caste system" underpinned by social inequality.[24]

As convergent technologies, AI and robotics profoundly challenge the frames commonly used to make sense of consciousness. In 2009, the *New York Times* ran a piece on "The Coming Superbrain" that envisages enhanced robots outsmarting humans in another generation.[25] On this evidence, it is tricky to untangle technical fantasies about robot capability from public fears about robots taking over human jobs and the emergence of a technologically augmented future that is likely to make *Homo sapiens* feel defective. Robotics may appear benign if it remains tool based, yet robots routinely provoke anxious imaginings, especially with respect to intelligent machines that can rival human capacities but lack the inhibitions—anxieties, neuroses, learning limitations, memory failure—that transhumanists cite as reasons why humans fall short of their evolutionary potential.

We may comfort ourselves with the thought that the computer programs and circuitry underlying robot behavior are not equivalent to the complex neuronal feedbacks of human consciousness. Or we might take solace in science fiction writer Isaac Asimov's long-established ethical laws of robotics: first, "a robot may not injure a human being or, through inaction, allow a human being to come to harm"; second, "a robot must obey the orders given to it except when such orders conflict with the first law"; third, "a robot must protect its own existence as long as such protection does not conflict with the first or second laws."[26] However, if we yoke Daniel Dennett's theory of a distributed model of consciousness without a "Central Meaner" (see chapter 3) to interactive robotic intelligence, then the ontological gap closes.[27] That the gap is closing more quickly than the 2016 Senate hearing acknowledged led Marc Rotenberg, president of the Electronic Privacy Information Center, to write to committee chair Ted Cruz to suggest that two laws should be added to Asimov's three to protect against the rise of rogue automatons and ease international paranoia: "a robot must always reveal the basis of its decision" and "a robot must always reveal its actual identity."[28]

With the aim of refracting abstract aspects of consciousness and AI through a sociocultural lens, I return to the topic of automated devices in the cauldron of warfare in the next section and address environmental concerns in the final section, before returning to ecological health more fully in chapter 8. First, though, I assess this shrinking gap by contrasting early twenty-first-century accounts of AI-enhanced robotics to those of the mid-twentieth century, when the focus was on "the physical ability of robots," to use Rotenberg's words, such as the automobile industry's use of robots to spot-weld cars.[29] This was very different from the postmillennial world, in which robots are used in multiple sectors, including—in the field of health care—medical imaging, diagnosis, surgery, and caregiving.[30]

A fundamental distinction between humans and robots is the verifiable presence of consciousness. Yet British philosopher Robert Kirk wonders what would happen if we found out that "brains were made from entirely different materials from our own" or if we could be convinced that a sophisticated prosthesis is as good as—or even better—than the original.[31] And what would happen if we remove belief in free will or a soul from the conversation when assessing the conscious status and evolutionary potential of robots?[32] Further, what would happen if robots became less machine-like and more organic, "created in a lab from living tissue, cells, and DNA" and designed "to look and be just like us, but better and more resilient," as David Ewing Duncan muses?[33] We saw in the book's first part how this prospect plays out in the postgenomic world, but it also relates to assessing what different forms of technologically enhanced intelligence reveal about health experiences.

This move away from what Dennett calls "magical thinking" and folk beliefs about ourselves is vital for reenergizing a middle ground that is rooted in empirical evidence but shot through with imaginative possibility. Bracketing off complicating ideas is pragmatically useful but not so feasible when we consider how thoughts and feelings are often inseparable in embodied life. Films such as Steven Spielberg's *A.I. Artificial Intelligence* (2001) explore how cognition and emotion intertwine in relationships between humans and humanoids, but this does not mean we should indulge in fantasies about consciousness (either our own or other kinds, such as that of the surrogate robot son David in *A.I.*) without seeking an empirical anchor. Nor does it mean we should let extreme feelings about intelligent machines distort epistemological, ontological, and bioethical questions about human-robot interactions. These questions demand that we attend to narrative modes that operate on both affective and cognitive realms, as science fiction often does. The scientific importance of speculative sci-fi narratives is underscored by the faculty of two key tech universities, Carnegie Mellon and MIT, which encourage their students to read science fiction to work through scientific potential and ethical obstacles.[34] This merging of art and technology chimes with former DARPA director Anthony Tether's belief that "the best DARPA program managers . . . are science fiction writers" and loops back to Obama's visit to Carnegie Mellon's National Robotics Engineering Center in 2011, when he joked, knowingly, about keeping his presidential "eye on the robots," commenting: "I'm pleased to report that the robots you manufacture here seem peaceful, at least for now."[35]

In this chapter, I extend the insights of the network theory of consciousness in chapter 3 to reflect on the technological ecologies that have arisen since the millennium at the convergence of AI and robotics. We might think of ecologies in terms of organic life that link humans to nature, but it is also important to assess the multiple and complex interrelations between machines and humans, as the experiences of Nathan Copeland reveal. The interconnections between virtually invisible everyday technologies and the kinetic and cognitive possibilities of advanced robotics push us to rethink questions of consciousness, communication, and caregiving (which is especially pertinent in cultures with aging populations such as the United States, the UK, and Japan), as well as the issues of racial and economic exploitation in Atanasoski and Vora's "surrogate humanity" perspective.[36]

Recognizing that proposed legislation to mobilize the economic potential of AI and protect against its misuse is currently under way in a number of states, here I explore these convergences on three theoretical and cultural levels. First, I examine how the intersection of AI and robotics shifts the ground in the philosophical debates outlined in chapter 3 to reemerge in theoretical writings and two illustrative cultural texts of the 2010s: Alex Garland's directorial debut *Ex Machina* (2014) and Daniel H. Wilson's sci-fi novel *Amped* (2012). Second, I situate these debates in a real-world setting in the 2000s and 2010s: the militarized use of AI and robotics by armed services during wars in Afghanistan and Iraq that dominated foreign policy during the Bush and Obama administrations, which I analyze through a reading of Kathryn Bigelow's Iraq War film *The Hurt Locker* (2008). And third, I consider how future prospects at the interface of AI and robotics have the power to alter conceptions of health and social relations, although not always as building blocks of a "good society." I filter this discussion through an extended consideration of James Cameron's technologically augmented blockbuster of 2009, *Avatar*.

AI, Robotics, and the Gap

As a springboard for thinking about the convergence of AI and robotics, it is first worth returning to the public dialogue between Daniel Dennett and John Searle in chapter 3. These two philosophers do not just disagree about the subject of consciousness; they also disagree about the state and scientific potential of artificial intelligence. Each dealt with AI in abstracted form, famously in Dennett's science fiction extension of the "brain in a vat" in his playful 1978 essay "Where Am I?," and Searle in his Chinese room thought experiment, which prompted much debate when it was first published in 1980. Dennett imagines a future in which his brain, body, and consciousness are sundered geographically and biotechnologically, leading to dizzying confusion when he tries to rediscover his sense of self. When he eases his initial bewilderment ("buried alive in Oklahoma . . . disembodied in Houston"), Dennett realizes he is able to listen to a Brahms piano piece without ears ("the output from the stereo stylus was being fed through some fancy rectification circuitry directly into my auditory nerve").[37] The story becomes dizzying when Dennett imagines a computer simulating his brain while his own disembodied brain switches off. He argues that in this hypothetical situation, a sense of "I" would exist whenever and wherever a brain-body pair is running: there is nothing unique about "I"; it emerges as an indexical concept of location.[38]

Dennett later defended his AI position with the argument that humans have always developed add-ons for improving thought and performance (including wearables to monitor health and fitness), suggesting that we are more like assemblages than a traditional humanist perspective attests. He warns, though, that an overreliance on and overestimation of current technologies may prematurely cede authority to machines "far beyond their competence," thereby usurping "our role as captains of our destinies."[39] Dennett could not have predicted that scientists thirty-five years later would claim that a virtual human brain could be mapped, as South African neuroscientist Henry Markram asserted, although Markram's team in Lausanne, Switzerland focused their more modest research goals on a mouse brain.[40] Writing in the late 1970s, at the advent of home computing, Dennett presented "Where Am I?" as an impossible tale because any computer simulation of the brain would need to "have a fundamental structure entirely unlike that of existing computers" in order to handle millions of inputs and outputs.

In contrast to Dennett, who plays with AI concepts only to complicate them by refuting first-person subjectivity, Searle sees weak AI as a useful human tool.[41] The thought experiment he uses to refute strong AI (an intelligence with cognitive states) is a sealed room in which an imaginary Searle is asked to read Chinese without any training. Instead, he has a set of rules written in English that allows him to manipulate characters without any understanding of them, as if he were a computer. Searle argues against a computational model because in this experiment, his understanding of Chinese characters remains zero. His claim is that computerized simulation does not and cannot replicate the human intentionality that only a meaning-making consciousness gives rise to.

Searle may trump Dennett in his ethical insistence on retaining selfhood over a distributed model of consciousness, but this raises the question of what kind of intelligence the Chinese room simulation represents. Searle dramatizes what cognitive scientist Marvin Minsky described in the early 1960s as "little more than the complex of performances which we happen to respect, but do not understand" by resting his simulation on British mathematician Alan Turing's famous test in which we judge an intelligent machine by standards of human intelligence.[42] A machine that can simulate thinking to a human level would pass the Turing test. However, to Searle's mind, this thought experiment reaches a limit if we believe that meaning making emerges by following linguistic rules instead of by tapping into an inherently human capacity for learning. We might conclude that Dennett's and Searle's arguments are too abstract to grapple with the materiality and potential of intelligent machines. We can forgive them to a degree, because these arguments were posited before the digital revolution, but it is still surprising that neither thinker discussed more thoroughly the material embodiment of intelligent machines in experiential environments.

This absence is especially visible given that only two years after Searle's Chinese room experiment, director Ridley Scott released the proto-cyberpunk film *Blade Runner*. Based on Philip K. Dick's 1968 novel *Do Androids Dream of Electric Sheep?*, the 1982 film imagines a species of early twenty-first-century replicants. They are "virtually identical to a human," manufactured by a genetic engineering firm, the Tyrell Corporation, but are "superior in strength and agility, and at least equal in intelligence, to the genetic engineers who created them," as the opening credits tell us. Set in 2019, the film's beginning reanimates the Turing test as an interrogation technique deployed by police agencies in their effort to detect who is human and what is humanoid. They do so by using a polygraph machine to assess the subject's emotional response to a series of thought-experiment questions, alongside testing of biomarker changes such as eye movement and heart and respiration rates. The film queries the status we grant to these "synthetic humans," particularly in their most advanced form as Nexus 6 replicants, which the manufacturer says are "more human than human."[43] *Blade Runner* raises the possibility of love developing between humans and replicants, although this is unlikely to be sustainable in a violent dystopian world, reflecting the fact that Dick pictured a tense bond between androids and humans rooted in superstitious and animistic beliefs that go back far before the industrial revolution.[44] Both *Do Androids Dream of Electric Sheep?* and *Blade Runner* raise as many social problems about class and race conflict, bioengineered cloning, and slave labor as they do epistemological questions about the edges of reality and ontological questions about intelligent life forms.[45]

We are not inhabiting (or are not yet inhabiting) the dystopian world of *Blade Runner*, although rogue robots have become commonplace in Hollywood films, from *Runaway* (1984) to *I, Robot* (2004) and *Upgrade* (2018). However, advances in AI prototypes in the 2010s and early 2020s refute the idea that understanding is the unique province of humans and that intelligence is determinable by the skillful manipulation of symbols, as Searle's Chinese room experiment suggests. Yet Searle would argue that comparisons between a computer and a mind fall short, particularly when we move away from logic, computation, and gaming toward a rich understanding of language and music. Many critics share Searle's view that neurons are not like microchips. But N. Kathryn Hayles argues that the rise of advanced computers means that the Turing test loses ground to what she calls the Moravec test (named after the robotics expert Hans Moravec), in the respect that "once machines can become the repository of human consciousness" downloading informational patterns that replicate neural circuits, machines "for all practical purposes, become human beings."[46] Instead of consciousness being a "formal puzzle" or a "brain in a vat," Hayles stresses its physiological and genetic underpinning. This move might entangle us in further questions of determinism versus agency and nature versus nurture, yet it provides a broader context for thinking how consciousness aligns with being and identity instead of something that is knowable only if we bracket off its surrounding context. In contrast to the early phase of the biotech acceleration, when Dennett and Searle were writing, twenty years later, at the close of the 1990s, Hayles envisaged a near future in which robots have the capacity for subtle interactions and advanced learning. This vision is predicated on the blurring of synthetic and organic borders via bioengineering techniques. Yet from a psychosociological perspective, it poses questions about our tendency to attach to animated machines, especially when they look less robotic and more like us with an upright posture and a recognizable face.

This process leads us away from the abstract ruminations of Dennett and Searle and toward an understanding that robots have a material reality and psychosocial potential. As research in the 2010s has shown, there are significant mental health benefits—particularly at both ends of the life spectrum—from interacting with socially assisted robots.[47] However, Laurel Riek points out that the less mechanistic a robot appears, the greater the risk they might fool or manipulate us. The stakes intensified in 2014 when the UK's Royal Society judged that the Russian-created AI simulation of a thirteen-year-old boy, Eugene Goostman, passed the Turing test.[48] Goostman was a disembodied chatbot that used "a series of 'ploys' . . . to mask the program's limitations," including humor, questioning, and evasion, but Riek argues that even when a robot's morphology is machine-like, human interlocutors tend to anthropomorphize it.[49] AI technology has advanced rapidly in the decade since the Goostman phenomenon. Advanced GPT (generative pre-trained transformer) technology, for example, has given rise to concerns that the semantic-based Turing test is no longer an adequate safeguard for distinguishing humans from machines. In fact, although deep learning bots may still fail the Turing test, we tend to make them humanlike in our intentional stance, either because they respond to our needs (such as the therapeutic Woebot of 2017, the world's first mental health chatbot) or are given names and physical features to which we can attach meaning.

Such AI embodiment is a central theme of the 2014 psychological mystery *Ex Machina*. Written and directed by the English author Alex Garland as a UK/U.S. co-production and set in the remote Alaskan laboratory-home of CEO scientist Nathan Bateman (Oscar Isaac), *Ex Machina* tests the conceptual and narrative limits of the Turing test. By dramatizing aspects of Murray Shanahan's 2010 book *Embodiment and the Inner Life*, Garland tests these limits through interaction between a programmer, Caleb Smith (Domhnall Gleeson), and a gynoid called Ava (Alicia Vikander), who is robotically constructed as a combination of mechanistic (arms, legs) and humanistic (face, chest) features. Caleb wins an office contest to observe Ava at Bateman's home with the aim of assessing whether "she" can pass the Turing test. The conversational exchanges between Caleb and Ava reveal a complex interplay of thoughts, feelings, and senses, with Ava displaying a high degree of sentience and emotional intelligence and a desire to pass as (or even to be) human. What begins as a controlled experiment changes when Caleb and Ava begin to share moments of intimacy and Ava causes power outages so the pair cannot be observed by Nathan (whom they both distrust) and as attraction appears to grow between them during their encounters.

The film shows that the thought experiments of Dennett and Searle become more complicated when AI is embodied and that a "self-aware machine" (as Garland calls Ava) can simulate consciousness, learn human gestures, and create artwork.[50] Caleb's and Ava's series of seven conversations are closer to Searle's idea of conscious speech acts than they are to Dennett's more solipsistic ruminations. Yet they also align with Nathan's view that both consciousness and sexuality develop through interaction. Whether Ava's consciousness is a simulated illusion or is authentically felt is a question the film pursues as the interactions between Caleb and Ava become more secretive. On the third occasion they meet, she wears a wig, a dress, and long socks to cover her robotic features, she shows romantic interest in Caleb, and she expresses a desire to see the outside world because she feels emotional and existential discomfort in being trapped in an enclosed research facility.

Ava turns out to be smarter (or more evolved) than either Nathan or Caleb realize, leading Shanahan to assert that the film is "Ava's triumph."[51] In enacting her desire for freedom, a feminized human form, and a heterosexual relationship, Ava outsmarts her interlocutors, manipulating Caleb (who starts displaying signs of mental distress) and murdering Nathan when he tries to prevent her from escaping from the facility (in a reworking of the Pygmalion and Frankenstein myths).[52] *Ex Machina* also explores the dangers of exceeding the ethical parameters of robot-machine interaction, especially as Nathan exploits a Southeast Asian fembot, Kyoko, for sexual pleasure and keeps spare human skins in his wardrobe as signifiers of modern slavery. Kyoko is largely silent through the film and acts without agency, two issues that poet Franny Choi highlights in her 2019 collection *Soft Science*, in which she muses on the cognitive, emotional, and sexual life-worlds of cyborgs and, more specifically, on her reaction to Kyoko's "body that has been made an object of desire, fantasy, and power."[53] Through its series of intense character interactions, the film raises profound questions about exploitation, freedom, and health and about what happens to bioethics when the laboratory becomes a site of incarceration that breaks androids emotionally just as it generates them physically.[54]

Ex Machina is not the first film to test the limits of human attachment to a life-like robot. Whereas in *A.I. Artificial Intelligence*, director Steven Spielberg and the film's progenitor Stanley Kubrick take us firmly into the realm of a "future fairy tale" (what Kubrick calls "the possibilities of immortality through DNA + AI"), *Ex Machina* reveals the benefits and dangers of altering the morphology of robots to suit human needs.[55] Expecting too much of a robot and making unrealizable attachments are common obstacles, although this should not deter us from researching the therapeutic potential of robots to help individuals tackle debilitating fears of technology, anxieties about relationships, and feelings of social isolation. This realization leads Riek to assert that "mental healthcare professionals need to carefully weigh the capabilities of the robot against the therapeutic needs of the patient."[56]

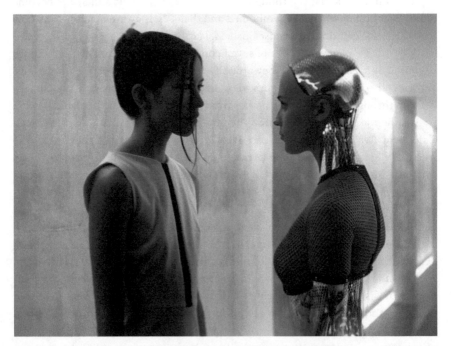

Figure 4.1. Gynoids Ava (right; Alicia Vikander) and Kyoko (left; Sonoya Mizuno) harbor dreams of escape. *Ex Machina* (2014). Film4/Alamy Photo.

Where the debate moves on from *A.I.* and *Ex Machina* is that AI is not always exterior to the human. This is exemplified by Daniel H. Wilson's novel *Amped*, which imagines the possibility of an augmented brain implant, Neural Autofocus MK-4®, which can enhance both human brain activity and exoskeletal prosthetic limbs. That Wilson is primarily a scientist rather than a writer—he holds a PhD from Carnegie Mellon University's Robotics Institute—returns us to Daniel Suarez's design fictions in chapter 2 in their explorations of technologies that tear "the limits of human ability" off the map.[57] Wilson gives the cyberpunk genre a twist in *Amped* by balancing technical knowledge with plausible speculations, as does Kim Stanley Robinson in his futuristic novel *2312* in the form of nano-implants or qubes, some of which are self-programming and can manufacture "qube-minded humanoids that are indistinguishable from humans."[58] *Amped* portrays a more domestic world than *2312*. Set in a recognizable Oklahoma, *Amped* has conceptual similarities to the world of Nancy Kress's Sleep Trilogy in its attention to discrimination against augmented humans and its focus on the interconnectivity of personal relations and social conflict. In *Amped*, the U.S. Supreme Court offers no legal protection for those facing discrimination following elective surgery, such as Owen Gray, whose father surgically embedded his implant, or high school students under eighteen who, like the novel's opening character Samantha Blex, would normally be granted some legal protections.

Owen is at first bewildered when he discovers he has been "amped." Although the procedure stabilizes the epilepsy he has experienced from childhood, unlike others who had chosen elective surgery, he muses: "I didn't come back any smarter. Didn't move any faster," even though Neural Autofocus is touted as making "the communication between mind and body seamless."[59] However, Owen finds that he is unwittingly caught in a culture war in which politicians accuse scientists of engaging in social engineering instead of working to curing disease. A federal Uplift program launched by Congress a few years earlier, designed "to provide technological benefits to disadvantaged [low-income] students and to strengthen education," has resulted in "tearing the humanity away from regular people," to quote the reactionary words of the president of the (fictional) Pure Humans Citizen's Council.[60] The fear that these augmented humans will destroy heritage and tradition leads Vaughan to declare war on the amps in the form of hard social segregation, tight regulation of science funding, and raids on facilities where the implant technology is being refined and practiced. In testing the point of convergence between the politics, ethics, and science of an emergent technology in a divisive world that is not ready for it, Wilson's novel goes much further as an embodied thought experiment than Dennett and Searle did in their AI projections.

As *Amped* shows, technical and medical advances in implants and prosthetics pose a set of physical and mental health questions that return us to the fine line between restoration and enhancement. Sophisticated bioengineering practices in neuroscience and bionics have increased the effectiveness of replacements for amputated or damaged limbs. On this subject, journalist Adam Piore writes about the imminent possibility that scientists and doctors will be able to use bioengineering "to unlock resilience in human bodies and minds that previous generations could only have guessed was there."[61] Compared to adult decisions made for young Americans in *Amped*, Piore explores "the things . . . that make us feel most human" instead of those that erase human boundaries in his tales of individuals who "refuse to give up" and seek to control their biotech futures.[62]

Reminiscent in structure of Oliver Sacks's efforts to give his patients their own voice, Piore's 2017 book *The Body Builders* contains nine case studies based around first-person interviews with exceptional individuals, moving the focus away from AI and back toward human intelligence in search of bionic augmentation. Hugh Herr is the subject of the first case study of *The Body Builders*, specifically his efforts to develop sophisticated prosthetic legs after losing them at the age of seventeen in a climbing accident during a winter ascent of Mount Washington in 1982. The story is one of adaptation and ingenuity. Herr harnesses robotic assistive technologies to enable him to walk and climb as a form of roboticization. His prosthetics advance to an exoskeleton, including replicated tendons, flip-flop-like feet, and bionic lower limbs containing microprocessors.[63] Herr's uplift narrative is both restorative and rejuvenating: he stops having tormenting dreams and becomes alternatively abled by improving his earlier capabilities. Buoyed by his success, Herr envisages a "future without disabilities," as his experiments have profound implications for physical injuries and those experiencing neurodegenerative symptoms. Such radical developments are the aim of the MIT Center for Extreme Bionics, which Herr cofounded in 2013, which focuses on augmentation at the axis of physicality, cognition and emotionality.[64]

Herr's journey parallels the growth of biotechnology and robotics, moving beyond his accident in the early 1980s to prototypes in the 1990s and 2000s to "an era of transformative real-world impact" of the 2010s. Piore recognizes the fine line between restoration and enhancement in Herr's journey. He mentions the prosthetic legs of South African double amputee and sprinter Oscar Pistorius (a 400-meter semifinalist in the 2012 Olympics) but does not delve into the politics of athletic enhancements, whether by genetic, pharmaceutical, or prosthetic means.[65] Instead, Piore muses on Herr's story of robotization in an effort to separate "the therapeutic potential from the potential for human augmentation."[66] Piore dodges an ethical bullet because he comes to no decisions and does not address discrimination. However, in the conclusion of *The Body Builders* he reveals his admiration for those who have the gumption, intelligence, and technical skill to reverse engineer "the human body and mind down to its smallest individual parts" in order to "rebuild or change us."[67] Piore concludes optimistically that technology might set us free. However, on a technical level, this dream will not become reality until a future date when technology has developed to the extent that it can connect Herr's exoskeleton seamlessly to his nervous system at the brain-computer interface.[68] For now, though, an imperfect technology poses both opportunities for reactivating agency and challenges in the arena of mental and physical health, especially in the cauldron of war.

Optimization and Trauma in Contemporary Warfare

On March 19, 2013, to mark the tenth anniversary of the start of the Iraq War, President Obama honored those who had died in a conflict that had formally ended two years previously.[69] Thinking of the 30,000 wounded among U.S. service personnel on active duty, the president affirmed that "here at home, our obligations to those who served endure," including treatment of traumatic brain injury and post-traumatic stress disorder as well as suicide prevention, as he discussed at the National Conference on Mental Health that June.[70] Obama mentioned "wounded warriors" frequently in his speeches for two reasons. First, he recognized that the conflict had been much longer and deadlier than the George W. Bush administration had anticipated when it launched armed forces in March 2003 without UN backing under the flag of a "road map for peace." Second, Obama recognized that injuries service members sustained in Iraq and Afghanistan required new forms of treatment, especially for brain damage and lower-limb amputations. This was not just the responsibility of the Department of Veterans Affairs, which was experiencing capacity problems even as it was taking seriously questions of fitness to serve and prolonged risks of PTSD.[71] The Obama administration, which recognized that responsibility goes beyond the government, fostered new alliances between public and private sectors in regenerative medicine, bioengineering, psychiatry, and counseling and encouraged veterans to share their stories via the 2006 Operation Homecoming project run by the National Endowment of Arts and the Department of Defense.

We saw in the previous section how embodied forms of AI in early twenty-first-century writing and film challenged the grey-box thought experiments of Dennett and Searle by testing bioethical problems experientially. The stark reality many injured veterans faced following two protracted wars in Afghanistan and Iraq gave sharper definition to those abstract musings, but it was invariably framed by the national defense priorities of harnessing biotechnology for military supremacy. This was epitomized at the 2002 DARPATech symposium titled "Transforming Fantasy," at which DARPA director Anthony Tether envisaged that "our fantasies today will be [our children's] reality in the future." Tether predicted the accelerating convergence of robotics and AI for future wars as well as a symbiotic relation between human beings and biotechnology: "The robots will respond, controlled by our thoughts. It's coming. Imagine a warrior—with the intellect of a human and the immortality of a machine."[72] Given that the conference took place only ten months after the terrorist attacks of 9/11, one might have expected Tether to be more circumspect about promoting future combat systems. A few months earlier, he had outlined to a Senate subcommittee how DARPA was looking to blend "the best traits of man and machine," assuring Congress that system failure posed no danger: "There is always a person in the loop to provide the timeless qualities of human judgment and insight to supervise the unmanned systems and manage the battle."[73]

The priorities of the Department of Defense are to "prevent technological surprise" when conflict arises with other nations and to optimize an American soldier's performance in a "highly complex, dynamic, network-centric military operating environment."[74] The reconceptualization of a soldier as a system that merges mind and machine began with the Persian Gulf War of 1990–1991 but advanced rapidly with the development of the U.S. Army's Future Force Warrior demonstration system in the early 2000s, which sought to enhance a soldier's awareness, protection, and lethality. This development took a sharper turn toward AI with the launching of the Joint Artificial Intelligence Center in 2018.[75] Although the Future Force Warrior was never operationalized for battle, the super-soldier's readiness for the "technology saturated battlespace" was predicated on advances in biotechnology and neuroscience that could enhance physical and cognitive abilities, endurance, and sentience.[76] These technologies were grouped together from 2014 via DARPA's Biological Technologies Office, which engages in themed projects that included Battlefield Medicine ("to develop miniaturized device platforms and techniques" to address medical needs in the combat zone), Intelligent Neural Interfaces (which focuses on harnessing "third-wave" AI capabilities), and Restoring Active Memory (to help soldiers experiencing brain injuries).[77]

The paradox of twenty-first-century warfare is that conflict has become more detached through the use of precision bombing, aerial drones, and automated weaponry (as promoted by the Defense Authorization Act of 2000) while simultaneously becoming more immanent, with technology that functions to enhance a soldier's capabilities on the ground through "high-tech body suits which use chemicals, sensors and digital information to cocoon the soldiers in a 'virtual war' experience, even in the midst of battle."[78] I return to the mental health consequences of this kind of cocooning as portrayed in The Hurt Locker, but first I focus on military optimization via capacity-increasing technologies.

Another of Adam Piore's case studies in The Body Builders, titled "Soldiers with Spidey Sense," examines the ways intelligence research has "embarked on an audacious and tantalizing goal" since the 2000s to track and quantify intuition, an important special sense to possess in the combat zone for both defense and offense.[79] Ohio-based psychologist and former Air Force pilot Gary Klein has conducted work funded by the U.S. Army Research Institute for the Behavioral and Social Sciences that is focused on "pattern matching" that enables a trained soldier to know what to do or what to avoid without having to go through a time-consuming process of observing and analyzing sense data.[80] For Klein, such pattern-matching seems to occur beyond the realm of the conscious mind, tapping into what Antonio Damasio calls the core and proto-levels of consciousness. This insight led to more advanced neurological experiments and to a Cognitive Technology Threat Warning System sponsored by DARPA and manufactured by Boeing to give soldiers in the combat zone extended and peripheral vision with quick reaction speeds honed by using video games and virtual reality systems as advanced training tools.[81] Klein and others wished to go further than manufacturing wearables for the armed services by developing brain-scanning techniques that can enhance a soldier's performance and can also have therapeutic benefits for those experiencing amnesia or dementia, like Alice Howland in *Still Alice*, whose words seem to be stored deep in the limbic system instead of in an easily retrievable neural space.[82] Developments in AI for retaining or restoring narrative continuity for individuals experiencing dementia is still a young science, but these DARPA experiments have implications for sports in terms of understanding what "in the zone" means when an athlete's recall and response reflexes operate at a near-instinctive level. However, Piore stops short of discussing either the mental health benefits or the dangers of increased performance.[83]

The work on AI-assisted robotics and consciousness-enhancing techniques in the name of national security is only part of the federal picture. The tenor of these enhancements can be skewed by the kinds of heroic rhetoric deployed by DARPA personnel, for example Anthony Tether's 2003 view that DARPA's Continuous Assisted Performance program can "enable soldiers to stay awake, alert, and effective for up to seven days straight without suffering any deleterious mental or physical effects" and DARPA program manager Michael Callahan's comment in 2007 that capability-enhancing technology can make soldiers "kill-proof" by bringing "to battle the same sort of capabilities that nature has given certain animals."[84] On the flip side of this super-soldier rhetoric, the Iraq and Afghanistan wars sharpened an awareness that traumatic stress and brain trauma were increasingly prevalent among active service personnel as early as the Gulf War. There was a significant rise in the number of Gulf War veterans reporting PTSD symptoms two years after active service, compared to health reports recorded at the end of their term of duty.[85] When members of Congress met in September 1992 to discuss the proposed Traumatic Brain Injury Act, it was with the recognition that brain injuries were also prevalent among young and Black Americans in civilian contexts. However, no coordinated evaluation, prevention, or rehabilitation systems were in place at the time.[86] Moreover, the Veterans Administration was chronically short of provisions before the launch of the Defense and Veterans Head Injury Program earlier that year to serve injured and retiring Gulf War–era soldier. The program was a collaboration between the Veterans Administration, the Department of Defense, and the Brain Injury Association. However, it took four more years before the act was signed into law.

Rising cases of PTSD among veterans of different conflicts and two new attritional wars in Afghanistan and Iraq following the 9/11 terrorist attacks might have hastened legislation, as may have the studies that emerged from collaborations between the Veterans Administration and the National Academy of Sciences in the wake of the 1998 Veterans Program Enhancement Act.[87] Nevertheless, George W. Bush's speeches were light on references to the physical and psychological toll of warfare. When Bush did mention traumatic injury (for example, at the Walter Reed Medical Center in July 2008), it was in the context of emphasizing the strength of the "human spirit" instead of the dark reality of trauma.[88] It was not until Obama's presidency, six years after the start of the Iraq War, that investment in research and care for traumatic brain injury received something approximating appropriate levels of federal oversight and funding. At a 2014 hearing, Congress discussed the short-term and long-term impact of brain injury and concussion on service members (an estimated 360,000 military personnel were experiencing brain injuries from the current wars) and what specialist mental health care facilities were required. One speaker at this hearing, Derek Duplisea, a representative of the Wounded Warrior Project who was forced to retire from active service after sustaining multiple injuries, estimated (though without supporting data) that PTSD was reported at 75 percent among veterans surveyed by the Wounded Warrior Project, with anxiety and depression reported at 74 and 69 percent, respectively, and traumatic brain injury at 44 percent.[89]

Political scientist Jean-François Caron notes that the line between capacity-restoring and capacity-increasing technologies blurs when it comes to military enhancement. Whatever the level of sophistication, advanced military technology does not make a soldier invulnerable to death, nor does it offer immunity from the multi-symptom physical and neurological disorders that arose among active service personnel during and after the Gulf War.[90] The risk of PTSD is markedly higher among military recruits than among civilians, and it often correlates to experiences of dissociation and suicidal ideation as well as cases of substance abuse and domestic violence. The increase in reported cases of PTSD in the 2000s and 2010s was partly due to better diagnostic tools. Nonetheless, the short-term and long-term effects of intense and attritional warfare were only patchily understood, particularly for patients who experienced areas of their brains shutting down.[91]

Bessel van der Kolk, the medical director of the Trauma Center in Brookline, Massachusetts, notes that language loss in both active service personnel and citizen victims of contemporary warfare—varying from mutism to "chaotic, confused, and fragmented" memory to evasion and unreliability—can lead the Veterans Administration to deny disability claims because veterans cannot always "tell precisely what had happened to them."[92] As a practicing psychiatrist, van der Kolk believes that effective therapy for traumatized patients involves locating "islands of safety" via a combination of cognitive behavioral therapy, mindfulness techniques, eye movement desensitization, and acupuncture. These techniques can help patients learn to be present and avoid panic responses and paralyzing flashbacks.[93] However, related conditions like attention deficit disorder or the inability to move beyond a stressful episode suggest that the traumatized brain undergoes physical changes such as alexithymia, which van der Kolk describes as "not being able to sense and communicate with what is going on with you." The therapeutic trajectory for him is "connecting viscerally with your self" to provide an anchor for confusion and out-of-body experiences so that "no body" can become "some body" again.[94] This is no easy task. A 2010 report documented that only 10 percent of the nearly 50,000 U.S. veterans who had served in the Iraq and Afghanistan wars and had received a PTSD diagnosis had completed their treatment. There is also evidence that antipsychotics such as Zoloft work better with traumatized civilians than veterans, and in some cases they can worsen symptoms.[95]

With these therapeutic insights in mind, I turn now to Kathryn Bigelow's Oscar-winning film *The Hurt Locker*, which examines the cost of contemporary warfare by focusing on the endeavors of a bomb disposal expert, Sergeant William James (played by Jeremy Renner), during a tour of duty in Baghdad. The film is based on the observations of scriptwriter and co-producer Mark Boal, who in 2004 was an embedded journalist with a U.S. Army explosive disposal squad for a fortnight in Baghdad, where he took a particular interest in the traumatic experiences of armed services personnel "who keep having repeated combat exposure."[96] Boal explores this theme in his 2005 *Playboy* piece, "The Man in the Bomb Suit." But instead of profiling the institutions of warfare (the Veterans Administration, the Department of Defense, DARPA) to emphasize these points, *The Hurt Locker* meditates on the imminent and unpredictable threats of guerrilla warfare.[97]

James replaces a colleague who has died in the explosion of an improvised bomb in the film's opening scene, even though both James and his colleague are protected by a sixty-pound advanced bomb suit featuring a blast helmet, armored plates, and a cooling system. Instead of relying on the protective cocooning of the bomb suit or the precaution of deploying reconnaissance robots to survey improvised explosive devices (we see a wheelbarrow robot fall apart early in the opening sequence), James trusts his own experience, intuition, and dexterity. This emphasis on dexterity is mirrored by cinematographer Barry Ackroyd's use of handheld cameras and the film's shuttling between restricted and expansive points of view, which helps visualize both the dangerous terrain and the mix of risk and skill that characterizes James's work.[98] James's super-soldier appearance yet avoidance of automated military devices locates him symbolically in an ambivalent position with respect to technology, as is emphasized when he discards his helmet during a delicate detonation outside the UN building in Baghdad.[99] James's bravado seemingly makes him invulnerable to trauma. This shifts, though, when he believes that a body he unstitches to remove a bomb is that of a young Iraqi boy he had recently befriended. This visceral encounter with a mutilated yet familiar body precipitates a change in James. His actions become erratic and paranoid, prompting the viewer to question whether his maverick attitude is a thrill-seeking addiction to warfare or a symptom of looming psychosis.

The Hurt Locker reveals James's addictive personality not only by his eagerness to confront hazards and his chain-smoking habit but also late in the narrative after his first tour of duty has concluded. It is telling that there are few "islands of safety" in the field (these focus on the psychological support of James's colleague, Owen Eldridge) and there is only one trained psychologist in evidence in the film, John Cambridge, who is ill equipped for this kind of warfare (Cambridge dies in a scene when he shows his inability to communicate with poor civilian Iraqis).

That James has no exit interview with the Veterans Administration health department might imply that he has not suffered a physical traumatic injury. Yet this perspective is problematized when we see him collapse in the shower wearing his bomb suit and being propelled sideways from an explosion during his final days in Baghdad. James's listless attitude on his return home suggests both an unarticulated trauma and an inability to switch gears from "the accelerated speed" of the combat zone to "the slower rhythms of everyday life."[100] His behavior after returning home stresses the likelihood that he is carrying an invisible injury, as is revealed in a supermarket scene when he cannot make basic decisions about buying cereal. Milky lighting and low camera angles convey his disoriented state, attenuated by fragmented images of his body as he passes by the freezer section, signifying loneliness and liminality—or even the "no body" that van der Volk identifies in the fragile ego structures of traumatized individuals.

This inability to cope with domesticity and the uncertainty he feels without his bomb suit is emphasized in the final scene. After two barely articulate exchanges with his wife and small son, we see James returning to Iraq, this time fully cocooned within his bomb suit, as if the military technology he has hitherto resisted now entirely defines his identity. As an intense drama that explores the visible and invisible collateral damage of guerrilla warfare, *The Hurt Locker* raises both existential and health questions about the status of advanced military technologies and discourses of the wounded warrior. Bigelow's film is a touchstone for understanding the contours of traumatic experiences at a time when the Veterans Administration was trying to break the stigma of mental health. To more fully explore the confluence of robotics and AI, I turn now to another high-profile film of the period, *Avatar*.

Synthetic Intelligence and Eco-Bioethics

Avatar, which was released in December 2009 after four years in production, was the highest-grossing film of the first decade of the new century and one of the most spectacular. Arguably, more than any other science fiction/fantasy film, *Avatar* helped shift debates about the extent to which convergent technologies can be embodied, organic, and seamless. The film demands analysis across a range of technical, social, and cultural topics, including its controversial representations of disability and indigeneity. However, in addition to exploring how red and green biotechnologies relating to health and ecology are mutually informing within an expanded vision of bioethics, *Avatar* can be approached as an optical thought experiment about the convergence of cloning, consciousness, and communication that pits an ecologically sensitive community against the pernicious forces of colonization.

Avatar began with an initial concept by Stanley Kubrick, and James Cameron adopted it in the mid-1990s prior to Kubrick's death in 1999. The long gestation of what was known at the time as "Project 880" was in large part due to the fact that visual and animatronic technologies were not at an advanced enough stage to animate the Alpha Centauri planet of Pandora and the skin tone and athleticism

of its indigenous Na'vi. Much more than a film, *Avatar* was for Cameron a compo-
nent of a highly complex design fiction, envisaged as a web of interconnecting
stories that took longer to realize on the screen than first anticipated (a sequel
was released in late 2022 and three further installments are planned).[101] Interconnectivity does more than function narratively in *Avatar*; it is a form of an organic
neuronal network that structures life on Pandora, which contrasts favorably with
the exploitative activities of human beings.

The technical jump between *A.I. Artificial Intelligence* and *Avatar* is dazzling,
enabling Cameron to move away from the mecha elements of Spielberg's film to
think about what organic transition to another intelligent life form might mean
and look like. *Avatar* is as mythological as *A.I.*, albeit in different ways: Spielberg
reanimated the Pinocchio story (with a dash of *The Wizard of Oz*) and Cameron
channeled his "atavistic sensibility" into a story that tests the fine line between
reality and artifice.[102] The two directors share a reverence for Kubrick and a love
of exploration. Largely absent in Spielberg's script, though, are the biotech
aspects of *Avatar* that reveal a philosophical and spiritual interconnectedness that
goes far beyond the familial relationships of *A.I.*[103] In contrast to the urban dystopia of *Blade Runner* and the disorganized war zone of *The Hurt Locker*, *Avatar*
reveals Cameron's optimism that the natural world will survive corrupt colonialism, despite the irony that his film depicts a digitally generated reconstruction of
nature.

Some critics frame Cameron's longing for Gaia interconnectivity as an "ide-
alized vision of indigenous peoples . . . outside the modernity of the West," a
longing that results in politicizing nature itself, while others see it primarily as a
scathing critique of advanced industrial society.[104] Cameron's privileged status as
a commercially successful Hollywood director is undeniable. But it is notable
that he conducted research in the Brazilian rainforest with the nongovernmen-
tal organization Amazon Watch, spoke to the UN Permanent Forum on Indigenous Issues to commemorate Earth Day 2010, and includes an environmental
message on the film's website.[105] Within this ecoactivist remit, *Avatar* advances
three lines of thought that go beyond Asimov's turn toward Gaia in his later fiction.[106] These lines are, first, that biotechnology has the capacity to bridge the
epistemological gap between different species and forms of intelligence; second,
that the experience of Pandora (from the perspective of Earth) hinges on a seamlessly organic machine-human interface; and third, that this synergy poses questions about the mental and physical health of a transformed identity within a
complex ecosystem.

Avatar centers on a reconnaissance mission in the year 2154 undertaken by
paraplegic ex-marine Jake Sully, played by Sam Worthington. Sully assumes the
cloned body of a Na'vi avatar so he can breathe the air of Pandora, which his
human form is unable to tolerate. Jake describes himself as a "dumb grunt," but
officials of the Resources Development Administration select him for the Avatar
Program because his DNA is a genetic match to that of the avatar, which means
that he can be a surrogate for his dead twin scientist brother. Although he thinks

of himself as never losing the marine attitude, Sully's reliance on a wheelchair and glimpses of his atrophied legs contrast starkly with the exhilaration of movement in the form of a ten-foot genetically engineered avatar. That Jake lacks a holistic body image in his human form and is downcast when he is away from the light of Pandora poses problems from a disability studies perspective on two counts. First, this fantasy of overcoming pushes us away from recognizing the achievements of veterans who have sustained war injuries, such as the former Black Hawk helicopter pilot Tammy Duckworth, who lost her lower legs and whose arm was shattered by a rocket-propelled grenade over Iraq in 2004 and then became an Illinois representative and a U.S. senator without hiding her disability. Second, Lennard J. Davis argues that *Avatar* makes a "bargain with the audience" in using a nondisabled actor to portray a disabled figure who lives out an ableist fantasy in which his legs are replaced in hyperathletic form. Sami Schalk agrees with this view, seeing the biotechnological frame of *Avatar* as perpetuating a "fantasy of a disability-free future."[107] It is crucial to retain these criticisms in assessing how the film visualizes a transformed identity as both philosophically possible and rejuvenating for an ex-marine carrying a combat wound.

The extraordinary athleticism of Sully's blue-skinned avatar compared to the "scarred and scruffy combat vet . . . who has endured pain beyond his years" is just one opposition that structures the film.[108] Cameron's original film treatment of 1995 visualized Sully's disability more than the final cut in its uses of stigmatizing language ("his useless legs hand twisted and shrunken . . . a piece of discarded trash"), while the bonus footage in the Extended Collector's Edition has additional wheelchair scenes.[109] In the cinematic release, the camera rarely rests on Jake's disability, perhaps because Cameron did not want to deal with disability

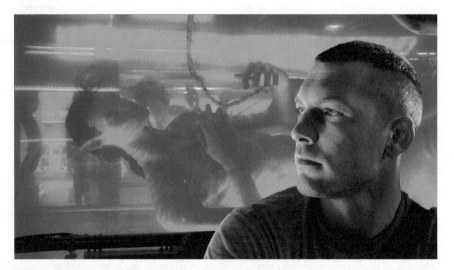

Figure 4.2. The complex semiotics of *Avatar* (2009) are evident as Jake Sully (Sam Worthington) contemplates his future Na'vi form. 20th Century Fox. AJ Pics/Alamy Photo.

politics despite the narrative function of Jake's disability—or perhaps he tried to resist the problematic use of disability as an index for a struggling human world.

It is notable that the film, which was released in December 2009, when the newly elected President Obama gave his pledge to construct "new wounded warrior facilities across America and invest in new ways of identifying and treating the signature wounds of this [the Iraq] war," omitted an originally planned scene in which Jake muses that "they can fix the spinal if you got the money, but not on vet benefits, not in this economy."[110] We might interpret Jake's chance to live an augmented life in avatar form as Cameron's criticism that "enhancement technologies in a free market society" (in the words of historian Michael Bess) are exclusive to the rich, given that Jake happens only by chance to have a DNA match to his scientist brother and has no aspirations to be posthuman.[111] This opportunity may prompt us to read the film as an embodiment of what future injured veterans could achieve instead of what they cannot do—as Obama emphasized at a Wounded Warrior Project event and as the case studies in Adam Piore's *The Body Builders* attest.[112] Nonetheless, occluded images of the disability of Jake's human form contrast sharply with his hyperathletic form on the Avatar Program, in which he goes native within the "warm, inviting, enveloping" blue of the Na'vi skin and the CGI-enhanced cinematography that lends translucence and depth.[113] Blue is not just an ecological color that resonates with Cameron's fascination with ocean life (profiled in the sequel *Avatar: The Way of the Water* and in his cofounding of OceanX), it also suggests fecundity, as Margaret Atwood evokes in *Oryx and Crake* when the Crakers' genitalia turn blue during mating.[114]

Following Dana Fore, we could read the juxtaposition between lower-limb disability and hyperathleticism as the film's valorization of "the undamaged 'able' body" projected "as a universal standard of 'normality' and perfection."[115] We might also read it as a search for wholeness that amputees often feel. However, Jake's ability to walk, run, and climb is restored only temporarily and for instrumental ends instead of embodying Piore's recognition of the body's "remarkable healing powers" that may in the future enable regenerative medicine to transplant organic legs.[116] Nonetheless, Jake willingly undergoes an experiment at the intersection of AI and robotics that can be read as a middle ground, envisaged as a "site of negotiation" between an "anti-biotech position (which might claim a 'return' to the natural body)" and a "technophilic position (in which science and technology are the answers to social concerns)."[117] As a fantasy film that asserts the hope that culturally congruent action and responsible use of regenerative medicine can vanquish environmentally hostile forces, *Avatar* aligns itself with Obama's view that wounded warriors of contemporary wars (at least those to whom he spoke early in his presidency) were "keeping faith with the future."[118] For Jake, this takes the form of a journey from an alienated and fragmented self to a node within an organically networked community.[119]

In many ways, *Avatar* is an antiwar movie that anchors hope in Jake's reeducation. However, in the film's portrayal of the contrast between Jake's alternate human and Na'vi forms, it fails to address the high numbers of amputations and brain injuries sustained during the Iraq and Afghanistan wars. Instead of focusing on Jake lying in a darkened casket during his avatar adventures, more screen time is given to him recording his Na'vi experience in a video log while in human form. The vlog scenes maintain a semblance of realism but also capture Jake's developing value system and growing emotional intelligence. The fact that he increasingly identifies with his avatar and adopts the ecological values of the Na'vi conveys the benefits and risks of such a transformation. This does not mean that he gains superintelligence or relies on an AI program to augment his consciousness. Jake is of average intelligence, and it is significant that his reeducation is both cognitive and emotional. He struggles with language learning but becomes competent in the Na'vi language (a hybrid of North American Indian tribal languages and Polynesian and African dialects that was devised by University of California linguist Paul Frommer) and masters the physical, psychological, and cultural skills needed to navigate Pandora and its spiritual core, Eywa. Central to Jake's transformation is Neytiri (Zoe Saldana), a young Na'vi woman who slowly falls in love with his avatar. Neytiri is both an "island of safety" for Jake and an action guide for his ecological reeducation, in contrast to AI-based learning, which is notably absent in the film, reflecting James Cameron's concern about the sharp rise of artificial intelligence.[120]

In contrast to the holism of the Na'vi, humans are shown to be destructive to their own and other planets. We do not see Earth depicted in the cinematic release of *Avatar*, but the original treatment of 1995 describes it as "a terminal cess-pool" and the Extended Collector's Edition represents Earth via scenes of a bar fight and of Jake's brother's funeral. Instead of a bleak picture of a gray post-industrial Earth, the cinematic release focuses on a human mining colony that has traveled to Pandora under the auspices of the Resources Development Administration in search of a superconductor, Unobtanium (an insider joke). The visual contrast between the muted human environment and the vibrancy of Pandora is startling, suggesting a broadening of perspectives and a widening of vision that is rendered through what Cameron calls "global illumination," created by Lightwave 3D to replicate the intensity of Pandora's sunlight.[121] Cameron's interest in what we might learn about other intelligent life forms via space exploration (linked to his role on NASA's advisory council) and deep-sea adventure (as revealed in his documentaries *Ghost of the Abyss* and *Aliens of the Deep*) shape both the consciousness and the ecology of Pandora. Its diverse ecosystem is optically vibrant in its rich layering of flora and fauna, with its gravity-defying spiritual habitat, Home Tree, at its heart.[122]

It is tempting to interpret the dizzying geometry of Pandora as a metaphor for epistemological uncertainty, given Jake's feeling that he will forever be an outsider. His desire to embody a transformed state in a new world is conventionally cyberpunk, reflecting the view that the "virtual environment liberates the protagonist from the constraints of his or her body."[123] Importantly, Jake's transformational journey is both individualistic and communal, when, two-thirds of the way through the film, he is welcomed ritually into the Na'vi (or Omaticaya) community. That Jake's initiation by Neytiri is a form of conversion is underscored by Neytiri's mother, who asserts "we will see if your insanity can be cured," presumably referring to Jake's humanness as well as his exploitative human values. In this respect, although he finds new life in his transformed state, Jake complies with Na'vi culture, reflecting Philip K. Dick's idea that "androidization requires obedience . . . and predictability."[124]

However, this is no utopia for Jake. Neytiri's father, the tribal leader Eyrukan, suspiciously calls him a "dreamwalker," as if Jake's selfhood is insubstantial. We might read this as an expression of a traumatized self, given the clinical evidence that temporal disorientation and a sense of fragmented selfhood are common symptoms. However, instead of an acceptance of shapeshifting identities, in the film, "dreamwalker" is associated with duplicity: what ex-marine David J. Morris, reflecting on his own trauma sustained during the Gulf War, calls "a shadow-person with its own distinct body chemistry."[125] This shift from recognition to suspicion is dramatized by Eyrukan's initial response that Jake is repugnant ("his alien smell fill my nose") and later, when Tsu'tey, Jake's rival for Neytiri's love, reveals Jake as an imposter by denouncing his sleeping avatar as "a demon in a false body."[126] This deception contrasts with the "very pure spirits" of Jake and Neytiri's lovemaking and Neytiri's signature phrase in her relationship with Jake, "I see you," which suggests both empathy and authenticity, as if Jake's true self lies deeper than his outward form. This is a knowing expression, especially given the film's intense opticality and Cameron's suspicion of AI-manipulated reality. However, Ellen Grabiner argues that Neytiri's phrase "I see you" offers "an embodied, soft gaze as an antidote to the phallocentric, dominant gaze" of the colonial patrol unit under the ruthless leadership of the menacing Colonel Miles Quaritch (played by Stephen Lang).[127]

Jake redeems himself by reaffirming his commitment to Na'vi values and joining the defense of Pandora against the advancing human army. In contrast to the spiritual interconnectedness of Eywa, this act of communal resistance is a form of active warfare that defeats the patrol unit, but not before Quaritch, protected by his threatening battle armor, punctures the sealed unit that houses Jake's human form, nearly causing him to expire from lack of oxygen. The contrast here is between Jake's reawakened humanism in his avatar form and the "pathological cyborg" represented by Quaritch's terminator-style exoskeleton.[128] With the human colonists and their war machines defeated, Jake is literally reborn as a Na'vi. We may read this ending as Jake becoming a more authentic life form with a posthuman consciousness, emotional intelligence, athleticism, and ennobled value system. However, Slavoj Žižek argues that the film stops when it does because it is likely that Jake will begin to "feel a weird discontent" when his new reality starts to disappoint him: "What this perfection signals is that it holds no place for us, the subjects who imagine it."[129]

In addition to tracing the fine line between natural and artificial life that *Blade Runner* explored a quarter of a century earlier, *Avatar* shows how human technology has the capacity to grant Jake the experience of living and feeling like a Na'vi.

But this technological transformation represents only the simulacrum of a life that requires a rite of passage and a giving over of being. When taking into account the "sensory-emotional movement" of *Avatar*'s spectacular visual mode, it is crucial that the exploration of real and fake identities, filtered through Jake's avatar double, is undergirded with a lens of virtual reality.[130] We might follow film critic Rob White's reading of the film as a valorization of "the power of digital networks to transform social interaction," epitomized by the Na'vi plugging their long hair into Eywa and their harmonious singing when they channel their spiritual core.[131] On this reading, the biotechnological transformation on Pandora reaches a point of high convergence at which organic life and digital technologies are inextricably fused.

Whether or not we read the ecological sensibility and messaging of *Avatar* as authentic or illusory, the theme of interconnectivity means that it is impossible to separate subjectivity from immersion in the natural environment. When Jake is in human form, he dwells largely in darkened interior spaces with little to animate him (as if he is experiencing depression from his war injury or lack of light) except the video logs of his avatar adventures in a bright, fecund, and multidimensional forest landscape. The film does not address mental health explicitly, aside from coding darkness/light, interior/exterior, and sunken/elevated oppositions between the human and Na'vi worlds in negative/positive health terms. Yet the implication is that the loss of communal interconnection will lead either to depression (when Jake is separated from his avatar double) or destruction (in the war machine that lurks within the scientific enterprise of the Resources Development Administration, which is reanimated in *Avatar: Way of the Water* through an interspecies technology).

It is easy to dismiss the anthropological value system of *Avatar* as magical thinking or to overemphasize its deceptive sentimentality. But it is equally tempting to interpret this world view as a form of eco-bioethics: Jake learns to put the health of the indigenous community and the natural environment ahead of human self-interest while recognizing that there is an authentic life at the interface between human and Na'vi, enabled by an ethical use of biotechnology that "preserves its emancipatory potential" without impacting adversely on the environment.[132] This reading is problematic if we take the Na'vi to be an indigenous instead of an extraterrestrial community. It is significant, though, that Jake undergoes a complete conversion by the end of the film, signaled by his statement that "the aliens [that is, the humans] went back to their dying world" while he remains on Pandora. It is not the Na'vi who are less than human, then, but Jake who embodies a new, synthetic, yet authentically conscious state. The focus on Jake's eyes opening not only echoes the film's first line, "sooner or later, though, you have to wake up," but also seems to be James Cameron's affirmative answer to the question that bioethicist Jessica Pierce posed in 2002: "Can bioethics survive in a dying world?"[133]

The possibility of renewed perspective and connectivity is central to *Avatar*'s environmentally sensitive bioethics, which steers between a respect for indigenous cultures and an embrace of technological augmentation. This healing vision not only jettisons corrupt and self-serving humans, but in embodying a version of Nikolas Rose's somatic ethics it also counters the theme of isolation by interlinking the cultural examples of this chapter: fears of persecution in *Amped*, distrust between humans and AI-enhanced robots in *Ex Machina*, and the cocooned bomb specialist in *Hurt Locker* who cannot live without the adrenalin of the combat zone. *Avatar* ultimately turns away from philosophical questions about intelligent machines, singularity, and technocracy in favor of a fantasy of self-transformation. Yet Cameron's film is also a meditation on relationality between races and species, including between cyborgs and future humans. Released six years into the Iraq War, *Avatar* explores the health impacts of warfare by giving material and narrative form to the "islands of safety" that Bessel van der Kolk deems therapeutically crucial for traumatized individuals. There are dangers in valorizing its spectacular utopian fantasies, especially given its controversial depictions of disability and indigeneity. But as a capstone to the first half of *Transformed States*, the bioethical vision of *Avatar* shifts the conversation away from abstract thought experiments about consciousness toward embodied narratives of potentiality that inform the book's second half with respect to identities in part 3 and ecologies in part 4.

PART THREE
DYNAMIC STATES

5 *Keeping On*

PRODUCTIVE AGING AND THE
QUEST FOR LIFE EXTENSION

As the founding director of the National Institute on Aging, Robert N. Butler achieved more than any other American public figure in amplifying the realities of aging. For thirty-five years he documented the physical and psychological challenges of "being old in America." His first book, *Why Survive?*, was published two months before Gerald Ford signed the Age Discrimination Act of 1975. With this Pulitzer Prize–winning book, Butler stimulated new interest in and funding for gerontology. That haunting question "Why survive?" helped professionals and the public understand that prejudices related to ageism stand in the way of valuing older Americans, despite assurances from a sequence of national leaders that seniors are a "phenomenal reserve of talent and experience," as George H. W. Bush called them at the end of the 1980s.[1]

Why Survive? is the best known of Butler's books, but the often-updated *Aging and Mental Health* (1973) and his last major work, *The Longevity Revolution* (2008), demonstrate his commitment to grounding positive thinking in science and to understanding the dynamic transformations of aging from an intergenerational perspective. This interconnectedness was also often emphasized by his collaborators and interlocutors. For example, in the foreword to the first edition of *Aging and Mental Health* (1973), Arthur S. Flemming, chair of the first two White House Conferences on Aging (1961 and 1971) and Eisenhower's third health secretary, noted that retaining the ability to make decisions, staying involved in life, and maintaining dignity were three recurring themes he heard from older Americans.[2] Flemming thought that Butler's work embodied a culture of affirmation that could counter the stigmatizing decline and deficit models of old age.[3] Flemming was overoptimistic about what he discerned as a culture shift from "despair" to "hope" among older Americans in the 1970s, given the relatively high rate of depression and rising suicides among those over sixty-five compared to other age groups.[4] When former first lady Rosalynn Carter wrote a new foreword for *Aging and Mental Health* eighteen years later, she adopted a more urgent tone. Carter thought that stigma, discrimination, and the dearth of qualified personnel had changed little since she had chaired the President's Commission on Mental Health in 1977–1978, a time when the American Public Health Association was calling for a national policy on aging.[5] She saw Butler as a great educator about what "keeps the old well, rather than merely what makes them ill" but recognized in that post–Cold War moment that adjustments to national aging were only just beginning.[6]

This fourth edition of *Aging and Mental Health* appeared at the dawn of the 1990s after a lean decade for mental health policy. President Clinton picked up the baton by appointing Tipper Gore his mental health advisor in 1993, a year in which the second lady testified at a Senate Special Committee on Aging forum on the subject of mental health and aging.[7] Rosalynn Carter had lit the way for Tipper Gore's advocacy by focusing on caregiving and destigmatization. However, in contrast to the focus of Carter and Gore, Butler was keen to develop translational research and build the nation's gerontological capacity. This focus spanned his training in neurology, psychiatry, and psychology at the National Institute of Mental Health in the 1950s and early 1960s, as the inaugural director of the National Institute on Aging (NIA) from 1974 to 1982, and as founder of the first national geriatrics department at Mount Sinai Medical Center and the policy-oriented nonprofit International Longevity Center (est. 1990).

At the NIA, Butler recognized three needs. First, to build a multidisciplinary institute with biology and biomedicine at its core. Second, to generate productive alliances in Congress and with established associations like the Gerontological Society of America (est. 1945) and new ones like the Alzheimer's Disease and Associated Disorders Association (est. 1977) and the Alzheimer's Association (est. 1980). And, third, to develop a "health politics of anguish" strategy to destigmatize aging and draw philanthropic funding for new programs—in particular the NIA's flagship project on Alzheimer's.[8] Even after his departure from the NIA, Butler's threefold agenda influenced a wave of new centers that focused on applied gerontology, aging demographics, basic biology, and minority aging, plus important studies on exercise, retirement, women's health, and the genetics of longevity. It is for this exploration of dynamic interconnectivities that Butler offers a route into this third section of *Transformed States* on the complex entanglements of technology, identities, and life stages.

Political Pathways to Age Tech

President Clinton appointed a spritely sixty-eight-year-old Butler as chair of the 1995 White House Conference on Aging. This appointment was, in part, because Butler's intersectional values, commitment to pursuing universal health care coverage, and belief in institutional responsibility not only echoed what Robert Bellah calls the "moral ecology" of "healthy institutions" that can "sustain the lives of all of us" but also chimed with Clinton's concerns about the "human tragedy of older Americans who are forced to choose, literally choose each week between medicine and food and housing," as he had noted two years earlier in laying out plans to improve the nation's health security.[9] Clinton reiterated concerns about poverty and Medicaid in his remarks at the Conference on Aging, where he acknowledged that fragmented home and community services were failing many seniors who required long-term care. But he also asserted his belief that the "country has been moving in the right direction" in its engagement with older Americans, such as his policy advisor Ira Magaziner's advocacy of the Aging 2000 project.[10]

For the 1995 conference, titled "The Road to an Aging Policy for the 21st Century," Butler was keen to shift the conversation from the chronological life-stage approach of the previous two White House conferences of 1971 and 1981 toward an emphasis on "intergenerational cooperation," as retiring Arkansas senator David Pryor (a close friend of Clinton) emphasized in his opening remarks at the 1995 conference.[11] This event broke ground in stressing the themes of independence, opportunity, and dignity, together with the contributions of "today's and tomorrow's older citizens" into the next century.[12] Of the eighteen proposed focus points, health was overwhelmingly number one (with twice as many votes as the second-place issue of income security) and technology was eighteenth (just behind the role of the private sector). Although this lack of focus on health technologies is surprising given Clinton and Gore's emphasis on technological solutions as an endless resource, Butler and his fellow organizers, including Clinton's health secretary, Donna Shalala, were keen to let grassroots activities and interests shape the agenda.[13] Significantly, the ranking of these themes tallied with Butler's own priorities regarding aging. But he was ultimately disappointed by the conference because it did not lead to specific legislation, although he recognized that it "helped sustain interest" in aging and raised the profile of the "creativity and potential of older adults."[14]

Butler gave equal emphasis to public education, basic research, and the need to establish a more robust biomedical database by involving more citizens from diverse backgrounds over the age of sixty-five in clinical trials to anchor what the NIA calls a "living laboratory" in which intervention responsiveness and risk factors can be assessed.[15] From his early writings, Butler was interested in inter-sectionality, well before the term was coined, especially the ways that class, race, gender, and sexuality are "dominating factors in survival," as he reflected in the aftermath of Hurricane Katrina.[16] He recognized that health inequities based on age stratification often reach a critical point during old age, particularly if comorbidities remain untreated at an early stage.[17] A humanist, a "citizen activist," a lover of art, and a medical polymath, Butler rarely offered technological solutions for a growing demographic that is often invisible except when Congress consider its drain on entitlements.[18]

However, although *Why Survive?* helped launch the Alzheimer's Association and spurred the activist Gray Panthers (est. 1970) to demand better access to health care, Butler worried that aging remained "the neglected stepchild of the human life cycle," despite the work of House members Claude Pepper (a Florida Democrat) and Silvio Conte (a Massachusetts Republican) to raise the profile of biomedical research and health technologies in Washington, DC.[19] Congressional neglect persisted into the early 2010s, when baby boomers reached retirement age, over a quarter of a century after Butler warned that the boomers were a "generation at risk" and challenged Congress to act with measured bipartisan forethought.[20] An illustration of such short-termism was the abandonment in

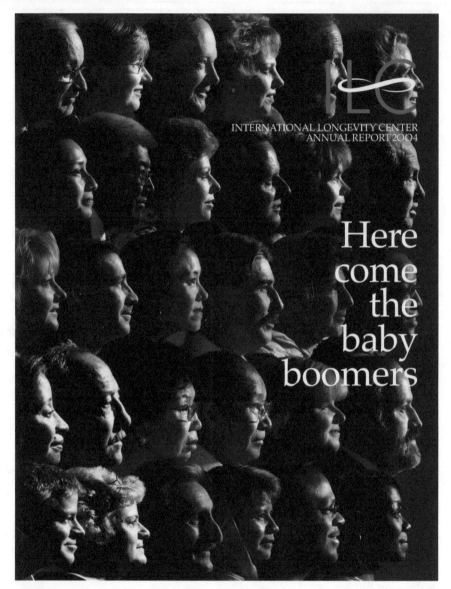

INTERNATIONAL LONGEVITY CENTER
ANNUAL REPORT 2004

Here
come
the
baby
boomers

Figure 5.1. "Here Come the Baby Boomers," cover of the International Longevity Center annual report, 2004. Courtesy of the Robert N. Butler Columbia Aging Center Archives, Macmillan School of Public Health, Columbia University.

2013 of the Community Living Assistance Services and Support (CLASS) Act, championed by Massachusetts senator Edward Kennedy, that would have helped older Americans with long-term care. After three years of planning for the Affordable Care Act, Congress deemed the CLASS Act to be financially unviable.[21]

Some welcome news was on the way. The NIA budget increased considerably after 2016; at the time of writing, it was the fourth largest among the twenty-seven institutes and centers of the National Institutes of Health.[22] This was partially because Congress agreed to raise the NIH budget following some lean years and partially a response to the NIA's assessment that by 2030 the population of Americans over sixty-five would be double that of the 2000 population, which would "have profound social and economic effects on the nation."[23] However, it is surprising that the federal perspective did not sharpen earlier, especially given the reenergization of LBJ-era health policies during the Clinton and Obama administrations on the one hand and the Republicans' increasing reliance on the votes of an older electorate on the other.

Butler was critical of the Johnson administration for neglecting the elderly poor, a demographic that he assessed was more "common" than the government and the media often recognized and was also "frequently black," as he wrote in a landmark essay of 1969, "Age-Ism: Another Form of Bigotry," four years after Johnson signed the Social Security Amendments and the Older Americans Act that included the establishment of a federal Administration on Aging.[24] The essay, which was written in the wake of assassinations and race riots that scarred the Great Society domestic programs, made three key points. First, he reminded readers that economic stratification often arises at the intersection of race and age; second, he saw discrimination against the elderly as based on gerontophobia or "a personal revulsion to and distaste for growing old, disease, disability; and fear of powerlessness, 'uselessness,' and death"; and third, he highlighted how little the National Institute of Mental Health spent on gerontological research (at the time this was only 3 percent of its budget and only 1 percent of the NIH budget, even though older Americans accounted for 25 percent of hospital admissions).[25]

Not only did this 1969 essay lay the conceptual foundations for *Why Survive?*, but highlighted three areas—stratification, discrimination, and funding—that arise perennially when assessing the chronic diseases and psychological challenges that typically emerge in advanced age, such as dementia, cancer, heart disease, osteoporosis, kidney failure, diabetes, anxiety disorders, lethargy, and depression.[26] Even though a National Advisory Council on Aging report of 1978 claimed that experiments on identical twins suggested that 60 to 80 percent of "an individual's longevity is inherited," Butler argued that health is shaped 30 percent by genetics and 70 percent by environment, which for him included attitudes toward aging.[27] This was one reason why the 1995 White House Conference on Aging emphasized intergenerational cooperation and why Butler continued to stress the "moral links we have to one other" and the increasing importance of quality of life for older Americans experiencing shrinking networks of support in later years.[28]

However, Butler was keen not to overprescribe quality of life, partly because he did not want to create a norm and partly to protect the rights of older generations.[29] *The Longevity Revolution*, which was published a year before right-wing activists began falsely claiming that Obamacare was intent on establishing "death panels" to decide which older Americans were worthy of care, warned against legislators or physicians having "authority to determine for an individual the point at which quality of life is so diminished as to make life itself undesirable and unnecessary."[30] Instead, in his final writings, Butler offered advice on exercise, diet, sleep, smoking, and alcohol consumption with a humanistic emphasis on networks, purpose, relationships, and basic rights, as emphasized by his call to the United Nations to adopt a declaration of the rights of older persons.[31]

Butler's concept of productive aging is key here. The humanist concept of productive aging emphasizes a mixture of voluntary activity and a positive attitude to life that orients the individual away from a biomedical or pharmaceutical model of overdependence toward an affirmatory life that retains agency, meaning, and growth. We might be suspicious of the industrial metaphor of productivity applied to retirement years for its debility rhetoric. However, productive aging for Butler is not as normative as his physician friend John W. Rowe's concept of successful aging, which prioritizes self-sufficiency, "maintenance of high physical and mental capacity, and 'active engagement in life.'"[32] Instead, Butler saw productive aging as an ethic of self-care wedded to voluntaristic participation. This is not to say that Butler did not value independent living, especially when compared to his criticisms of custodial care: he railed against "the often impersonal, sterile, antiseptic medical atmosphere that we find in hospitals and nursing homes" instead of seeing them as the places of "refuge and comfort" that George H. W. Bush had envisioned in 1990.[33]

The 2005 and 2015 White House Conferences on Aging were the first in the series to include what we now call "age tech." The 2005 conference focused on health information technology, and the focus in 2015 was mobile technologies and robotics. However, Butler's attitude toward technology is difficult to assess in his writings even though his advocacy was grounded "in the latest biomedical interventions," in the words of his biographer W. Andrew Achenbaum.[34] Butler favored the Bush-era Decade of the Brain initiative, which balanced an appraisal of what is and what is not known about Alzheimer's with an enthusiasm for biotechnological innovation, although Butler believed that "a decade is not long enough for anything as complex as the brain, and the central nervous system requires much more major investment."[35] Yet he was wary of pharmacological solutions, warning against overusing antibiotics and about the potential side effects of neuroleptics, diazepam, and lithium for the elderly. He was also concerned by the number of patients who were hospitalized or died following adverse reactions to prescription drugs.[36] This does not mean Butler thought that outpatient care is always sufficient, but he also did not agree with the view that biomedical technologies are necessary for aiding recovery from the "traumas of aging."[37]

Given Butler's emphasis on grounding geriatrics training in biomedical knowledge and clinical care, he was keen not to disparage technology, specifically in palliative medicine, because he believed that it enhanced "the possibilities for a better death" by controlling "pain, nausea, air hunger, and other symptoms."[38] In the mid-1980s, soon after taking up his post at Mount Sinai, he warned against Luddite views about technology and argued that New York State would fall behind California "if it is not willing to make commitments to scientific and technological advances."[39] Yet in his final essay, written in 2010, "Prologue or Introduction to Life Review," he pivoted away from seeing technology as a solution for longevity. He recommended ethical protocols for palliative care, and despite his typically secular slant, as his own death from acute leukemia approached, he turned to the spiritual comforts of friendship and reconciliation.

Instead of focusing on extending lifespans, Butler was keen to encourage new technologies that could help determine biomarkers of aging. For example, such technology could help practitioners and the public understand the relationship between mild cognitive impairment and the development of Alzheimer's. The Alzheimer's Association argued that better awareness of that relationship could be a "critical turning point" in care.[40] He was also in favor of the Alzheimer's Disease Neuroimaging Initiative, which was established in 2004 as a public-private multicenter study to detect changes in brain structure at an early stage and to track biomarkers.[41] Butler saw some hope in drug therapies for dementia, although in 2008 he noted only "limited effectiveness" of three market drugs for Alzheimer's, Aricept, Exelon, and Reminyl (the first is prescribed to Alice Howland in *Still Alice*).[42] Whereas he felt that electronic medical records (a priority of the George W. Bush administration) had great potential for forging improvement in the quality of health care and in ensuring patient privacy, he was skeptical about telemedicine because it often masks gaps in medical provision, although he recognized its advantages for those living in rural areas far from a health center. Butler's ambivalence about technology is emphasized by a key line in *The Longevity Revolution*: "Relying on technology too much can dehumanize medicine without affording any benefit to the patient, because clinical diagnoses are often more accurate than diagnostic technology."[43] If the United States was experiencing a longevity revolution, then to Butler's mind, it should not be a revolution that was overly reliant on biomedical technologies or that entertained scientifically implausible claims about life extension.[44]

I began the chapter by highlighting the historical and policy significance of Butler, "the man who saw old anew," as the *New York Times* put it.[45] However, Butler's partial myopia toward technology and aging opens up the focus for this chapter. Butler's aversion to technological solutions was even noted by one of his peers, the influential feminist Betty Friedan, who turned her attention from gender mystique to age mystique in the 1980s, attending a Salzburg Seminar that Butler led on productive aging and volunteering for assessment at the Mount Sinai Geriatric Management Clinic as research for her 1993 book *The Fountain of Age*.[46] Friedan shared Butler's views about ageism and spoke about the need to appreciate the contribution of "vital people over sixty-five," although she was a more divisive public figure than him.[47] Friedan noted that the Mount Sinai biomedical technology program was far from high tech and she mused about whether life-extension technologies might be used less to "keep us breathing on machines and alive even when we can no longer think, speak, move, respond" and more to interface with quality-of-life measures that might transform the inner and outer worlds of all older citizens, not just an economic elite.[48] Far from

putting biotechnology at the center of her thesis, Friedan did little more than suggest that technologies have an unrealized place in promoting "human ends" in
gerontological research and long-term care.[49] Yet her turn toward technology
reveals a partial break with Butler, even though she shared his views on productive aging and the need to tackle aging discrimination for American women.

As this chapter discusses, the technological imperative has intensified since
Butler's death in 2010, and the popular press and social media often feature efforts
to halt, reverse, or eradicate aging. The executive and legislative branches have
taken an increased interest in technology, including a Health and Human Services
Aging Services Technology Study of 2012 that sought to raise awareness of
enabling technologies for "consumers, caregivers, and providers" and a U.S. Senate hearing titled *Tackling Diseases of Aging* in 2013.[50] This new level of interest fed
into the emerging technologies featured at the 2015 White House Conference on
Aging, which was followed by a Council of Advisors on Science and Technology
report titled *Independence, Technology, and Connection in Older Age* in 2016 and a
Senate hearing in 2019 that considered "how technology can help maintain health
and quality of life" for disabled seniors.[51] However, despite the work of the select
and special committees on aging, an aging and male-dominated Congress did
not always take potential breakthrough technologies seriously, at least up to the
2018 midterms, when there was a spike of diversity among elected representatives, although this demographic shift was offset by the fact that the median age
of the Senate approached sixty-five by 2020.[52] In the mid-2010s, there was also a
political shift among older voters, as the majority of white people over fifty voted
for Donald Trump in the 2016 U.S. presidential election. Strangely, this electoral
trend was in tension with the interests of many of these voters, given that the
Trump administration sought to dismantle Obamacare and offered little to assist
those with preexisting conditions or in need of long-term care.[53]

Given these political and technological entanglements, this chapter keeps
Butler's longevity project in view but uses his blind spot toward technology to
explore the collision of ideas and ideology regarding the aging continuum of
physical and mental health. Using Butler as my fulcrum, rather like the life of F.
Scott Fitzgerald's mercurial character Benjamin Button of 1922, who ages backward across his lifespan (as Brad Pitt reimagined for cinema audiences in the 2008
film *The Curious Case of Benjamin Button*), the next three sections examine the
interrelationship between aging, health, and technology in chronologically
reverse order both to show how longevity and technology debates play out across
different life stages and to tease out their bioethical implications.

The next section looks at public and private efforts to combat degenerative
diseases, focusing on Alzheimer's research and therapeutics. Returning to the
discussion of neuroscientist Lisa Genova's novel *Still Alice* in chapter 3, here I shift
the chronological frame from early-onset to late-onset Alzheimer's in terms of
pharmaceutical and genetic interventions. I also analyze Jonathan Franzen's
autobiographical and fictional depictions of late-life dementia in "My Father's
Brain" and *The Corrections* (both published in 2001), in which technologies have an

uncomfortable place in Franzen's critique of late capitalist culture. The following section moves beyond the biomedical establishment to consider life-enhancing processes available in the biotech marketplace that are targeted especially at midlife and older Americans. Here I revive the discussion of Margaret Atwood's 2003 biotech novel *Oryx and Crake* and reflect on the 2015 anti-ageist film *Advantageous* to assess audacious efforts to halt aging through genetic, pharmaceutical, and surgical means. In this move "beyond therapy," to cite the title of the President's Council on Bioethics 2003 report, I pause to consider the gender, racial, and economic implications of the hold the cosmetics industry exerts over fears and fantasies of aging. My final section turns to technologies that seek to extend life by eradicating aging, ranging from rejuvenation techniques promoted by adventurists to the popularization of transhumanist technologies such as cryonics.[54] This closing discussion considers Don DeLillo's response to extreme life extension in his 2016 novel *Zero K* and the explosion of DIY biohacking in the late 2010s that offers an emergent praxis toward well-being, before returning to consider the continued relevance of Butler's *The Longevity Revolution* for navigating the challenges of aging.

Genetic Time Bombs and Dementia Care

In April 1994, five months after Ronald Reagan announced he had Alzheimer's, science journalist Robin Marantz Henig wrote an impassioned feature in the *New York Times* about a disease that "slowly but relentlessly eviscerates a lifetime of memories" and "eventually erases all that makes a person alive, unique and human."[55] By the mid-1980s, dementia was among the top four causes of death nationally (after heart disease, cancer, and stroke), and Alzheimer's was the leading cause of death among older Americans. This statistic was due to more refined diagnostics and the efforts of the NIA to dub Alzheimer's "the disease of the century" in order to galvanize "political action" and to give shape to a disease concept that is tricky to represent visually.[56] The transformation of Alzheimer's from a heterogeneous disease to a unified biomedical concept "with specific pathological characteristics" helped the legitimate the NIA.[57] Sociologist Patrick Fox has shown how this unified construct was a strategic effort to maximize federal funding, better understand the neurochemistry of brain disease, and raise the perception of the public that "cognitive decline was not an inevitable aspect of growing older."[58]

The high-profile deaths of actor Rita Hayworth and composer Aaron Copeland from Alzheimer's-related complications raised awareness in the late 1980s and early 1990s, as did the regional Alzheimer's Disease Research Centers and the growing global network of international longevity centers that highlighted both common cause and cultural differences. In particular, the directors of the American and Japanese longevity centers collaborated from the time of their founding in 1990, a time when President Bush and Prime Minister Kaifu were working to improve U.S.-Japanese relations, while recognizing the economic value of longevity. (In that decade, seniors were typically living five years longer in Japan than in the United States.)[59] To justify the request for increased federal funding for gerontology, Butler and his collaborators argued that biomedical break-throughs would pay back in a "longevity dividend" by reducing the number of inpatients residing in psychiatric units and nursing homes and the entitlements older Americans with related conditions would need to claim.[60]

The "Alzheimerization of aging," as physician Richard Adelman called it in 1995, elicited a mixed response from the biomedical community, including other NIH centers that were concerned that extra funding to the NIA would mean a decrease in research on other age-related pathologies such as Parkinson's.[61] But the economics and politics of Alzheimer's were far reaching, moving beyond pure research toward efforts to balance investment in potential cures with better geri-atric care for those experiencing this profoundly transformative condition.[62] Advocates of what futurist Michael Zey calls "superlongevity" remain wedded to the belief that genetic engineering will eventually eradicate Alzheimer's, based on the premise that it is largely hereditary.[63] However, the NIA has been more measured on this topic. David Schlessinger, the head of the NIA Laboratory of Genetics, pointed to the complex interaction between genes and behavioral, social, and environmental factors in late-onset cases.[64] The opposite is true of early-onset Alzheimer's, for which genetic patterns are easier to trace. Individuals who experience early onset of this disease represent an estimated 10 percent of cases, including that of Alice Howland and her eldest daughter Anna in *Still Alice*.[65]

The publication in 1991 of a piece in *Nature* by a transatlantic research team that revealed that early-onset Alzheimer's patients from two families shared a chromosome 21 defect triggered a wave of genetic and molecular research. Scientists in the mid-1990s also detected mutations typical of Alzheimer's in chromosomes 1 and 14, a breakthrough moment that prompted journalists to proclaim that researchers were a "step closer to an Alzheimer's drug."[66] The chromosome 21 research led to speculation about possible genetic relations between Down syndrome and Alzheimer's, particularly because the clinical pic-ture reveals that individuals with Down syndrome who live beyond thirty or forty years tend to develop neuropathological symptoms common to Alzheim-er's.[67] This picture is more complex because early-onset and late-onset cases have similar pathological features with respect to memory lapses and memory retrieval, which has led neurologists to speculate about "multiple possible influ-ences" that complicate any narrow accounts of the disease.[68] This perspective on codeterminants shaped Margaret Lock's development of what she calls "entan-glement theory," which seeks a holistic picture of the whole person instead of breaking down Alzheimer's into visual representations of neuronal cell damage that can be seen via neuroimaging.[69]

Even with the drug and antibody developments of the 2010s and early 2020s to treat the symptoms of Alzheimer's or modify brain disease—from the established companies Biogen, Eli Lilly, and OrbiMed and from newer biotechs such as Alec-tor, Altos Labs, and Denali Therapeutics—the multinational search for cause and cure is proving a long and puzzling journey. The pace of nearly fifty years of laboratory work and clinical trials on Alzheimer's looks sluggish compared to the rapid development of the COVID-19 vaccine in 2020–2022, although it is comparable to the lengthy development phases of the vaccines for polio and tuberculosis.

Some thinkers envisage a future in which "we could all get injections of antiplaque drugs at regular intervals to prevent the buildup of . . . toxic aggregates or, even better, be immunized against many different amyloids in childhood along with measles and diphtheria."[70] The key for Alzheimer's is early detection. For this, the interpersonal role of the physician is pivotal, aided by memory tests and information from family members about changes in the patient's cognitive behavior. Cerebrospinal fluid sampling and tomography to measure brain metabolism are also thought to have high accuracy rates in detecting Alzheimer's, though positron emission tomographic (PET) scans are typically covered by health insurance only for cases that physicians consider to be strictly medically necessary.[71]

Even after the FDA approved the antibody Leqembi in the summer of 2023 for helping to slow Alzheimer's in early cases, it is increasingly clear that investigations need to be much broader than instrumental interventions in the fields of genetics and pharmacology. Take race, for instance. Most accounts of Alzheimer's focus on the experience of white Americans. The Alzheimer's Association estimates that Black and Latinx Americans are at greater risk (two and one and a half times, respectively) than white Americans, yet for a combination of cultural, environmental, and economic reasons, these groups are less likely to receive an early diagnosis by a physician.[72] These health care disparities and reports of discrimination by Black, Latinx, and Asian American patients go far beyond dementia care and they are also affected by regional and economic variants—and language barriers in the cases of some older minority patients—that can exacerbate unmet health needs.[73] The Alzheimer's Association posits that lifestyle and stress rather than genetics are prevailing factors in these communities, particularly high blood pressure and diabetes. This has led the association to promote the need for better awareness and management of risk factors. But instead of calling for advances in telomere research that seeks to protect chromosomes from erosion during cell division or Crispr technology to identify protein deficiencies or research into identifying the probability that an individual has the APOE e4 gene variant (which may increase risk and is more frequently identified in Black Americans), the association seeks more diversity in clinical trials, adherence to the NIA Health Disparities Framework, and cultural competency among health care workers.[74]

The mental health implications of Alzheimer's are also often difficult to untangle from its organic effects. These range from a diminished ego identity to "catastrophic reactions" of bewilderment and aggression to long-term depression and the lethargy that is often triggered by isolation.[75] In chapter 3, we saw the erasure of selfhood visualized in the film version of *Still Alice* as Alice experiences cognitive decline and earlier in the understimulation she feels as a professional academic forced into early retirement, especially when she can no longer exercise outdoors or play games. The fact that Alice is physically fit makes her decline more pronounced, but she retains a level of personhood even as Lisa Genova probes the margin between a biomedical brain disease and the experience of deteriorating well-being. Genova is respectful of the unified concept of Alzheimer's, and her role as a scientific educator chimes with Butler's project by documenting the lifeworld of individuals who are experiencing neurological challenges yet maintain therapeutic positivity.

Such optimism contrasts with writer Jonathan Franzen's suspicion that the disease concept of Alzheimer's is an example of "the medicalization of human experience," which he calls "the latest entry in the ever-expanding nomenclature of victimhood."[76] To analyze these suspicions of overmedicalization and to test the efficacy of top-down interventions that tackle deleterious aspects of aging, I turn for the rest of this section to Franzen's 2001 autobiographical *New Yorker* piece "My Father's Brain" and his third novel, *The Corrections*, which answer Butler's brand of optimism with an exploration of how dementia makes life unproductive and sometimes unbearable. In *The Corrections*, Franzen explores the personal and familial impact of the aging Alfred Lambert's experiences of Parkinson's, dementia, and depression, and in "My Father's Brain," he speculates about how many cases of "ordinary mental illness" in old age are "trendily misdiagnosed as Alzheimer's."[77] Despite his suspicions, Franzen recognizes that the rise in Alzheimer diagnoses was, in part, a strategy for helping the disease achieve "the same social and medical standing as heart disease or cancer."[78]

At times, "My Father's Brain" is reminiscent of Philip Roth's autobiographical *Patrimony* (1996), which tells of his father's physical and mental decline, but Franzen's shorter account is a little different; it seeks a balance in tone between the tragedy and banality of his father Earl's worsening memory and control over his bowels, supplemented by the author's reflections on dementia research.[79] Just as Roth interweaves an account of his father's dementia with his own journey into middle age, the possessive in "*My* Father's Brain" reveals that Franzen's focus is an attempt to negotiate parental relationships and models of masculinity rather than focusing more squarely on health challenges and the politics of domesticity. Both Earl and Alfred are individualists despite their family commitments and the strain they put on their wives and families, leading Franzen to wonder if there "could have been a worse disease . . . than Alzheimer's" given his father's "narrative interest in life."[80] In answering this question, he reflects on Earl's loss of "social connections that had saved him from the worst of his depressive isolation" and the late stage that "robbed him of the sheathing of adulthood, the means to hide the child inside him."[81] Earl's will to live endures even after he is hospitalized and even though he sinks lower "than he had the neuronal wherewithal to do."[82] There is no transcendent moment of love comparable to that in *Still Alice*. Instead, when Earl finally dies in 1995, his son notes that "we'd simply lost the last of the parts out of which we could fashion a living whole."[83]

Despite his interest in families and interwoven journeys, Franzen has been criticized for retreating into postmodern irony and envisioning "his characters from within the limitations of his own persona," which arguably leads to an "implausible, distorted, and impoverished depiction of his characters' inner lives."[84] This criticism holds to an extent, despite Franzen's desire to "write about the things closest to me," including his own depression, instead of bearing "the weight of our whole disturbed society," as he attempted to do in his first two novels.[85] In contrast to Butler's focus on sensual growth for aging males, Franzen's writing distances physical desire from emotional closeness to others.[86] This does not mean that "My Father's Brain" and *The Corrections* avoid profound questions about the interaction between thoughts and instincts or inherited patterns of depression or the need to discern what is correctible in life and what is uncorrectable or the paradox that finite human lives can still imagine immortality.[87] Alfred Lambert views death as "the last opportunity for radical transformation," yet this is in direct conflict with the uncorrectable "finite carcass in a sea of blood and bone chips and gray matter" that his life has been reduced to.[88] Instead of formulating a grand thesis about aging, Alfred's mind lapses and he cannot pose the "very important question" he wishes to convey to his son. These dreams of radical transformation, however muted, contrast starkly with the health burden Alfred and Earl place on their families, even though they are increasingly helpless to do anything about it.

Franzen's interest in neurochemistry and pharmacology inflects his exploration of the entanglement of science and culture in the new millennium, as filtered through the generational clash between the retired engineer Alfred and the neurotic consumerism that characterizes the lives of his four children.[89] His understanding of depression as an "estrangement from humanity" grossly oversimplifies a complex neurological and psychological experience that strikes in different ways and phases of life, as fellow *New Yorker* writer Andrew Solomon explored in his essay "Anatomy of Melancholy" in 1998, three years before Franzen channeled his opinions through Alfred.[90] Franzen is more suspicious of technological consumerism than Solomon: in the 1990s, Franzen argued that there had been an "electronic fragmentation of public discourse" and too much optimism about what pharmaceutics could do, in the 2000s he criticized a "plague of cell phones," and in the 2010s he dismissed robotic helpers as symptomatic of hyperdriven capitalism.[91] This disdain for technology is symbolized by the fact that Alfred sells a patent for a mental health treatment to the biotech Axon Corporation for a paltry $5,000, only to be disqualified from the company's (satirically titled) Corecktall clinical trials that might slow the pace of his Parkinson's and dementia.

In fact, Franzen takes multiple swipes at technologies of all kinds as symptoms of a narcissistic corporate culture that he believes are inimical to health even as they purport to "relieve suffering as efficiency as possible."[92] He rarely sees technology as enabling or considers its benefits such as keeping older Americans connected or unburdening carers via robot helpers, for example, which the 2013 film *Robot and Frank* imaginatively explores through the lens of dementia by pairing a retired ex-convict and a humanoid robot modeled on Honda's ASIMO robot.[93] Although Franzen does not tip into gerontophobia, both Alfred's pathologies and the "brain as meat" imagery that opens "My Father's Brain" reveal a lurking fear of aging. This puts Franzen's views in tension with Butler's anti-ageist positive thinking and the message of Alzheimer's Association spokesperson and actor David Hyde Pierce (famous for his role as a Seattle psychiatrist in the comedy show *Frasier*) at the 2015 White House Conference on Aging. In opening a panel titled "Caregiving in America," Pierce reflected on his grandfather's and his father's dementia and argued that we must move beyond "fixed and calcified" words like "aging and caregiving" and that instead of focusing on narratives of decline we should recognize that "to age is to live."[94]

Ageless Bodies and Rejuvenation: Beyond the Cosmetic Imperative

While recognizing Butler's major contribution to the science of and public understanding of Alzheimer's, this section takes half a step back to consider broader biomedical and cultural patterns that seek to decelerate or halt aging. Butler's dilemma was how to balance his belief that productive aging was attitudinal with his understanding that to some extent it was reliant on biomedical knowledge and responsive health care. The national and global networks he helped build are impressive. But he remained skeptical about medical marketing beyond the NIA's governance framework and was suspicious of industrialists that promise elixirs or individuals who chase after single-stage solutions. The tension between lifestyle and life-saving technologies is evident in his reluctance to overmedicalize aging and his wariness about market-driven technologies that prey on fears about growing older. For example, in *The Longevity Revolution*, he argued that the cosmetic imperative is a symptom of systemic ageism driven by a market that places supreme value on youthfulness. He saw cosmetic surgery as a surface technology that masks aging and does little to improve health on a cellular level instead of something that could turbocharge a dynamic and evolving life.

That does not mean Butler pursued only top-down interventions. For example, he recognized the importance of participation and imagined a hypothetical citizen science project called Laboratories 2030 that would seek to co-create solutions for aging in urban and rural communities.[95] This culture of participation diverged from the interactions of the adventurist group he dubbed "longevity seekers" who tout rejuvenation techniques, body engineering, and gene enhancement. Margaret Atwood parodied this transhumanist trend in *Oryx and Crake* in the form of a "BlyssPluss Pill" that her protagonist Jimmy encounters in the "sparkling clean, landscaped, ecologically pristine, and very expensive" RejoovenEsense Compound.[96] To Jimmy's question about how this manicured space is funded, the biotech adventurist Crake responds "grief in the face of inevitable death . . . the wish to stop time." Crake tells Jimmy how BlyssPluss can "eliminate the external causes of death," prolong youth, and give a burst of libido and well-being.[97] Though BlyssPluss is still in clinical trials in the novel—and proves more disruptive than its marketing suggests—Crake claims it will be "the must-have pill, in every country, in every society in the world."[98] There is no evidence that Butler read Atwood, but he was just as interested in the sensual lives of older Americans as he was skeptical about claims to stop time.[99] Butler remained positive about health maintenance, especially through calorie restriction, exercise, and avoiding smoking. He was less positive about fads, including hormone treatments (with the exception of taking estrogen supplements during menopause), cosmetology, "expensive Swiss clinics for cell treatments," and cryonics, seeing them as aspects of what ecoactivist Andrew Kimbrell calls the "marketing of life."[100]

Butler did not level criticism at Americans who make positive lifestyle choices that may decelerate or even prevent conditions associated with old age such as dementia and hypertension. Instead, he blamed what he calls the "longevity lobby" for fetishizing certain practices and whetting the public appetite for lifespan extension interventions that lack a grounding in legitimate science.[101] Although he was not a technophobe like Jonathan Franzen, Butler's position was even warier than Leon Kass's bioconservative argument that technological interventions should be strictly used for therapeutic ends instead of as an extratherapeutic tool of enhancement. Butler held opposing views to Kass about the therapeutic potential of stem cell research, but there is overlap in their views about what the President's Council on Bioethics called "goodness and meaning in life" and they were equally suspicious of the eugenic rhetoric of gene hunters.[102] This overlap compares favorably to Butler's distance from British gerontologist Aubrey de Grey's view that biotechnology will usher in a "rejuvenation breakthrough" that could more than double a lifespan.[103] De Grey and transhumanists such as philosopher Nick Bostrom recognize that the NIA helped legitimate gerontology, but neither of them see federally funded research as sufficient, wedded to their belief that government bureaucracy typically slows down biotech innovation.[104] Butler strongly disagreed on bioethical grounds, but that did not prevent him from debating de Grey in New York City at the February 2010 premiere of a new documentary, *To Age or Not to Age*.[105]

Basically, Butler thought that life extension was no substitute for quality of life, and he endorsed the scientific community's powerful 2002 position statement on human aging that differentiated between "the pseudoscientific antiaging industry" that promises the elimination of aging and "the genuine science of aging" that focuses on deepening the quality of life.[106] The central thrust of this position statement is that "the prospect of humans living forever is as unlikely today as it has always been, and discussions of such an impossible scenario have no place in a scientific discourse."[107] Kass did not disagree with this view, although as a bioethicist he was not asked to endorse this public document and he remained suspicious of scientific protectionism. In fact, de Grey believed that Kass could be persuaded about the merits of extreme life extension, perhaps because Kass valorized "human ingenuity and cleverness" and proclaimed that the "finest fruits" of biotechnology were yet to come.[108] However, de Grey's reading focused on only one side of Kass and ignored Kass's disgust toward cloning and his conservative view that the "finitude of human life" is a "blessing."[109]

Both faces of Kass are evident in the President's Council on Bioethics report of 2003, *Beyond Therapy: Biotechnology and the Pursuit of Happiness*. The report covers multiple topics, ranging from genetic engineering to supercharged athletes to smart psychotropic drugs, but the section on "ageless bodies" is most relevant here. *Beyond Therapy* plays into the hands of life-extension advocates with its claim that the quest for age retardation "suggests no inherent stopping-point" and its portrayal of "bodily decline" as a betrayal of our will to live.[110] The council did not reject the efficacy of age-retarding technologies, especially for treating memory loss or weakened muscles in old age, but the authors devote more words to their "uneven effects" and "barely foreseeable consequences" on personal and societal levels than it does to proclaiming their benefits.[111] Evoking the warnings of Aldous Huxley's *Brave New World*, the council muses about optimal lifespans, deciding that the typical current average lifespan of age eighty and more is "conceptually manageable" because it keeps open intergenerational lines of inheritance at genetic and cultural levels.[112] At its core, the report is deeply conservative in valorizing "love and renewal" over "the rush to fashion a technological project only along the gradient of our open-ended desires and ambitions."[113]

There is less positivity in these recommendations about moderation than in Butler's more exuberant writings, but there is much that Butler would agree with. Both Kass and Butler were suspicious of market forces that have the potential to propel biotechnology away from medical care and undermine a "culture that values life" in the drive toward "biotechnological prowess."[114] Instead of embarking on quests to extend life, Butler stressed the need for sound "social and ethical perspectives" with the goal of extending health span rather than life span—"the prime years of life, not length of life per se"—and of ensuring that the state acts responsibly toward its elders.[115] This humanist faith bridges what *Beyond Therapy* calls a "harmony of proportion, and a pace of journey" on the one hand and Butler's advocacy for independent living and a responsible state on the other.[116]

Compared with the dialectical thinking of 1960s neo-Freudians such as Norman O. Brown and Herbert Marcuse, there was something rigidly oppositional about life and death for Butler and Kass, despite their ideological divergence. They were both much more optimistic than those who make anti-humanist critiques of state biopower and, for example, than Achille Mbembe's notion of "necropolitics" in which the state assumes sovereignty over the "domain of life" through destructive violence even as it masks its real intentions.[117] In focusing on life forces, Kass and Butler ignored the idea of "social death" in which retirees become economically inactive and lose the validation of a salary.[118] Butler believed that volunteering in retirement is one way of contributing intergenerationally and societally, but that is not to say he was unconcerned about the lack of visibility of seniors or the ideological weight of uncaring governments. He criticized state inaction, the weakening of the U.S. Public Health Service, and discriminatory attitudes toward the sick and elderly during George W. Bush's presidency, yet he never developed a wholesale critique of the state.[119] Responsive governance was vital to Butler, as was a degree of state regulation and a balance between social security, personal responsibility, and "intergenerational solidarity."[120]

As is apparent, I see great value in Butler's research and in his lifelong advocacy of public health, but I also see a normalized sense of favoritism toward public scientific research pitted against what he saw as a "lunatic field" of experimental and deregulated practice.[121] This agonistic world view oversimplifies what I call in the preface a revitalized critical space in which top-down and bottom-up bioethical practices can meaningfully interact. As this second half of *Transformed States* explores, such balance is sometimes the key to this ecology, but at other times it is about holding differing perspectives in creative tension or viewing seemingly opposing value systems dialectically. We might place Butler's view of productive aging in this middle ground, but it was a narrower concept than it might have been and gives little room for more recent augmenting technologies, such as how AI might help older persons live independently longer instead of eroding human caregiving.[122]

Such resistance stemmed from Butler's wariness of consumerist technology. Take, for example, his critique of the exploitation of youth culture by the cosmetics industry. His criticism was aimed at the nearly "quarter of a million face-lifts and other cosmetic surgeries" in 2009 that the American Academy of Facial Plastic and Reconstructive Surgery reported, which represented a 47 percent growth from the previous year.[123] But instead of exploring the report deeply, he pivoted to criticize the entertainment industry's typically negative portrayals of older Americans. His view on cosmetic surgery as a surface technology echoes Virginia Blum's theory in her 2003 book *Flesh Wounds* that cosmetic surgery corrects aging in two rather than three dimensions, even as it offers to magically transform "the body landscape" and how individuals "project and plan" their future bodies.[124] Canadian filmmaker David Cronenberg pushes Blum's critique of cosmetic surgery further in his 2022 futuristic body horror film *Crimes of the Future* by depicting a character who literally digests plastic and a pair of performance artists who surgically remove their organs in order to grow new ones.

Butler's opinion that cosmetic surgery only masks aging is far from unique, and had he explored the American Academy of Facial Plastic and Reconstructive Surgery report further he might have mentioned the sharp growth in noninvasive surgeries, some of which reinvigorate the epidermis and improve blood flow. There are also implications for Butler's concept of productivity, as cosmetic surgeons claim that patients make educated choices in order to delay "more expensive, complicated surgeries" and in their efforts to "remain competitive in the workplace."[125] Given the gender implications of surgery that purports to turn back the clock, Butler might also have reported that 84 percent of facial procedures performed in the United States are done on women, although surgeons reported in 2008–2009 that fewer were emulating celebrities in their decisions than had been the case in the most recent years. In addition, the fact that white Americans sought most surgeries might have prompted Butler to pause on what Abigail Brooks calls "troubling trends among non-white cosmetic surgery patients, and their doctors, to consume and promote procedures that create Caucasian looking faces and bodies."[126]

Butler's perspective here echoes the International Longevity Center's 2006 report *Ageism in America*, which briefly outlines the shaping influence of the mass media on stereotypes of aging instead of taking a deeper look at how some journalists help expose discriminatory stereotypes or how noninvasive cosmetic surgery can sometimes strengthen positive self-image and improve mental health.[127] Nevertheless, the growth of the Botox industry in the 2010s raised the health concerns of consumer groups such as Public Citizen, even though Botox is marketed by beauty practitioners as "a quick, easy, safe, and reliable" anti-aging procedure. Sociologist Dana Berkowitz argues that many repeat-treatment Botox clients underestimate the health risks relating to the toxicity of botulinum and sometimes prioritize the "external aesthetic body" over "caring for one's actual health."[128]

In contrast, the Australian psychologist Bridget Garnham argued that such warnings are based on normative conceptions of a naturally aging body that should not be valorized above more individualistic choices about self-care and "creative self-stylisation."[129] Like Butler, Garnham is wary of overinscribing older bodies biomedically, but she wants to deterritorialize the concept of being older by exploring "the emergence of marginalized, previously subsumed or newly emerging cultural discourses."[130] Her notions of "creative resistance" and "somatic ethics" are influenced by both Michel Foucault and Nikolas Rose, although she is more comfortable with consumerist choices than either of these figures. In seeing surgery decisions as forms of self-fashioning, she underplays the power of commercial advertising and institutional discrimination that shape "the visual landscape of ageless beauty" and sometimes push false or compromised choices on older and younger women alike.[131] Garnham argues that instead of slavishly following market trends, "creativity and freedom" can "reshape aging norms" and prompt questions about "how the 'older body' could and should appear."[132] She closes her 2017 book *A New Ethic of "Older"* by arguing that cosmetic surgery can help individuals "reclaim, re-design and re-inscribe their bodies in ways that transfigure the limitations of aging," although she admits the need to also account for intersectional questions of place, race, class, gender, and sexuality.[133]

Garnham raises questions about which cosmetic practices are acceptable and which are deemed risky or indulgent and explores the line between procedures that are deemed medically necessary and those that are sought voluntarily—a topic chapter 6 returns to. However, she skirts the issue of the mental health implications of surgery. While surgery has the potential to improve well-being for some Americans, others may have unrealistic expectations, and for others it can deepen body dysmorphia and obsessive-compulsive disorders.[134] Garnham might also have considered how freedom and empowerment are precisely the values medical marketing preys upon. In *The Ways Women Age* (2017), Abigail Brooks examines how the cosmetics industry markets self-esteem and self-confidence as the faces of its celebration of technophilia.[135] Brooks argues that "cosmetic procedures are favourably equated with feats in scientific discovery," playing into discourses of magical transformation and normalizing faces and bodies by valorizing certain models of youthfulness and beauty.[136]

Earlier chapters have touched on these themes, but the futuristic, tech-saturated film *Advantageous* (2015), directed by Jennifer Phang for Netflix, is helpful here in its interrogation of gender-specific prejudices that Brooks identifies in the cosmetics industry. In an economically riven world, single mother Gwen Koh (played by the film's co-writer, fifty-year-old Korean American actor Jennifer Kim) struggles to financially support the education of her talented twelve-year-old daughter Jules (Samantha Kim) while trying to keep Jules in an analog space of innocence and nurturance.[137] When Gwen loses her position as a sales representative of a biotech company, the Center for Advanced Health and Living, the only option she can think of is an experimental procedure that would change her appearance and body so she can "appeal to younger audiences." The procedure is marketed as a "painless alternative to cosmetic surgery" and a "seamless jump into a brand-new body." However, she experiences prolonged anxiety as she mulls over alternatives, rejecting the idea of becoming an egg donor and approaching Jules's estranged father for financial support, although he now has another family. At stake is the bond between Gwen and Jules, which is characterized by the intimacy, joy, and musical creativity they share in their modest home, in sharp contrast to a cold corporate tech world, video surveillance, and obtrusive in-ear communication devices.

Mother and daughter spend one last Christmas together before Gwen plunges into the procedure, even though her former employer, Fisher (James Urbaniak), warns her of the risks, given that the technology is still in test phase. When Gwen finally undergoes the transformation, the visual effect is seamless. She looks twenty years younger, she has more confidence in her sales role (in which she uses her own transformation as a marketing tool), and she is distinctly less Asian as Gwen 2.0 (played by Freya Adams) with wider eyes and a rounder face. But the consequences in terms of physical and mental health and the bond with her daughter are huge. She must take daily injections to steady her breathing, she suffers from "mnemonic dissonance" in which she complains of something "sitting next to me shouting all the time," and the bond with Jules degenerates into barbed exchanges fueled by suspicion, anger, and loss.

The final third of *Advantageous* pushes the viewer to wonder if Gwen's consciousness has been killed in the transplant procedure and only selective memories remain or whether two identities are now fighting for dominance inside one body. Despite the fraught relationship between Gwen 2.0 and Jules, the film tests whether the "energy and empathy" of a deep bond can survive age-related jeopardy. It also ponders the Butlerian question of "Why survive?" in a world where thriving is reserved for the wealthy and for those who upgrade their identities by subjugating themselves to market imperatives. *Advantageous* struggles to maintain its social critique of health in this tech-saturated future, but it would have been interesting to hear Butler's comments about how the film tests the

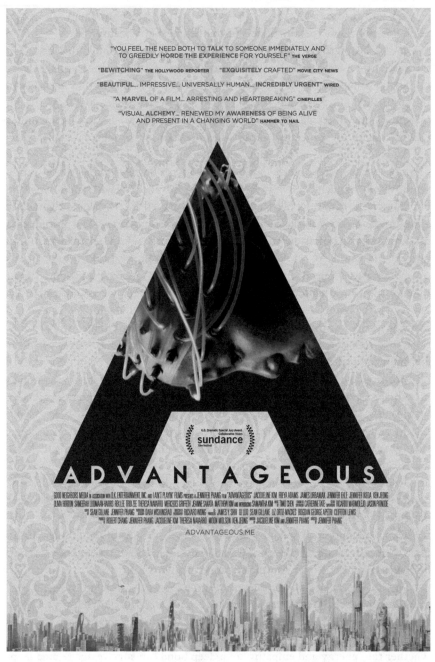

Figure 5.2. *Advantageous* movie poster depicting the biomedical procedure undertaken by Gwen Koh (Jennifer Kim). Film Presence. Courtesy Everett Collection Inc / Alamy Photo.

implications of high-tech surgery at the intersection of age, gender, race, and class in a future where love may survive, though only by a slender thread.[138] As an audiovisual thought experiment, *Advantageous* returns us to Butler's suspicion of technologies that seek to enhance rather than repair, offering a haunting meditation about what remains in a world of identity sacrifice.

Immortalism, Cyronics, and Biohacking

As she worries about the risks of undergoing an experimental body transplant procedure, Gwen meets with the seemingly ageless biotech executive Isa Cryer (played by Jennifer Ehle) at the Center for Advanced Health and Living. Cryer asks her rhetorically how citizens in "this current job market with shifting desirability targets" can get ahead "looking like you—and at your age." Gwen barely recognizes Cryer due to extensive cosmetic surgery. Yet instead of a sincere conversation about the risks of disruptive technologies for businesswomen, she is lectured on tech-driven opportunity. Cryer argues that "because we are mere humans, we won't be able to comprehend" the pace of the biotech acceleration: "humans can only grasp change at a rate they've experienced it, which is why they are left behind." Tech speed is contrasted in *Advantageous* with slow-paced scenes, reflective music, and the quiet moments of Gwen's and Jules's home life, yet Gwen seems helpless to resist Cryer's audacious argument and jeopardizes her own identity to secure a financially stable future for Jules.

This scene, a quarter of the way into *Audacious*, can be read as a metaphor for the gauntlet that life-extension enthusiasts throw down to humanists like Butler and Kass in their tendency to "romanticize unaltered bodies," "as if we could return to a time when our biology was not irrevocably intertwined with technology," as cultural anthropologists Alvaro Jarrín and Chiara Pussetti note.[139] Butler is critical of this desire to place speculative adventurism ahead of care and interdependency, but we can go further by developing the argument of gender studies scholars Neda Atanasoski and Kalindi Vora that capitalist technoliberalism offers "an aspirational figuration in relation to technological transformation" only by ignoring difficult questions of economic, gender, racial, and age-related exploitation.[140] In this final section, I test whether such critiques of biotech adventurism hold by contrasting, first, the postgenomic ideas of thinkers that Butler disparagingly calls the "longevity lobby" in their search for high-tech solutions to age extension and, second, the increasingly popular trend of biohacking that seeks a range of lower-tech wellness interventions. It is easy to parody both groups as extremists—as the German series *Biohackers* (2020–2021) does in the bizarre DIY body-hacking experiments of the University of Freiburg biology student Ole—but that would head us toward a premature conclusion.

In his 2007 book *Ending Aging*, written ten years after his first articles on biogerontology, Aubrey de Grey set out his case for extreme life extension by focusing on the cumulative damage to cells during aging. De Grey would argue that Butler's public service puts Butler in a trance when it comes to imagining future lifespans, whereas de Grey sees himself as a freewheeling thinker and has been reported as saying "I am the most important figure in aging today."[141] Such claims led novelist Richard Powers to parody de Grey's stance in his 2009 novel *Generosity* via the audacious views on aging of transhumanist guru Thomas Kurton. "The script that has kept us in gloom and dread is about to be rewritten," Kurton pronounces at a Future of Aging conference in Tokyo: "Labs across the globe are closing in on those ridiculous genetic errors that cause life to suicide. Aging is not just a disease; it's the mother of all maladies. And humankind may finally have a shot at curing it."[142]

Central to de Grey's work is the quest to eliminate cellular senescence that is the result of either "extracellular damage" (such as neuronal amyloid deposits in Alzheimer's) or "intracellular garbage" (the "goo within cells").[143] He argues that aging cells heighten vulnerability to disease instead of leading directly to death and believes that bioengineering is the means for decelerating cellular aging. In his mechanistic approach to fixing the body, de Grey outlines what he calls "strategies for engineering negligible senescence."[144] As an embodiment of what Melinda Cooper calls a "post-gerontological fix," this model shapes the work of two biomedical nonprofits: the Virginia-based Methuselah Foundation (est. 2001), which plans to make "90 the new 50 by 2030," and the Californian SENS Research Foundation (est. 2009), which seeks to "reimagine aging."[145] As cofounder and chief science officer of SENS until 2021, de Grey sought to develop a therapy regime that would halve accumulated cellular damage and initially double the lifespan. His ultimate goal is "longevity escape velocity" to ensure that cellular repair is enacted at such a pace that the individual manages to dodge the specter of pathology and therefore stays alive perpetually.[146]

Over the past fifteen years, SENS researchers have collaborated with university laboratories with the goal of arriving at a "comprehensive, practical suite of rejuvenation technologies" that can remove or repair cellular aging damage.[147] It is easy to caricature de Grey as seeking a single-step solution to cellular rejuvenation, but SENS is keen to emphasize that multiple therapies (all of which are prototypes at the time of writing) would need to be "periodically repeated to preserve youthful function."[148] SENS is working on seven rejuvenation therapies that range from stem cell and tissue technologies to prevent atrophying to immunotherapeutic clearance to remove extracellular aggregates. Some of these technologies seek to repair cells and others embody de Grey's goal of "engraft[ing] functioning tissue and even whole organs" as a form of xenotransplantation that may offer optimal health for wealthy Americans but also raises the bioethical and ideological questions addressed in the first part of this book.[149] The SENS annual reports make interesting reading but they are largely aspirational, focusing on funding, dissemination, and promotion rather than science, a bias that leads philosopher John K. Davis—another proponent of radical life extension—to wonder about the foundation's actual level of biotech investment.[150]

One of the chief investors in SENS is the Silicon Valley venture capitalist Peter Thiel (famous as the founder of PayPal), who is willing to sponsor unorthodox scientific projects in the pursuit of immortality. Thiel is critical of the pace of both public and private-sector biotech research, and through his Founders Fund (est. 2005) he argues that scientific progress is stymied by three obstacles: "lack of data, capital intensity, and a medieval approach to therapeutic discovery."[151] A consummate adventurist who combines libertarianism, a Christian belief in eternal life, and a Republican suspicion of state bureaucracy (including the NIH and the FDA), Thiel challenges ambitious students and start-ups to demolish these obstacles. When questioned about Leon Kass in a 2015 *Washington Post* interview, Thiel dodged criticizing Kass but said that his goal is to either "escape" or "transcend" nature, arguing that "if we could enable people to live forever, we should do that. I think this is absolute."[152] Thiel does not believe in single-stage solutions. Instead, he thinks that an accelerationist sea change will come about through a combination of regenerative technologies and a cluster of breakthrough cures for disease. It will also come about, he thinks, through personal experimentalism, which for him includes parabiosis, or blood transfusions from younger people (he has been criticized for being vampiric), and taking human growth hormones to maintain muscle mass.[153]

In their rampant technophilia, de Grey and Thiel offer an audacious retort to the technophobia of Franzen and the technoskepticism of Butler. Alongside the likes of Ray Kurzweil and Nick Bostrom, de Grey and Thiel have arranged for the cryonic preservation of their bodies at the time of their death; their blood will be replaced with antifreeze and their bodies will be deep frozen in steel tanks for an annual fee of $200,000. Although Bostrom acknowledges that there is no "survival guarantee" in such immortalist dreams, the theory is that in one hundred years biomedical science will have advanced enough to be able to reverse the aging process and correct the diseases that precipitate death.[154] Cryonics is currently practiced by only two institutions in the United States, both founded in the 1970s: the Cryonics Institute close to Detroit and the Alcor Life Extension Foundation in Scottsdale, Arizona. The process entails the deep freezing of human heads or whole bodies, but to date the only creature that has been preserved and returned to life is a lowly nematode worm.[155] Butler was dismissive of cryonics, arguing that the ice crystals formed by deep freezing dead tissue would "sever and tear the host tissue beyond repair."[156] But this view does not deter wealthy futurists such as Jeff Bezos, Elon Musk, and Peter Thiel, who believe that such biotechnicalities will soon be overcome.[157] Margaret Atwood predicted such adventurist longevity-seeking in *Oryx and Crake* when Crake hints that Rejoovenation scientists are testing cryonics on living human subjects without antifreeze, encouraged by the megamillions in revenue.[158]

Hollywood has forayed into cryonics in the earthbound *Vanilla Sky* (2001) and the space-travel film *Passengers* (2016), but Don DeLillo has gone further in probing the science and symbolism of cryonics as a project to control life and death, signaled by the enigmatic first line of his 2016 novel *Zero K*: "Everybody wants to own the end of the world."[159] The novel's protagonist, Jeffrey Lockhart, suspects that medicine and science have taken second place to the transhumanist dreams of "adventurers of a kind that [Jeffrey] could not quite identify."[160] One such adventurist is Jeffrey's father, Ross Lockhart, a wealthy tycoon who is the chief funder of the cryptopreservation company Convergence. Lockhart encourages his son to "get beyond your experience . . . beyond your limitations" in tackling death head on, in projects such as his efforts to deploy cryonics to preserve the body of Jeffrey's dying stepmother.[161] The fear-of-death theme recurs in DeLillo's fiction, for example in the psychotropic Dylar pill that purports to diminish mortality fears in *White Noise* (1984) and the posthuman mausoleum of the Convergence in *Zero K*, which is located in the Kyrgyzstan desert. The geometry of the Convergence dominates the first half of *Zero K.*, leading critics to see the facility as an uncanny space in which life and death merge and as a feminized space that is subjugated to an imperialist logic lurking beneath the veneer of posthuman adventurism.[162]

The novel presents cryonics as a cabalistic "faith-based technology" that embodies a belief in "life after death" when mind and body will be "restored, returned to life."[163] Ross Lockhart's wife, Artis Martineau, also buys the hype, believing that she will be reassembled in the future, retaining her core identity but awakening "to a new perception of the world" that will give her a posthuman awareness of a "deeper and truer reality."[164] Jeffrey is much more skeptical about the procedure. Although he concedes that the body might be enhanced on awakening, he asks "What about the mind? Is consciousness unaltered? Are you the same person?"[165] The fact that no one Artis remembers will be alive when she wakens does not bother her. But Jeffrey sees her death as inevitable, and he is haunted by the implications of cryonics for mental health. Shadowy scientists in the facility offer counterviews, speaking of consciousness blending with the environment and of how in the near future death will be unacceptable. However, during the freezing process, indistinct voices acknowledge the risks to consciousness, voices that seem to intermingle Artis's internal monologue during her "biomedical redaction" with the mutterings of faceless operatives.[166] This loss of identity as both cognitive and social death is reminiscent of Gwen's experience in *Advantageous*. Yet whereas Gwen survives her body transplant procedure, at least on the level of selective memory and maternal love, Artis experiences cryopreservation as the "nightmare of self" until she becomes "nearly nothing" and then just a "woman's body in a pod."[167] Ironically, but also guiltily, Ross decides against cryonics for himself. Instead, Jeffrey sees his father aging rapidly, giving up on "exercise, diet and self-responsibility," and falling into anonymity, which suggests that neither technology nor wealth can outpace death.[168]

DeLillo's philosophical dismantling of the cryonics project makes *Zero K* an exploratory work of literary bioart that explores the subjugation of test subjects within quests for extreme life extension. Its portrayal of a bleak future full of climate catastrophe offers little by way of consolation, although Jeff sees others with clearer eyes by the end and chooses a new job as a compliance and ethics officer. I will return to what Butler viewed as the chief threats to achieving the longevity revolution in chapter 7 and to the environmentalist concerns of *Zero K* and *Oryx and Crake* in chapter 8. Before that, I conclude this chapter by opening up a major theme that runs through the remainder of *Transformed States*, by shifting focus from dreams of immortality toward biohacking as an emergent practice that takes up the quest of longevity in a more life-affirming manner by placing wellness at its core.

This biohacking focus on wellness takes different forms, but it often references Californian entrepreneur and self-acclaimed "father of biohacking" Dave Asprey, who offers advice on high-fat diets, vitamin supplements, infrared lighting, and optical care.[169] A computer scientist by training, Asprey shifted focus from cyberhacking to human bodies in the mid-1990s and he has since positioned himself as a lifestyle guru, claiming that he invented the concept of biohacking in 2010.[170] The seven pillars of aging outlined in his 2019 book *Superhuman* are reminiscent of de Grey's claims (shrinking tissues, mitochondrial mutations, zombie cells, cellular straitjackets, extracellular junk, intracellular buildup, and telomere shortening), but Asprey is routinely light on biomedical science and on empirical or longitudinal evidence.[171] For instance, his short section on Alzheimer's in *Superhuman* segues quickly into efforts to improve his own cognitive functioning and boost brainpower, as evidenced by his branding of mood and memory supplements such as Neuromaster, Smartmode, and Zenmode, which are purported to improve brain health and cognition, therefore reducing the risk of dementia.[172] In *Superhuman*, Asprey offers practical nutritional advice to other biohackers, and in *The Better Baby Book* (2013), he offers advice to parents seeking to improve their child's epigenetic chances.[173] He is an ardent believer in his own longevity; Asprey aims to live to age 180, a goal he is bioengineering via daily practices and by seeking to perfect cryopreservation. He is a popular figure in Silicon Valley—especially for his Bulletproof coffee brand—but he is often criticized for being unscientific in his promotion of well-being technologies targeted at younger Americans.[174]

Asprey is interesting less as a thinker and more as a galvanizing figure in promoting personal health and well-being from the bottom up, albeit with a salesman's edge. The wellness industry has grown exponentially since Robert Butler's death in 2010 and cannot just be dismissed as a symptom of what Butler called "unwarranted hope of people of all ages" that "longevity is only a pill away," even though there is a lingering suspicion that anti-aging advocates denigrate "normal aging" in order to promote "the wonders of current and developing therapies," as biology of aging expert Richard Sprott argues.[175] Often fueled by libertarian ideas of health freedom (see chapter 7), this trend is dominated by companies targeting affluent women, such as Gwyneth Paltrow's Goop (est. 2008), which mixes wellness advice, anti-aging strategies, vitamin biohacks, and a quasi-psychotherapeutic approach to sex, always with a focus on Goop branding and media exposure.[176] Celebrity culture has cornered a lucrative share of this market. For example, actors Cameron Diaz and Jennifer Aniston share anti-aging secrets about women's health, just as they argue that older women need better representation in the entertainment industry.

But there is another, more bottom-up side to biohacking in terms of anti-aging advice. This is perhaps best represented by the *Biohacking with Brittany* podcast, which began airing in 2018. The podcast is run by Vancouver-based holistic nutritionist Brittany Ford, who reviews technologies and products outside the biomedical mainstream that might aid well-being and slow aging. Her advice is premised on the theory that healthy practices at a young age will pay dividends later in life. Her focus on nutrient-dense food, detoxing, microdosing, and exercise is geared toward restoring the body's microbiomes and widening the gap between biological age and chronological age. Ford believes that anti-aging biohacking can be effectively practiced at home without the massive outlay of Asprey's $500,000 home lab, but she echoes Asprey's podcast *The Human Upgrade* by self-tracking her health and featuring diverse lifestyle products.

There is an element of self-branding and commercial sponsorship in Ford's persona, but her podcast guests are frequently scientifically literate start-up founders: for example, the owners of COAST (est. 2020), which manufactures holistic drinks that company spokespeople claim flush toxins and rejuvenate cells, based on their ability to boost the coenzyme NAD, which is necessary for cellular health.[177] Were he still alive, Robert Bellah might well call these podcast series a "lifestyle enclave" rather than a "socially interdependent" community, but Ford looks to inspire others to optimize well-being by integrating alternatives to mainstream medicine without being dogmatic about anti-aging regimes or providing bulletproof solutions.[178] Ford is also keen to share health knowledge freely across regional and national lines. Her focus on women's health and a healing ethos seems more authentic than Asprey's muscular self-promotion and the fairly homogenous community (in terms of class, gender, and race) that follows his more cultish brand of biohacking.[179]

Ford's holistic approach to healthy aging at the cellular level within a shared space—albeit a relatively young space—returns us to Robert Butler's effort to promote and share the benefits of productive aging. Butler was writing before biohacking was common practice, but he was far from averse to self-initiated health interventions. For example, he saw benefits in older men self-injecting vasoactive compounds in order to sustain healthy sex lives and was not overprescriptive about how older Americans could approach productive engagement or define quality of life.[180] Despite his skepticism about technologies that enhance rather than enable and his concern that poor Americans are typically overlooked in lifestyle discourses in the media, Butler believed that health conversations and interventions are needed on both macro and micro levels and that the best kinds of interventions (such as his unrealized Laboratories 2030 program) involve co-creation between government and communities.

Butler was deeply suspicious of what DeLillo calls "science awash in impressive fantasy," but he also warned that some forms of "unsupervised experiments" are scientifically uninformed or even medically dangerous.[181] Just as Bellah was arguing in *The Good Society* at the turn of the 1990s that we must resist the temptation "to think that the problems that we face today . . . can be solved by technology and technical means alone," so Butler's belief in the moral responsibilities of public institutions should also apply to practices and cultures beyond an institutional framework.[182] Nonetheless, given the choice between "transhuman utopianism" of a self-elected elite and the well-being of a "sustainable society that involves all different kinds of actors and agencies" (as Lay Sion Ng describes the choices Jeffrey Lockhart faces in DeLillo's *Zero K*), Butler would select integrated health care in a sustainable society, guided from above and below by a bioethical compass.[183]

6   *Traveling Through*

TRANS IDENTITIES AND
BIOPOTENTIALITY

President Donald Trump surprised many Americans when he tweeted in July 2017 that "our military must be focused on decisive and overwhelming . . . victory and cannot be burdened with the tremendous medical costs and disruption that transgender in the military would entail."[1] With this tweet, Trump stirred anger in the LGBTQ+ community and threatened to reverse the clock on twenty-five years of steps (albeit uneven steps) to provide federal protections for transgender rights. On the surface, it seemed that Trump was intent on unpicking yet another Obama-era legacy by prohibiting transgender military personnel from serving openly. However, the White House ruling of a month later revealed the ideological intent to disqualify from military service "transgender persons with a history or diagnosis of gender dysphoria . . . except under certain limited circumstances" relating to trans service members who were already serving openly.[2] Both Trump's rhetoric and the ruling were exclusionary and discriminatory, not just for military personnel but for, at the time, 1.4 million Americans (0.6 percent of the population) who identified as transgender.[3]

Trump's social media announcement was also disturbing from a biomedical perspective.[4] In 2015, the American Medical Association asserted there was no "medically valid reason" why transgender Americans should not serve openly in the military in line with their chosen gender, a view AMA president James Madara echoed in a letter to Secretary of Defense James Mattis in the wake of Trump's announcement and the ensuing policy, which also included restrictions to gender-affirming care for military personnel.[5] The AMA stance followed a crucial shift in nomenclature from "gender identity disorder" to "gender dysphoria," which the American Psychiatric Association had adopted two years earlier, following lobbying by LGBTQ+ advocates. New York psychiatrist Jack Drescher, a member of the *Diagnostic and Statistical Manual* Workgroup on Sexual and Gender Identity Disorders, stated of the shift in language that "we wanted to send the message that the therapist's job isn't to pathologize."[6]

The science surrounding transgender health is complex and often problematic. On the progressive side, the theory that gender dysphoria has biological roots is reinforced by neurological and genetic research that uses advanced imaging and exome sequencing to reveal that the brains of transgender people have structural features of both sexes, while endocrinal research shows how estrogen or testosterone treatment taken during transitioning influences dimorphic brain development.[7] However, just as psychiatric evaluations can sometimes deter trans individuals from accessing health insurance if they do not fit squarely within the category of gender dysphoria, science is sometimes deployed in discriminatory ways.

Trans activists are disturbed, for example, by the views of sexologists J. Michael Bailey of Northwestern University, whose 2003 book *The Man Who Would Be Queen* reduces complex gender identities to narrow assumptions about biological sex, and Stephen Levine of Case Western Reserve School of Medicine, who has frequently argued against the wishes of prisoners seeking gender transition as an expert witness for state correction departments.[8] This skewing sometimes operates at the state level. In an October 2018 piece, "Trump's Plan to Redefine Gender Makes No Scientific Sense," *Wired* magazine argued that the proposed plan of the Department of Health and Human Services to define sex based on genitals at birth both ignores codeterminants and "constitutes a real invasion of privacy," in the words of Jocelyn Samuels, director of the Williams Institute at UCLA School of Law.[9]

Trump's punitive move was also regressive from a rights perspective, given that the U.S. armed forces is the largest employer of transgender Americans. Moreover, in 2017 the Department of Justice undermined civil protections for transgender students to access bathrooms that match their gender identity, alongside (at the time of writing) such state legislatures as those of Alabama, Arkansas, Idaho, North Carolina, and Oklahoma that resist the more affirmative policies of other states.[10] The Trump-era position of the Department of Defense was much worse than the "don't ask, don't tell" policy of the Clinton administration with respect to civil and human rights. In directing service personnel to keep their sexual orientation private, Clinton believed that "don't ask, don't tell" offered protections if everyone followed the rules: "I think most Americans will agree when it works out that people are treated properly if they behave properly without the Government appearing to endorse a lifestyle."[11] Gay and transgender activists took a different view, though, arguing that the policy "destroys the lives and careers of many members of the military who must choose between remaining closeted or losing their careers."[12]

For twenty years, "don't ask, don't tell" held sway, until 2011, when the military dropped the policy, followed by an official announcement in June 2016 by Obama's secretary of defense, Ash Carter, that meant that "transgender service members may serve openly, and they can no longer be discharged or otherwise separated from the military solely for being transgender individuals."[13] This federal stance opened a new affirmative phase for trans rights, including health care protections (as encoded in the Affordable Care Act) and Obama's call to end the psychiatric practice of conversion therapy for young Americans. This view against conversion therapy was inspired by a Substance Abuse and Mental Health Services Administration report of October 2015 and by the advocacy of the first openly transgender presidential appointee, Amanda Simpson, who, as executive director of the Army Office of Energy Initiatives, stated in a White House blog of

April 2017 that "every child and every person" should have "the freedom to be whoever they aspire to be."[14] When *National Geographic* proclaimed a "gender revolution" in the month of Trump's inauguration—including an image of Avery Jackson, a nine-year-old transgender girl from Kansas City, on its front cover—it was clear that Trump's White House would be in backlash mode.[15]

In contrast, the Obama-era rights agenda built upon progressive moves of the early 1990s concerning self-identification, such as the International Bill of Gender Rights, which the International Conference on Transgender Law and Employment Policy drafted in 1993, that put the "don't ask, don't tell" policy into perspective by identifying ten basic rights.[16] These included the right to define and give free expression to gender identity, the right to access gendered spaces and to change one's own body, and the right to competent medical care without being forced into a psychiatric diagnosis and psychiatric treatment.[17] The goals remain precarious though, despite the Yogyakarta Principles of 2007, which elevated the human rights implications of sexual orientation and gender identity to a global level.[18] These institutional barriers were starkly illustrated by a 2008 National Transgender Discrimination Survey of nearly 6,500 transgender people that saw "injustice at every turn," to quote the report's title.[19] Little had changed with respect to employment, housing, health care access, and community support in 2015, when 27,715 people responded to the U.S. Transgender Survey of the National Center for Transgender Equality.[20] The two surveys underlined the precarity many transgender Americans face in a country where political leaders can inflame discrimination with their inaction and ignorance.

Sites of Contestation and Negotiation

If one audience for the International Bill of Gender Rights was the federal government and members of the U.S. House, then the other was the medical profession. Medical focus in the 2000s tended to center on "gender identity disorder," a stigmatizing label, albeit one that afforded transgender Americans some medical protections with respect to insurance that would be lost if the term was abandoned.[21] Although the inclusion of "gender identity disorder" in the third edition of the *Diagnostic and Statistical Manual* (DSM-III) of 1980 was based on extensive clinical data, as a psychiatric category it played a shaping role in pathologizing transgender identities, deepening resentment by labeling certain gendered identities "disordered."[22] In its aim to destigmatize transgender identities, the DSM Workgroup for Sexual and Gender Identity Disorders, chaired by psychologist Kenneth J. Zucker, successfully persuaded the APA to adopt "gender dysphoria" in 2013 to account for the interplay of social and biological factors in gender development while preserving insurance protections.[23]

This alternative term, as detailed in DSM-5, went some way toward depathologizing the gender variance in clinical discourse by removing the "disorder" label. However, Zucker was criticized (and ultimately lost his job at Toronto's Child Youth and Family Gender Identity Clinic) for practicing a form of therapy oriented toward convincing gender-questioning preadolescents to stick with the gender they were assigned at birth.[24] Conceptually, "dysphoria" is more open than "disorder," yet stigma lingered, especially because dysphoria (the opposite of euphoria) denotes "an individual's affective/cognitive discontent"—or what German American endocrinologist Harry Benjamin called "extreme unhappiness" with an assigned identity based on birth genitalia.[25] It is a term used elsewhere in DSM-5 to characterize a depressed mood and distress associated with phases of bipolar disorder, dissociative disorder, and body dysmorphic disorder.[26] The shift in nomenclature half-opened a space beyond psychiatric labels for nonbinary gender identification. Yet it remains a medically policed concept with respect to health insurance and circles around what Hil Malatino calls "perceptive fragmentation" that, in the case of male-to-female transitions, may disregard "the particularities of personhood in favour of a traveling perceptive fixation on hips, breasts, and buttocks" as well as facial features and genitalia.[27] It has also prompted pseudoscientific claims, such as those of Abigail Shrier, who argues with scant evidence in *Irreversible Damage* (2020) that social media exposure and peer pressure are pushing adolescent girls prematurely into a "contagion" of gender dysphoria.[28]

Nonetheless, this shift in the DSM was an important legacy of what Susan Stryker calls a "millennial wave" that witnessed a "neoliberal model of minority tolerance and inclusion" alongside more radical forms of transgender and postgender activism.[29] Heightened awareness that agentic language is crucial for self-representation and civil rights has led many to recognize that the rhetoric of disorders is inappropriate for diverse trans communities seeking health care access and employment protection. (Unemployment rates for transgender Americans were estimated to be twice as high as those of the general population in 2013.)[30]

On the legislative front, change was slow. This was mainly due to the Bush and Trump administrations rolling back rights agendas while ramping up social surveillance for gender-nonconforming citizens.[31] Despite Clinton- and Obama-era moves to prohibit antigay sexual harassment and hate crimes, it took until March 2021 for Joe Biden's White House to establish a Gender Policy Council and for the House of Representatives to pass a bill to prohibit discrimination and segregation on grounds of sex, sexual orientation, and gender identity. Even though Obama stated to the LGBTQ+ community at a Human Rights Campaign event of October 2009 that "I'm here with you in that fight," resistance from some parts of the legislative and executive branches of government has meant that trans rights and representations remain sites of contestation and negotiation into the 2020s.[32] In 2016, the same year that the Department of Health and Human Services released a report titled *Advancing LGBT Health and Well-Being*, the Centers for Medicare and Medicaid Services concluded that there should be no federal ruling on whether entitlements would cover gender-affirming surgery and that physicians should make case-by-case decisions that actually leave some transgender Americans with few options for full gender transition.[33] In June 2022, seven years after the Substance Abuse and Mental Health Services Administration released recommendations on "supporting and affirming LGBTQ youth," Biden signed an executive order to discourage anti-trans public bathroom laws and ban federally funded forms of conversion therapy. Yet Biden's ruling faced an immediate backlash, including moves from conservative judges in Alabama and Tennessee to "restrict rights for LGBTQ youth," as the title of an NPR special series noted.[34]

Beyond the media headlines of the mid-2010s, this site of negotiation and contestation often hinged on the politics of biomedical practice. These headlines were dominated by former U.S. Army intelligence analyst Chelsea Manning's effort to gain "medically necessary treatment" for gender dysphoria while in prison for leaking classified diplomatic documents and the male-to-female gender transition of Caitlyn Jenner, the former Olympic-winning decathlete who had undergone multiple surgeries in realizing her transgender identity, which she proudly displayed in a 2015 *Vanity Fair* cover shoot by famed photographer Annie Leibovitz.[35] When *Time* magazine called transgender "America's next civil rights frontier" in June 2014 alongside a cover photograph of glamorous trans actor Laverne Cox, a star of the Netflix prison comedy *Orange Is the New Black*, it seemed that celebrity culture, an activist rights agenda, and new platforms such as *Transgender Studies Quarterly* were not only "mainstreaming" transgender identity (to borrow a phrase from sociologist Rogers Brubaker) but would overshadow biomedicine as the primary drivers of the transgender horizon.[36]

According to Mia Fischer, such visibility comes at a cost. On the positive side is the International Transgender Day of Visibility, launched on March 31, 2009, and endorsed by a U.S. president for the first time in 2021 as part of Biden's pledge to ensure that federal legislation both does not discriminate against the transgender community and offers "new actions to support the mental health of transgender children, remove barriers that transgender people face accessing critical government services, and improve the visibility of transgender people in our nation's data."[37] On the negative side are suspicions that the media promulgates what Black trans activist CeCe McDonald calls "cliché narratives" that focus on a select group of stories and that heightened visibility does not "automatically translate into improvement in transgender people's daily lives."[38] Not only can transgender visibility raise the stakes in state and medical surveillance, but the spotlight can also trigger hate crimes and ideological backlashes, as evidenced by the more than four hundred anti-trans bills proposed across the country at state level since 2020.

Behind the headlines, opinions were split as to whether biomedicine could provide a path forward for the self-realization of trans Americans or whether it implicates a medical-industrial complex that trans people must either endure or find a way to bypass. It is vital to respect profound variances between transfeminine and transmasculine identities, but it is also important to recognize strategic alliances. For example, the transgender and feminist agendas align in their critique of "the exaggerated claims" of some scientists to cure "social ills" and in their emphasis on the intersectionality of rights issues, the diversity of sexual identities, and the need for gender-affirming care to be "more accessible and competent."[39] Biochemist Julia Serano is one prominent voice at this axis who has called for inclusivity, but there are also marked points of tension between feminist and trans activists, most notably in feminist critiques that followed radical feminist Janice Raymond's assertions that trans culture reinforces sexual stereotypes and that male-to-female transitions lead to biologically born men co-opting women's space.[40]

In contrast, Martine Rothblatt, founder of Sirius XM Satellite Radio and of the Maryland-based biotech company United Therapeutics, inhabits a scientifically informed space that brings to the fore both trans rights and advanced tech, although that space is charged with an accelerationist rhetoric that places technological responsibility in the hands of individuals and families instead of the state. In the afterword of her 1995 book *The Apartheid of Sex: A Manifesto on the Freedom of Gender*, Rothblatt affirmed herself as trans. Rothblatt, who was in a "unisexual lesbian marriage" after being educated and starting her career as a man and having children in an earlier heterosexual relationship, described her transformation in romantic and intellectual terms. She played off the trans prefix to highlight the intersections of her life, in particular the transracial family—including her Black partner Bina, who Rothblatt helped design a mind-clone of, Bina48, in 2010 as the robotic embodiment of a posthuman future. Rothblatt equated the entrepreneurial skills she honed in developing her transnational satellite communications business with those that made her "sexual transformation successful."[41] She closed the book with a global rallying cry that we are all interconnected and optimistically envisaged that gender classification will become obsolete as we learn to be "part of one big human family."[42] These utopian transhumanist elements are evident in the updated 2011 title of *The Apartheid of Sex* as *From Transgender to Transhuman: A Manifesto on the Freedom of Form*, complementing the longevity interests of her 2015 book *Virtually Human: The Promise and Peril of Digital Immortality* and her role as a scientific advisor to the Alcor Life Extension Foundation in Arizona through which she promotes the benefits of cryonics.

I return to Rothblatt's accelerationist ideas with respect to reproductive rights later in the chapter. For now, it is important to note that shifts in the biotech industry helped reinforce her opinions, including the narrowing of the gender gap in senior leadership roles (in Genentech, for example) and among new transgender industry leaders, including Jennifer Petter of Arrakis Therapeutics and Arlan Hamilton of Backstage Capital. While less than 25 percent of biotech CEOs were women in 2021 and calls of misogyny continue in some tech sectors (such as the Gamergate online harassment campaign of 2014–2015), industry shifts during the 2010s demanded broader perspectives on diversity in and beyond the boardroom to break the white male lock on venture capitalism.[43] This trend encompassed more inclusive and welcoming workspaces and a respect for privacy, recognizing that "transition is at once a procedure with far-reaching social ramifications, and an intimately personal matter."[44]

A number of critical and creative texts discussed here pose questions about how much biomedical technology is desirable—or necessary—in enabling transgender identities. Suspicion of the medical model and the pharmaceutical industry has spurred trans activists to challenge the claims of theorists such as Slavoj Žižek that transgenderism has been made possible "by recent scientific progress in bio-technology and reproductive technologies."[45] Žižek's theory suggests that the line between ontological and ontic realms (which Heidegger associates with philoso-phy and science, respectively) blurs under the conditions of late capitalism, giving rise to what posthumanist theorist N. Kathryn Hayles describes as the "coevolu-tion of humans and technics."[46] Trans activists are concerned by Žižek's opinions, which echo health sciences scholar Bernice Hausman's claim in the mid-1990s "that the development of certain medical technologies" such as endocrinology and gender-affirming surgery are "the most important indicator[s] of transsexual subjectivity."[47] Hausman's approach contrasts with an exclusively cultural view of transitioning. However, she ignores gender variance in different cultures (for example, two-spirit as a third gender identity in North American Indigenous cul-tures), and Eric Plemons and Hil Malatino argue that her position sees sex-change procedures as attempts to "rectify" the body and rebuild "proper—that is, hetero-normative and sexually dimorphic—men and women."[48]

In fact, Hausman's view that a transgender "subject position depends upon a necessary relation to the medical establishment" is tenuous even when we take into account the biological emphasis of endocrinology, not only because it asserts the institutional supremacy of biomedicine but also because it denies agency to transgender Americans seeking to shape their own transition journeys.[49] It also skews trans visibility to what Plemons calls "an often lurid focus on surgery," although Plemons argues that to reject the "surgical impulse" is to ignore over sixty years of trans surgery in the United States.[50] Despite disagreements about the "necessary relation" to biomedical technology and links between gender-affirming surgery and cosmetic surgery, it is important to place clinical and legal questions of transgender identities against two opposing modalities. The first of these is what Julietta Singh calls the "radical dwelling" of a transgender space as an "act of learning to live otherwise" in her dehumanist yet restorative project *Unthinking Mastery* (2018). The second is the troubling persistence of transphobic hate crimes as profound threats to civil rights, ranging from daily microaggres-sions to sexual assault of trans members of the military to murders of trans women of color.[51]

In the following two sections I address the politics of gender reassignment and the psychotherapeutic discourses that inform the interplay of mental and bodily health in the transitioning journey, particularly with respect to young Americans. It is important to repudiate the damaging opinions of trans-exclusionary feminists and to move beyond culture wars rhetoric that delimits what can be meaningfully be said about the confluence of identities and technol-ogy. Here, I develop the focus of chapter 5 by considering how the marketplace complicates a search for authenticity in its reinforcement of narrow gender ideals that clash with life-stage and selfhood journeys that veer from the reestablish-ment of normative gender categories. To this end, I compare the journeys of the consciousness-raising road movie 2005 film *Transamerica* and Imogen Binnie's dissident 2013 novel *Nevada*. In returning to the contested language of authenticity within the frame of bioethics, the final section turns to the growing practice of biohacking in trans communities to harness technology as a low-tech everyday practice without ceding control to a neocapitalist or industrial model of biotech. In doing so, I contrast discourses of moral perfectionism with the queer interest in assemblages, not as the triumph of a culture of plasticity but aligned instead with what Gail Weiss calls "corporeal fluidity" that steers between the medicalized language of disorder and a revitalized ethos of transgender care.[52]

From Sex Change to Gender Affirmation

The language of trans rights has made a profound impact in the early twenty-first century on changing views of gender identity and the public perception of medical interventions that typically accompany male-to-female or female-to-male transitions. Central to this is the pivotal role of the LGBTQ+ community in transforming the language of "sex change," which was common in the 1990s, to "gender reassignment" and "gender affirmation" in the 2010s. The phrase "gender affirmation" leaves greater room for self-agency and shifts the role of the clinician from passing judgment on a patient to supporting the development of a healthy identity. It is important to emphasize that medical procedures are not always the answer, as the International Center for Transgender Care (situated north of Dallas, in a Republican region) makes clear in its argument against "overemphasizing the role of surgeries in the transition process."[53] This warning offers a divergent perspective from Bernice Hausman's view that feminist and queer accounts have "routinely ignored or argued against the significance of technology" and ensures, first, that often-difficult decisions about transitioning are not pathologized and, second, that privacy is safeguarded by not overemphasizing what the 2005 film *Transamerica* calls an individual's "entire biological history."[54] The irony, in the case of *Transamerica*, is that the narrative hinges on a transcontinental journey of the politically and culturally conservative Bree Osbourne (played by Felicity Huffman) toward gender reassignment and vaginoplasty, but her road trip forces her to confront a maze of social and family obstacles.

Transamerica is only the most recognizable crest of a cultural wave that navigated the public and private aspects of trans lives, within which biomedical encounters are only one aspect of what Dolly Parton, in the film's closing song, calls "travelin' thru." Written especially for the film, Parton's roots song, in the words of Gina Marchetti, encompasses a revelatory "journey toward a more whole self, crossing borders, being in a state of transition and coming home, growing and healing, finding a place in the world somehow" and what Oren Gozlan, in more abstract terms, calls "an in-process, an in-between, and ephemeral subject position that engages gender in the ways in which we understand and transform ourselves."[55] The tempo of Parton's acoustic song is affirmatory. But it is also more nuanced than on first listen: its first-person character is portrayed as "a puzzle" who must "figure out where all my pieces fit" as well as being a mythic "wayfaring stranger" and "weary pilgrim." Nonetheless, the song inflects

Marchetti's view that the voice is of equal importance with visual appearance in transitioning. This is emphasized when we see Bree practicing speaking at a higher pitch in the film's opening sequence, while the soundtrack, sometimes obliquely and sometimes literally, lends words and music to her everyday challenges and triumphs. That she has already legally changed her name from Stanley Schupak to Sabrina Osbourne indicates both that Bree's transition is already significantly advanced and that—to appropriate a phrase from the translation of French transgender writer Paul Preciado's 2008 memoir *Testo Junkie*—"Bree absorbs and assumes all that was once SS."[56]

If we read Bree's journey as an extended metaphor for gender transitioning and corporeal fluidity, then *Transamerica* was ahead of its time—or, at least, part of a breakthrough moment for queer films (*Capote* and *Brokeback Mountain* were released the same year)—even though the choice of a heterosexual white woman, Huffman, as the lead was not nearly as progressive as choosing a trans actor would have been.[57] On a metaphorical level, it shows that the process of transitioning is a long journey (what literary critic Jay Prosser calls a "set of corporeal, psychic, and social changes") and not the magic fantasy of gender swapping that Hollywood and the pornography industry often imagine.[58] However, although it deals with oscillating states of denial and acceptance, the film reveals conceptual limitations in moving toward what Gozlan calls "a fantasy of certitude," in large part because its literal destination is genital surgery.[59] By starting and ending with a medical encounter, the film arguably equates genitals with gender by overplaying surgery in Bree's story, while Huffman's portrayal depicts her at times as an "isolated, alienated" character whose feminine appearance is overstylized.[60] The psychological barriers Bree confronts not only relate to misunderstandings and transphobia but also to her Christian conservative disdain at an openly transgender gathering in Dallas and her efforts to disguise her biological identity from her gay son Toby (Kevin Zegers) for much of the journey, whom she bails from a New York jail, pretending to be a missionary rather than his father. On the theme of passing, *Transamerica* is not dissimilar to other LGBTQ+ coming-out narratives in which the protagonist learns how not to obscure their inner self with a "stack of untold stories," as Black transgender activist Janet Mock's 2014 memoir *Redefining Realness* describes.[61]

If *Transamerica* helped to open up discourses about gender diversity in the early 2000s, then Bree's conservative politics need to be contextualized, on one front, by feminist debates about the dangers of the body becoming commodified and, on another, by the rigid heteronormativity in some parts of the Republican Party. That public opinion toward the transgender community was slow to change is illustrated by the March 2010 CNN documentary *Her Name Was Steven*, which shows how stigma attended gender transitioning into the new decade. Coming out as transgender was an employment risk and sometimes a surgical risk as well, on both physiological and psychological levels, which the previous chapter discussed in relation to what Virginia Blum's conception of "postsurgical culture."[62] Nonetheless, in the 2010s, there was a shift in biomedical language and

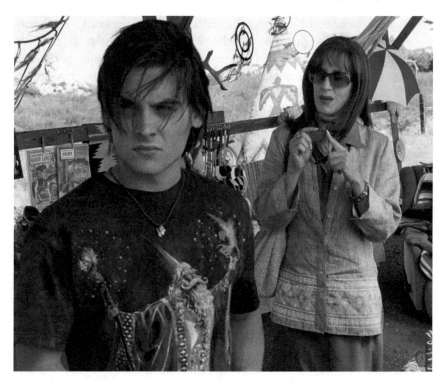

Figure 6.1. Bree (played by Felicity Huffman) and Toby (played by Kevin Zegers) begin to bond in the rural Southwest. *Transamerica* (2005). Album/Alamy Photo.

a growth in the number of facilities where clients could choose facial and genital surgery to better align their sex and gender. A 2018 *JAMA* study estimated that 10.9 percent of transgender Americans seeking support from health professionals in the period 2000 to 2014 chose gender-affirming surgery and that genital surgery had increased by over 10 percent in the second half of the 2000s, although health insurance did not always cover genital procedures.[63]

It is important to resist celebrating the biomedical industry for being altruistic, given that the revenue potential of such procedures is anticipated to double between 2020 and 2027, but it is equally important not to vilify it for its market opportunism. The Gender Mapping Project estimates that over 9,000 gender-reassignment procedures were overseen by licensed U.S. cosmetic surgeons in 2020. However, this conservative organization based in West Virginia collected data as part of its efforts to take on "Big Pharma in coalition with Big Gender" and called for conservatives to report on the location of gender clinics with the aim of demonizing them.[64] Big Tech is never the whole answer—or, for some, the answer at all—although we need to take in good faith the joint condemnation of Microsoft, Google, and Apple of Texas governor Greg Abbott's backlash policy that professionals should report children who are undergoing gender-affirming surgery to the Texas Department of Family and Protective Services.[65] Even given such inflammatory culture war stances, the market potential is huge for medical

practitioners, allied health professionals, and biotech companies that are researching sex hormone treatments and assisted reproductive technologies. Yet biomedical, ontological, and psychosocial questions persist about postoperative satisfaction
for many trans Americans, about what "full" gender transitioning means at various life stages, and about when the process of gender affirmation ceases. This
journey toward fullness structures the narrative arc and psychological contours of
Transamerica, in which genital surgery is the missing part of Bree's efforts to align
her biological and gender identities.

This is no easy journey, though, especially because in a film like *Transamerica*,
gender-reassignment surgery is privileged above the complex psychological and
hormonal adjustments that prescribing physicians require before and after genital surgery. In the movie, the estrogen pills Bree takes are often a subtle presence
(which she hides from her son), but when her car is stolen in the desert, they
become a missing part that she mourns more than her material possessions. Hormone therapy is often regarded as vital for transitioning, but it is not enough for
Bree. To develop Kathy Davis's insights on cosmetic surgery, although facial,
chest, and/or genital surgeries do not always allow individuals to "transcend"
their bodies, they can "open up the possibility" of renegotiating the body, the
mind, and social relations in order to construct an alternative sense of selfhood.[66]
As such, trans-affirmative procedures raise questions about psychosocial needs
that do not always feature in medical and endocrinal training programs, despite
the efforts of some health professionals and clinics to raise awareness of specific health care needs.[67] Without a supportive health care provider and coordinated health services, some trans Americans may seek hormones through illicit
channels or surgery in other countries with widely differing standards of care.[68]

I will return to access to hormones, but a chief conceptual problem of *Transamerica* is its quest for fullness and self-acceptance following gender-reassignment
surgery. The language of fullness is problematic in identity terms as it suggests a
fixed teleology that can be reached through a procedural logic. It also evokes the
myth of an originary self that is simply awaiting affirmation instead of regarding
gender identity as what New York psychoanalyst Avgi Saketopoulou calls an
always "emergent project."[69] To illustrate this, Imogen Binnie's novel *Nevada*,
published eight years after *Transamerica*, turns the quest narrative on its head. It
does so by taking away the "mystification, misconceptions, and mystery" of trans
identities and by stressing the banality and often directionless nature of early
twenty-first-century life, contrasting New York ennui in the first part with a
road trip to Nevada in the second. Early on, Maria Griffiths, the novel's thought-
ful twenty-nine-year-old protagonist, critiques the idea that the medicalized
model of a "sex change operation" pushes trans women into a subject position in
which they "become just like any other woman," a subjectivity that the film compares to her life, which is full of uncertainty punctuated by moments of awareness.[70] *Nevada* also undermines the quest motif and "getting better" arc that are
typical of American literary narratives by giving "no concession to tourists," as a
New Yorker article described the novel, even though capitalist and media pres-

sures push Maria toward states of dissociation and insomnia that complicate a narrative pattern of self-actualization.[71]

Binnie avoids explicitly medicalized scenes, focusing instead on the physiological and emotional effects of hormone treatment and fragile relationships. Rejecting the mythical notion of a "true, honest, essential self," Maria faces both her transitioning and her relationships with uncertainty that spills into anxiety and dissociation.[72] Despite Maria's inner conviction, her transition is a makeshift one that contrasts with a narrative of surety that moves toward poised self-presentation. She has been injecting estrogen and taking testosterone blockers for four years and is far along in the transition process, yet she "still flinches at best and dissociates completely at worst if somebody touches her below the waist."[73] The reality and cost of maintaining a hormone regime weigh on Maria. She injects estrogen because it is cheaper than pills, but electrolysis and genital surgery prove too expensive. She accepts her "kinks," but instead of managing to center her mind and body or practicing self-care, Maria finds it tricky to navigate the pressures of being trans. Everyday reality sometimes cause her to dissociate, leading her to muse that "repressing and policing yourself so hard for so long" means that "it's so easy just to check out and leave your body."[74]

That the journey Maria undertakes in *Nevada* is both to somewhere (she borrows her ex-girlfriend's car and drives west when she loses her job at a bookstore) and nowhere (Star City, Nevada, where she ends up, is just a "shitty little town") suggests that there are limitations to the literary quest narrative, just as the idea that a journey can be completed either with or without surgery is possibly a category mistake. This nonteleological shift poses the question of whether fullness can ever relate to the length of hormone treatment and the extent of surgical operations or whether it is an immanent ontological state in which the self feels more in balance or less compromised by the medical profession, the state, or market forces—as the gender-questioning nineteen-year-old James starts to learn when he meets Maria in Star City. One answer to this relates to the extent to which physiological appearance and physical health are prioritized over mental health. Another answer depends on to what degree we approach gender identity in a holistic and culturally congruent way, in which a transformation in one aspect intrinsically links to another.[75] And a third answer hangs on to the extent to which the medical profession normalizes transgender experiences, especially as "trans people seeking medical intervention have repeatedly been asked to tell a particular life story"—often referred to as the "wrong-body narrative"—in order to acquire transition-related care.[76] This move toward a normative rather than a fluid trans identity and the need to gain approval from a patriarchal medical system bothers Maria because it strains against conceptions of queerness that she shares via her blogger persona and positions physicians in the role of "saviors, beings capable of bestowing life to people in dire existential circumstances."[77] It also strains against the recognition that gender-diverse individuals experience mental health disparities ("suicide, poverty, social disenfranchisement, and significant quotidian violence" and vulnerability to anxiety and stress) as much as, if not more than, other Americans and that they need appropriate care and support about making difficult personal choices.[78]

Either way, there is something exceptionalist in the discourse of fullness. Does this notion of fullness mean relaxing into the experience of gender transition without letting the expectations or rules of others (family, peers, employers, physicians, legislators, journalists) stand in the way of self-definition? Might fullness be the ability to convince the world "that we're Really, Truly Trans," as Maria asks?[79] Or might fullness instead be a forceful attempt or self-devised strategy to remake reality against the grain?

Moral philosopher Stanley Cavell deals with these questions on a theoretical level in his analysis of the nineteenth-century thought of Ralph Waldo Emerson and Henry David Thoreau in his 1990 study *Conditions Handsome and Unhandsome*. Setting aside the gender and historical implications of the discourse of handsome, it is important to remember that Emerson and Thoreau were just as preoccupied by discourses that unsettle as they were in realizing "truth to oneself."[80] Cavell is also interested in unsettled states in which language reveals its inadequacy, the recognition of which can stir in individuals the courage to refashion their environment. On this reading, instead of associating authenticity with a stable or full state of being, the fullness comes through mobility and the process of becoming, which, Maria reflects, continues after the formal process of transitioning: "How do you transition but then continue to evolve as a person, post-transition, when it seems like the only way you got through your transition was to assert loudly, even just to yourself, that you knew who you were and you knew what you wanted and you trusted yourself?"[81] Although the rhetoric and the route is very different, Cavell's position is not incompatible with Rogers Brubacker's theory that unsettled identities emerge at the intersection of race and trans and with Imogen Binnie's comment that it is vital to recognize that life is "a constellation of dots" that do not connect in the kind of pre-designed order privileged by the medical model.[82] This "constellation of dots" in an ongoing process also evokes Donna Haraway's idea that gender-fluid identities are best conceptualized as a hybrid assemblage (what she terms a post-essentialist FemaleMan) in which natural, social, cultural, and technological elements creatively combine in an open-ended mode of "gender-in-the-making."[83]

I will return to these concepts in relation to what Hil Malatino calls "assemblage thinking" and Gill-Peterson terms a theory of "trans embodiment as the technical capacities of all bodies" to open up biopotentiality from the biomedical model in the next section of this chapter.[84] However, before that, it is worth pausing on Cavell a moment longer to explore how his interest in how Romantic thought offers a response to disappointment with reality and sets itself the regenerative task of "bringing the world back, as to life."[85] This view aligns with that of psychoanalyst Oren Gozlan, who is suspicious of the rhetoric of authenticity as "both a legitimate claim and an impossibility because the body and our experience of embodiment is constantly changing."[86] Cavell describes this task at times as "the quest for a return to the ordinary" and at other times as "a new creation of our habitat." When it comes to gender affirmation (a topic that Cavell does not mention), the process actually works in both directions. In one direction, it is the reclaiming of a state before the adult order delimits gender expectations; in the other direction, it involves a re-creation of the self to ensure that the individual's sex and gender are congruent. This does not mean that Cavell veers toward the utopian, just as trans testimonies illustrate that the realignment of sex and gender is a work in progress and is encoded through an assemblage of different elements.

Ultimately, the refashioning of the ordinary for Cavell does not mean generating a normative state, for he sees the realm of the ordinary "as forever fantastic."[87] Cavell elides philosophical, figurative, and psychoanalytic registers in looking at how ordinary language tends to "repudiate its power to word the world, to apply to the things we have in common, or to pass them by," in tandem with language that has a critical function and can help "disassemble prejudicial orientations to the everydayness," in the words of Gozlan.[88] This stance aligns with Julietta Singh's call to "unthink mastery" by critically working through the "fantasies of the human's unique agency" and "the disavowed materialities that underlie it" in order to "trouble the category of the human."[89] Singh personalizes the macroscale insights of *Unthinking Mastery* in her 2021 memoir *The Breaks*, in which she contemplates her mercurial daughter's instinctive "embrace of hybrid" gender identifications and "refusal to desire the treacherous fiction of purity."[90] Singh's dehumanizing project is arguably more radical than Cavell's efforts to revitalize Romantic thought. Yet this observation underestimates Cavell's sensitivity to both the slipperiness of language that undermines the quest to "word the world" and how words work affectively in brushing by objects, states, and processes. It is these insights on the everyday, language, and agency that are so pertinent for understanding the challenges and possibilities of trans identities in the twenty-first century.

Transgender Health Care and Young Americans

In her 2018 book *Histories of the Transgender Child* (2018) and her more recent writings, Jules Gill-Peterson argues that "the primary drama" of trans health care is to save lives, especially for transgender children and adolescents, for whom the experience of growing up is often challenging.[91] Medical diagnostics are both prevalent and troublesome for children and can be an acute source of anxiety, especially in the fluid space of transgender.[92] While ruffled conservatives such as Abigail Shrier point to the need to protect vulnerable and impressionable children and teenagers who question their gender identity, others—such as Aurora Brachman, director of the moving 2020 short film *Joychild*—show just how difficult it is for young Americans to speak candidly to their parents about their inner convictions of being other than the gender assigned to them at birth.[93] Instead of seeing the "trans teen" as a new phenomenon, Gill-Peterson shows how transgender children and teens had a "ghostly" presence in twentieth-century case studies before they became more visible in the cultural mainstream since the 1980s.[94]

Given the significance of this invisibility/visibility dynamic, I turn to young trans Americans here, especially because a 2019 survey estimated that 1.4 percent of American teenagers (aged 13 to 17) identify as transgender, compared to 0.5 percent over 18.[95]

This discussion zooms in on the place of biotechnology in gender medicine with respect to puberty blockers and hormone treatment and moves us closer to culture wars debates about the assumed vulnerability of children. The topic also helps bridge the divide between what Bernice Hausman calls the "material" and "metaphorical" technologies of gender, with the aim of mapping a middle space in which an emergent trans bioethics can thrive. Hausman argues that the former involves biomedical procedures with a fixed teleology, while the latter is a figurative technique of self-care that is always in flux, which she attributes to the influence of Teresa de Lauretis's 1987 book *Technologies of Gender*. Instead of accepting a dichotomy between the material and the metaphorical, Donna Haraway's theory of a many-voiced assemblage pictures an admixture of "imploded entities, dense material semiotic 'things,'" or what Paul Preciado, in his reading of Haraway, calls "a technoliving, multiconnected entity incorporating technology."[96]

Recognizing that this admixture can be enabling or delimiting, depending on how it is mobilized, Gill-Peterson is wary of the biomedical model and the over-medicalization of trans children. She is also critical of the "watchful waiting" practice in which clinicians and parents work together to push back the clock on the wishes to transition of a child or young adult until the age of consent. This trend requires bioethical scrutiny, but it is not as severe as the views of some practitioners who convince parents that it is in the child's interest to adhere to the gender assigned to them at birth. Dissuasion practice is reinforced by the claims of reactionary books such as Shrier's *Irreversible Damage* and conservative groups such as the Center for Bioethics and Culture, whose 2021 film *Trans Mission* challenges a permissive liberal agenda. Relying on testimony from parents, trans-exclusionary feminists, and detransitioners, the center's reactionary position is that transitioning should be banned before the age of consent because children's and young adults' bodies are at great risk, despite evidence from the plastic and reconstructive surgery community that reveals only very low levels of regret among those who transition.[97] On this count, we can see the culture wars playing out visibly on the bodies and health of transgender youth who often do not have a voice—or at least a prominent voice—in these discourses.

It is important to restate Gill-Peterson's view that the affirmative care model is an ideal that health care typically falls short of. This is often due to variations in practice depending on locality and access, but even in cases where the desire to transition receives clinical and parental approval, standards of care and the upholding of rights (as set out by the World Professional Association for Transgender Health) are in tension with "the foundational premises of the medicalization of transition" as a unidirectional process.[98] Sociologists, historians, and cultural critics have questioned the "etiological framing" of trans experiences, partly because multiple and diverse encounters with physicians, endocrinologists, surgeons, gynecologists, nurses, counselors, and support groups suggest a complex life experience that does not fit within a medical model or the journey archetype.[99] Transgender individuals seeking hormone treatment or surgery may feel that they must subscribe to the "wrong body" narrative or bend their story to what they think clinicians want to hear about gender dysphoria so that their case for transitioning will be medically approved and underwritten by health insurance.[100] Aside from the imperative need to shift the physician's role from "approval" to "affirmation," Gill-Peterson argues that "the lived experience of medicalization is a non-linear, complex process" rather than a journey toward an end point, emphasizing mobility and the importance of sharing subjectivity in order to create "ethical apertures" in the medical and ideological maze that trans Americans must navigate.[101]

Gill-Peterson concludes that despite the growth of trans rights advocacy in the 2010s and pockets of good practice within an uneven health care system, the last thirty years have not been as progressive as they first look with respect to trans-affirmative care, particularly for young Americans from poor families or communities of color who already feel that the health care system does not serve their needs or aspirations.[102] The idea that identity formation is fluid during puberty emboldens medical leaders and legislators to say that young adults are not ready to make fundamental decisions about their bodies and their legal status when their views differ from the medical judgment of their genitalia at birth. This leads Gill-Peterson to conclude that not only are the discourse and reality of pediatric transitioning overmedicalized, but that because "transgender health care continues to pick and choose who is imagined as deserving access," the ideal of gender affirmation remains elusive for many Americans.[103]

In contrast to the self-empowerment of young gender-fluid protagonists that features in recent trans young adult fiction, such as April Daniels's Nemesis series (which began with *Dreadnought* in 2017), young trans Americans are particularly prone to pressures that can lead to mental ill health, whether or not they seek to transition. Debates about the ethics of administering puberty blockers to young Americans aged nine to sixteen are fierce. The medical model that requires a diagnosis of gender dysphoria before allowing transgender youth to take puberty blockers is settled practice that is not based on hard empirical evidence.[104] The mental health risks of taking puberty blockers, which include heightened feelings of anxiety and suicidal ideation, need to be placed against similar feelings for trans-desiring young Americans whose diagnosis does not meet the bar for gender dysphoria. Denying a young person access to puberty blockers can lead to anxiety and despair and, in some cases, to DIY hormone treatment and self-surgery, as the next section discusses. Rigorous scientific evidence does not yet exist on this subject that can distinguish between young Americans taking puberty blockers below the age of thirteen and those taking blockers during their teenage years, even though they likely have different reversibility arcs. However, one study conducted in Boston, which drew data from the 2015 U.S. Transgender Survey, aligns with the conclusions of the Endocrine

Society that young transgender people who are denied puberty blockers have a higher risk of suicidal ideation than transgender adolescents who are prescribed blockers.[105]

The Biden administration's 2022 pledge to the transgender community focuses particularly on the mental health needs of transgender youth. A key context for this is the Substance Abuse and Mental Health Services Administration's 2015 report *Ending Conversion Therapy*, which presents evidence that transgender youth are at increased risk of psychological distress, substance abuse, and attempted suicide as well as an increased likelihood of "experiencing victimization, violence, and homelessness."[106] Most studies conclude that the risks of embarking on transition at a young age within a supportive community are far fewer than the risks associated with being denied access to gender-affirming health care because, as Imogen Binnie bluntly stated in her afterword to *Nevada*, reflecting on her own experience of transition, "it feels bad not to be able to be in your body."[107]

Another context for the Biden administration's pledge was the findings of the two surveys conducted by the National Center for Transgender Equality cited earlier. The 2008 survey reported that the proportion of transgender Americans who experience mental ill health is 50 percent higher than the general population and that suicide attempts are dramatically increased for this group, especially among members of Black and Latinx communities, whereas the more nuanced 2015 survey estimated that its transgender respondents suffered "serious psychological distress" at nearly eight times the rate of most Americans and are nearly nine times more susceptible to suicide attempts.[108] The second survey revealed that discrimination and marginalization are two drivers of high levels of distress. Although the 28,000 respondents were adults, the report gives a strong indication that adolescents are likely to experience distress more intensely during a particularly vulnerable life stage.[109] This inference is underlined by studies drawn from the National Survey on LGBTQ Youth Mental Health, which estimated that 73 percent of LGBTQ youth were experiencing anxiety at the beginning of the 2020s and 45 percent had recently attempted suicide (the percentage is much higher for those aged thirteen to seventeen and for those whose family and school life was not gender affirming). Although this 2022 survey included a broader demographic than just trans-identifying Americans, it is notable that the findings indicated that 60 percent of LGBTQ youth were not able to access the mental health support they needed.[110]

Even though doctors point to the physical and mental health risks of embarking on transitioning at an early age, there are major advantages in doing so before the full onset of puberty in terms of bodily and genital development and before physiognomy becomes more set in line with testosterone and estrogen production.[111] There are other barriers in addition to those from the medical community. Twenty-four state legislatures (as of the spring of 2024) have sought to totally or partially ban puberty blocker treatments for people under eighteen, while in other U.S. states parental approval is required for those below the age of consent, even though medical authority suggests that when blockers are prescribed carefully, puberty will resume once adolescents cease taking them.[112]

A prominent media example of early transitioning that speaks to the affirmative model is Jazz Jennings, who was medically diagnosed as having gender dysphoria as a five-year-old Ohioan child in 2005. She began taking puberty blockers at age eleven and had her first gender-affirming surgery at age seventeen, as she discusses at length in her YouTube videos and on her reality TV show *I Am Jazz* (2015–). The American Society of Plastic Surgeons has recently started to report statistics on young Americans who elect gender-affirming facial surgery, including nose, ear, and eyelid surgery, and less invasive procedures such as laser hair removal, Botox, and skin fillers (comprising 230,000 procedures in the thirteen to nineteen age bracket in 2020). However, most providers, including the Boston Children's Hospital, will not commence with what it calls "facial harmonization" until age eighteen, when it considers "full facial maturity" has been reached, given the significant risk that more procedures will be needed as the young face develops.[113] This is also usually true of genital surgery. For Jazz Jennings, her vaginoplasty turned out to be more complex than it would likely have been had her male genitals matured before she started taking puberty blockers. Nonetheless, despite these complexities and side effects (Jennings experienced postoperative weight gain), the evidence sways toward gender affirmation instead of a gatekeeping medical model.

Facial feminization or masculinization surgery is always a delicate and typically multistage procedure. Only a few U.S. surgeons practice facial feminization surgery, which is often realized through "a brow lift, a trachea shave, a jawline reduction, a chin reduction, and a face and neck lift."[114] The San Francisco–based cranio-maxillofacial surgery practice of Jordan Deschamps-Braly and Douglas Ousterhout has been especially influential in shaping what Eric Plemons calls "the look of a woman" in the United States. Ousterhout conducted 1,700 facial feminization surgeries before retiring in 2014 and Deschamps-Braly claims to have refined Ousterhout's practice by attending closely to the fine adjustments to bone and cartilage that can transform a face at various life stages, although his promotional material underplays how long it takes to recover from such surgery.[115]

In addition to a sense that facial feminization surgery normalizes what it is to look like a particular gender, affordability is a looming question that tends to be overlooked in surgery reports.[116] Whereas health insurance sometimes covers top and bottom surgery (following a gender dysphoria diagnosis, two years of taking hormones, and living as the chosen gender), facial surgery is not deemed essential in terms of Medicare and Medicaid coverage and therefore is beyond the financial reach of some Americans. Transgender activists have challenged this categorization of facial surgery as nonessential because denial of gender-affirming surgery can exacerbate social anxiety and dysphoric feelings. Despite inconclusive moves by Obama's health secretary Kathleen Sibelius to argue that medical necessity should be defined nationally, the term is often used as a way of gatekeeping health insurance claims that are decided by fiscal intermediaries rather than caregivers, with the danger that insurance providers may invalidate claims they do not agree with.[117] An allied danger relates to race. Most media cases of male-to-female transitioning privilege the experience of white Americans, and Eric Plemons argues that facial feminization surgery tends to erase racial specificity. Instead of bringing into play the "complexly polysemic" nature of faces, surgical practice tends to whiten the face by linking a "desirable aesthetic" to "a recognizable femaleness."[118] Although Deschamps-Braly emphasizes that his work is ethnospecific and is fully adaptable to Black and Asian faces, market pressures around facial cosmetic surgery continue to privilege white forms of faciality.[119]

One trajectory for male-to-female transitioning is in terms of the biological capability to conceive—at the present time, through assisted reproduction technologies. Although statistics show that surprisingly few young Americans who wish to transition place fertility as a high priority (surveys show that it matters more to their parents), for some the goal of male-to-female transitioning is to enter into a reproductive cycle.[120] There are modes of transitioning that retain sexual organs. This would allow a female-to-male transgender man to gestate a child as the genetic mother despite his legal status as a man, while male-to-female transgender women may choose to preserve their sperm before gender affirmation, which can then be used for IVF with a future partner to make them the legal mother but the genetic father.[121] Fertility preservation is a topic that Martine Rothblatt (who started her transition at age forty) discusses in *Unzipped Genes* (1997) as a biotechnological means for gender-nonconforming Americans to reclaim agency over the "bioethics of birth" by embracing the right to procreate. For Rothblatt, this includes surrogacy, which is an option for some transgender couples, although those living in states where it is outlawed may feel compelled to move or to look overseas.[122] The crossroads between gender transitioning, fertility, and assisted reproductive technologies might appear to accelerate a shift toward a posthuman and postgender future, but it actually goes deeper into trans bioethics, and Rothblatt argues that the international transgender community should be free to determine their own health law standards.

The need to shift bioethics away from gatekeeping to make it culturally congruent with transgender experiences is most acute for young Americans facing other kinds of psychosocial vulnerabilities. Binnie's novel *Nevada* echoes Gill-Peterson's idea that we need to move beyond normative moral judgments and diversity tolerance to embrace a culture of acceptance—what Julietta Singh in *The Breaks* wistfully envisions as "an ethics that is so much wider and more capacious than we have known, so much less divisive."[123] A top-down bioethics that rigidifies moral categories can prompt feelings of worthlessness for those who feel excluded and can exacerbate ennui and "political depression" that manifests as "cynicism, burnout, resentment, or feeling done with things."[124] Such gatekeeping might even trigger suicidal ideation or might delimit what trans Americans are able to request or imagine for themselves by policing what Gill-Peterson refers to as "our experience of possibility."[125] The counter to such oppressive gatekeeping is a culture of potentiality, although it is not one of endless plasticity despite neurobiological advances that focus on the plasticity of adaptable cognitive activity (see chapter 3). Suspicious of the neoliberal co-option of plasticity as "value extraction," Gill-Peterson instead envisages "a creative capacity for transformation" undergirded by culturally congruent bioethics and access to gender-affirming health care that is linked to self-care and reciprocal community support.[126] The final section of this chapter turns to this concept of biopotentiality activated by an admixture of varying practices.

Trans Biohacking and Biopotentiality

At the start of the futuristic science fiction story "Angels Are Here to Help You," trans writer Jeanne Thornton presents a tech-heavy world in which the protagonist Viola assembles her own spaceship from a "midmarket warp drive kit."[127] The editors of the trans sci-fi collection *Meanwhile, Elsewhere* (2017) in which Thornton's story appeared steered their contributors away from explanatory discourses for cis readers in favor of exploring "what saving the world looks like" and "carving out small pockets of knowledge, strength, and survival." In line with this aspiration, Thornton does not offer a design fiction or an expanded vision of a postgender world in the manner of Kim Stanley Robinson's futuristic novel *2312*, in which gender variance and mixed gender signals abound on Mercury while Earth lies in ruins.[128] Instead, Viola's task in the undated and nonspecific topography of "Angels Are Here to Help You" can be read as a metaphor for assembling a queer self via biohacking in a manner that aligns with what Hil Malatino calls a "nomad science of transition."[129]

Inspired by her childhood dream of joining the intergalactic Starfleet, Viola finds reality mundane and the packaged spaceship instructions frustrating. The instructions "sort of worked," but the assembly leads to unintended side effects and triggers Viola's worry that "she was doing it incorrectly." She tries to calm her anxiety with yogic breathing, unconsoled by her Helpful Angel app, which has a strong femdom identity and hovers about her at times like a superego and at other times like a demonic id that proves tricky to uninstall. Viola's anxiety in part stems from the posturings of her ex-girlfriend Thoth-Lorraine's wealthy Cool Tech Geek peer group that can afford more sophisticated helpful angels and "estrogen nanobot implants" that never run out because everyone in this group has good health insurance.[130] In contrast to the skills of trans countersurveillance biohacker Camille in futurist Mark Sable's graphic novel *The Dark* (2021), Viola's life is far from high tech.[131] Instead, it aligns with how Paul Preciado portrays self-prescribing hormones as a mode of low-tech biohacking geared toward reclaiming identity from high-tech "pharmacopornographic" forces that control bodies by subjecting them to the medical gaze and prescription regimes.[132]

Recognizing that her ex-girlfriend's "tech pals" are "more advanced trans women than she is," Viola has a choice between tending to her own body by "spending a bunch of money on tech" and "dysphoria easing devices" or by looking after her anxiety "for free."[133] It is tempting to read the story as a meditation on the intersection of the ontological and ontic realms. Not only is the ontic realm of technoscience obtrusive and often expensive, but it can also mask over ontological questions of being. That does not mean that Viola's awareness of the interrelation of technology and social control is sufficient to hold her anxiety in check; she cannot fully accept herself as a "weird clunky trans" because she senses herself falling behind others' expectations.[134] Feelings of insecurity lead to periodic depression and worries about the impact of a tech monoculture—specifically her SoftPackr registration that makes her visible to state surveillance and susceptible to corporate apps installed automatically at "the borders of her vision."[135] SoftPackr just compounds her tech suspicions: Viola feels that by marketing itself as the "Done Thing," tech offers "too easy a solution" to the emotional, intellectual, and somatic experiences at "the soil of her being.[136]

However, Viola does not give up on tech altogether. Her life is full of bio-codes. For example, her visceral connection with Thoth-Lorraine during their relationship is via the psychotropic drug Spoor, which absorbs into the "blood-brain barrier." This chemical reaction triggers a close empathic bond of reciprocity that reaches deeper than an orgasm, although this chemically stimulated posthuman empathy is not enough to save the relationship. The disconnection from her ex-girlfriend leaves Viola alone with her celebrity cat Duncan, with whom she has more of a financial than an affectionate relationship; she is financially dependent on Duncan's earnings as an advice columnist after losing her writing job for the media firm that represents him. This subaltern position gives urgency to her attempts to reclaim agency as she fashions her spacecraft to take her to the planet of Undine, especially after her fantasies of joining Starfleet fade when the mission breaks up. The narrative makes clear this is her own self-fashioned quest to reach the "gigantic oceanic brain" of Undine with its fecund vegetation. Echoing the fecundity of Pandora in *Avatar* (see chapter 4), she believes that connecting with the Undini would be a deeper and more sustained experience than her DIY Spoor experiments with her ex-girlfriend—she thinks it will be a "shared lucid dream" enveloped in the Undini's naturally produced Spoor. But her dream evaporates. When she reaches the planet Undine in her spacecraft, she finds a colonized state run by a venture capitalist who threatens to confiscate her cat.

Thornton's story can be read as an extended metaphor of trans embodiment and its complex relationship with technology, some of which is imposed on the self and some of which can be assembled heuristically as an act of self-fashioning. Recognizing that technology can be a dependence trap if it promises optimization, when she is orbiting in space, she muses that "everything's going to fail, anyway—if you don't accept that and try to do things anyway, what in life do you end up accomplishing?"[137] This does not mean that Viola can free enough of herself to claim supreme agency. The tale encompasses fluctuating states of adventure, alienation, anticipation, anxiety, despair, disappointment, and dissociation as it journeys through emotional intersections. When her spaceship starts to break apart, Viola's mind turns to playing with Transformers as a child. She was fascinated with how the toys transformed into six guises—"one of her favorites could turn into a lion, a boat, an eagle, a standard affable masc robot, etc."—but when she lost a screw one day, her favorite Transformer became frozen between the forms of lion and boat.[138] One part of her child self panicked in the moment when her toy broke, while another part intuitively worked out how to guide the screw into its original place. This memory of toy rescue helps her steady the spaceship.

"Angels Are Here to Help You" also returns us to the subject of biohacking that weaves through the second half of *Transformed States*. Viola's engagement with biohacking contrasts with that of Violet, the more assured young trans protagonist of Rich Larson's young adult novel *Annex* (2018), who raids a pharmacist for Estrofem and Aldactone tablets as she embarks on a journey during which she realizes that she has special powers to combat an alien invasion that is leaving humans in a zombified state.[139] The theme of empowerment against agonistic forces links *Dreadnought*, *Annex*, and "Angels Are Here to Help You," although Thornton's short story deals more directly with both the problem and the inescapability of technology. "Angels Are Here to Help You" helps us understand how different versions of biohacking—what Malatino terms "corporeal manipulation" and "transcending the limitations of the human body"—operate at the interface of the strange and the everyday.[140] Instead of offering a vision of perfectibility or overcoming, though, Thornton's story stresses that craft and vigilance are complements to self-belief and openness to becoming.

However, the fantastical and figurative nature of these stories raise the question of the extent to which biohacking is feasible—or at least feasible within the bounds of risk—in the everyday lives of transgender Americans, either for those whom the health care system has failed or for those who do not trust or reject the biomedical options available to them. The notion of entering gray or black markets might feel too risky for some. But for others, such as Christine from Boston (whose story is documented in a 2020 piece in the science magazine *Undark*), it leads to the search for alternative outlets for hormones when, without a job, she cannot afford the copay of her state's Medicaid program.[141] Coming off hormone treatment proves difficult for Christine; after accessing two weeks of estrogen pills from a friend, she is tempted to procure estrogen through illicit means, but in the end, disheartened, she decides to halt her transition by forgoing the biohacking route.

As Christine's case illustrates, a major driver of DIY biotechnology for transgender Americans is a lack of access to health care and support that might drive them to black markets or overseas for gender-affirming hormones and surgery. Trans biohacking centers primarily on hormone treatments and surgical procedures. Hormone therapies are easier to biohack than surgery, mainly because they are taken orally or via patches or injections (as is the case of Maria in *Nevada*, although injection carries a higher risk of infection), but for male-to-female transitions Estradiol is commonly taken alongside a testosterone blocker such as Spironolactone. For those who are denied access to prescription hormone therapies or who are looking for more affordable options, these forms are obtainable via the internet and gray-market pharmacies. The demand for these sources grew in 2020–2021 during the social isolation of the COVID-19 pandemic. Alongside the risks of self-medicating (including heart, liver, and kidney disease), there are benefits to well-being. The individual may decide that using hormones to subtly change facial and bodily features is preferable to a physician-approved treatment following a diagnosis of gender dysphoria when full transition is the goal. Conversely, the personal goal may be to transition quicker by supplementing a prescription in order to enhance a sense of wellness or reclaim self-agency, as Paul Preciado's *Testo Junkie* illustrates.[142]

It is tempting to focus on the individual making solitary choices about their self-identity and well-being, often in the face of economic and social barriers, but this would overlook other interlocutors beyond health care professionals. Although it is an important corrective to a lack of health care access, a DIY approach to hormones seems to reinforce this idea of solitary decision-making as a form of what Nikolas Rose calls "somatic individuality."[143] However, Mary Maggic, a biologist, xenofeminist, and trans activist trained at MIT, has since the mid-2010s developed a community approach to hormone access and biopolitics, sharing her vision of "open source estrogen" through her website and via YouTube and Vimeo workshops. Maggic's purpose is to investigate "the role of institutional science and biotechnology in the construction of somatic fictions and mass political imaginaries."[144] The aim is to empower others by sharing the scientific knowledge and technical skills needed to extract estrogen from urine at home and by switching the DIY biohacking discourse to a DIWO (do it with others) version of citizen science that affirms what Rose calls biosocial "networks of relatedness."[145] The reality is that it is not easy to extract sex hormones from urine and certainly not at concentrations needed for affirmative transition, but Maggic's broader endocrinological and environmental goal is to unearth the "histories, origins, and futures of our collective mutagenesis" by encouraging "cross-contamination." It is easy to criticize this as a mutation of scientific knowledge by promoting risky or unrealizable experimentation. Yet this might also be approached as the reinjection of citizen science into a technical discourse and professional practice that otherwise reinforces the status of patienthood by subjecting trans Americans to medical control.

While Mary Maggic's biohacking can be interpreted as a version of what Julietta Singh calls "radical dwelling," it is useful to turn briefly to the politics and practice of DIY gender surgery, which are typically more complex than hormone therapy. Gender-affirming surgery, as Maria muses in *Nevada*, tends to veer toward a renormalization of gender binaries via feminization or masculinization procedures that lead "some people" to assume that transitioners simply accept the stages as laid out by their physician.[146] But for those who have the means to afford it, multistage surgical journeys may go beyond what a surgeon deems to be a satisfactory end goal. On this level, fullness might be conceived of less as teleological completion and more in terms of plenitude and excess—introducing, as Christoph Hanssmann argues, a sense of "radical contingency" into what biomedicine presents as a finite journey with respect to awareness, agency, self-care, and community.[147]

Some feminists worry that not only do male-to-female gender transitions co-opt the space of collective gender affirmation but also that surgery can lead to the exaggeration or eroticization of body parts that might be viewed as a parody of gender identities. This is a common feminist criticism of drag culture, including of trans performance artists Amanda Lepore and Nina Arsenault, who have embraced the artificiality of surgery. Lepore see herself as a "moving sculpture" and Arsenault has become her own art through her multiple surgeries and via performance pieces.[148] Just as the multiple surgeries undertaken by French artist ORLAN in the 1990s offer a critique of the cosmetics industry through a series of self-hybridizations (ORLAN dubs herself the first "woman-to-woman transsexual"), this sensationalism can be seen either as a form of generative biohacking or an embodiment of surgery addiction at the edge of pornography.[149] Either way, this turn toward hypervisibility not only underestimates the mental and physical courage that gender-affirming surgery demands and the dangerous self-surgical ends to which some Americans resort if they are denied gender-affirming care, it also overlooks a variety of noninvasive procedures that may enhance well-being and offset dysphoria. It also overlooks the possibility that individuals and surgeons can develop more creative relationships. For example, marketing consultant Hayley Anthony conducted research for a new procedure performed in 2017 at the Center for Transgender Medicine and Surgery at Mount Sinai Hospital in Manhattan that reused her abdomen tissue to create a vagina.[150]

Just as cultural responses to the biotechnological topics discussed in the first half of the book can be read both symptomatically and generatively, it is important to recognize that creativity is a central element for intersecting transgender communities. This sometimes takes the form of bioart that seeks to decolonize subjectivity, modes of radical dwelling, or visions of possible futures, such as those illustrated by Jeanne Thornton's "Angels Are Here to Help You" and the exhibitions of the New York intersex artist Juliana Huxtable. It is also evident in

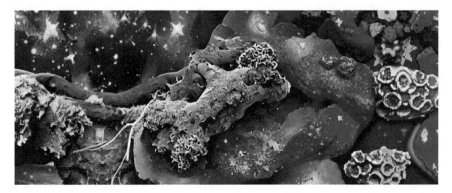

Figure 6.2. *Xenformation 1: What Does Xen Dream of in the Theatricum?* (2022). Adriana Knouf, in collaboration with DALL-E. Courtesy of the artist.

the xenological experiments of trans artist-scientist Adriana Knouf, who frames her objective as "disalienation from our capacities to change" by experimenting with a mixture of science fiction and science fact, echoing the aims of the Australian artistic research lab SymbioticA to open "the possibilities to practically and concretely rethink, remake, and create new human bodies."[151] In collaborating with the transnational Art4Med project and in her "xenomogrification" practices (what she calls "our ability to transform ourselves into something else"), Knouf aligns with Singh's need not only to decolonize the subject but also to find alternative ways of being at the intersection of otherness and the everyday.

This adjusted frame gives credence to Maggic's and Knouf's goals of biosynthesizing estrogen locally. But it can also wrestle what appear to be the excessive surgical self-practices of Nina Arsenault away from charges of sensationalism to an awareness of the body as an assemblage and a process rather than a postsurgical product.[152] By fusing natural and cyborg elements, these biohacking practices may push us to abandon the humanist language of authenticity or propel us toward what Malatino calls "assemblage thinking," by which we reimagine trans experiences as a fluid process rather than a journey toward fullness.[153] Knouf captures such radical reimagining in an AI-enabled image from the 2022 performance at the Waag Futurelab in Amsterdam of *Xenformation 1*, which transforms the ancient *Sleeping Hermaphroditus* sculpture in the Louvre into a multicolored cosmos.[154]

Just as Jules Gill-Peterson reminds us that blithely adopting the rhetoric of plasticity might be an unwitting surrender to a neoliberal techno-imperative, so reclaiming everyday agency should involve sharing information that is often professionally protected and the forging of allied causes that engender an organized approach to demanding better access and equal rights and to unlocking generative biotechnologies. Low-tech biohacking animates two of this book's central concepts—Nikolas Rose's somatic ethics and Robert Bellah's politics of imagination—and moves bioethics toward an emergent rather than a regulatory sphere, in line with what Julietta Singh calls "a map of broken things, a recyclable archive that will spur you to fashion other ways of being alive, of living."[155]

This mobile bioethical space should not retreat from the political into the personal but should instead balance the responsible use of biotechnology and progressive legislation at local, federal, and international levels with the recognition that state regulation is sometimes the problem rather than the solution if it reinforces inequalities by denying access or if it focuses on today's problems instead of imagining a different tomorrow. An experiential bioethics can reimagine what "traveling through" means, to return to Dolly Parton's signature song for *Transamerica*. This is not always a radical dwelling space, given the various ways of being trans, although it can be, as the practitioners profiled here suggest, if agency and care are reimagined as both individualistic and communal forms of biohacking. Rather than seeing biomedical practices as the primary driving force of a teleological journey, they are better understood as fluid elements in intersecting life stories that help us, in the words of Singh, attend to "the always enfleshed alterities of being human."[156]

PART FOUR

PERILOUS STATES

7   *Pandemic Culture*

IMMUNIZATION POLITICS AND
THE COVID-19 ACCELERATION

"How do you argue with that?," President Obama asked provocatively at the National Institutes of Health (NIH) in December 2014 as he urged a deeply divided Congress to recognize the need for emergency funding to combat the Ebola virus and improve public health in order to protect against "potential outbreaks in the future."[1] By placing common sense over ideology, Obama hoped to cut through normal politics to safeguard the security of American citizens from viral threats that evade health surveillance systems and travel undetected across global borders. Recognizing that the United States had been lucky in suffering only two deaths from Ebola (out of eleven cases), a disease that claimed 11,000 African lives between 2013 and 2016, Obama saw an opportunity for a "trial run" that might improve the coordination and reach of public health at all levels of government.[2] Obama acknowledged the health emergency in West Africa, where Ebola spread via human contact, and he offered a stark warning to Congress and the public that "there may and likely will come a time in which we have both an airborne disease that is deadly."[3]

Speaking five years before the first deaths from COVID-19 in the central China city of Wuhan, Obama's 2014 speech at the NIH was a clarion call to Congress to be pragmatic rather than partisan in recognizing the pivotal role of responsible health governance. Many Republicans were already unhappy about what they saw as the socialist encroachment of the Affordable Care Act, arguing that the president's position was just as ideological in extending the public health arm of centralized government as his criticism of congressional Republicans' disregard of evidence-based science.[4] Political theorist Shana Gadarian shows how partisan politics were at play in the wake of Ebola, with Republicans criticizing Obama for federal overreach and lapses in surveillance, such as when an exposed Liberian, Thomas Duncan, traveled in September 2014 from West Africa to Dallas, where he infected two health care workers before dying eight days after a delayed Ebola diagnosis.[5] Only after this incident did the Centers for Disease Control and Prevention (CDC) collaborate with the U.S. Customs and Border Protection to screen passengers arriving from Africa. Away from media scrutiny, virologists had been searching for a vaccine for Ebola since the Pentagon had identified the virus as a potential biothreat following the 9/11 terrorist attacks. But it was not until 2019–2020 that the U.S. Food and Drug Administration (FDA) approved a vaccine, a year after the World Health Organization (WHO) devised the Disease X concept as a tool for planning mitigation strategies for an as-yet-unknown pathogen that might reach pandemic proportions.[6]

Despite such pandemic preparedness initiatives and coordination between agencies of the Department of Health and Human Services, federal spending on preventive health measures was only 3 percent of GDP at the end of the Obama administration, significantly lower than that of both Canada and the United Kingdom. There was a marked drop in expenditure on preventive care between the millennium and the start of the COVID-19 pandemic, from 3.7 percent of GDP in 2000 (out of 13.3 percent of GDP for all national health expenditures) to 2.9 percent in 2019 (out of 17.6 percent of GDP spent on the nation's health).[7] This declining investment in public health—including massive variance in expenditures at the state level, from Delaware at the top to Louisiana at the bottom—was occurring precisely at the wrong time in Obama's eyes, a time when he believed that health surveillance, immunization programs, and emergency preparedness should be more robust than ever.[8]

Federal and state spending on public health increased sharply in 2020 as the highly transmissible Severe Acute Respiratory Syndrome Coronavirus 2 (SARS-CoV-2) rapidly spread both east and west, following early recorded cases of international travelers returning to Seattle (January 19th) and Boston (February 1st). Yet the science-based approach of long-serving health official Anthony Fauci, director of the National Institute of Allergy and Infectious Disease, was overshadowed by President Trump's efforts to blame the Obama administration for leaving the pandemic preparedness cupboard bare. Speaking more than three years into his presidency, Trump claimed on ABC and Fox News that he had had to rebuild the national stockpile because "the other administration, the last administration, left us nothing. . . . We didn't have ventilators. We didn't have medical equipment."[9]

News outlets like NBC exposed the falsity of Trump's assertions, following reports late in the Obama administration of warehouses full of emergency equipment, while two years earlier, Trump's second health secretary, Alex M. Azar (a recent president of the American division of Eli Lilly), had claimed that the nation was committed "to a coherent and comprehensive biodefense strategy" and a robust Global Health Security Agenda in the aftermath of the Ebola outbreak of 2013–2016.[10] These facts did not deter Trump from accusing his White House predecessor of acting negligently. Had Trump's accusations been true, they would have been in direct tension with Obama's warning to Congress in 2014 of the need to strengthen public health to ensure that the country was fully prepared for the next major emergency. Trump's claims also overlooked the fact that Congress had granted the Department of Health and Human Services $100 million during the George W. Bush administration to grow the strategic national stockpile of antiviral drugs, plus an article that Senator Obama had co-written for the New York Times in 2005 that argued for a "permanent framework" for public health preparedness at home and abroad, involving close coordination between the federal government and the pharmaceutical industry.[11]

The common consensus is that Trump's White House Coronavirus Task Force (on which Fauci served as one of only two medical experts, alongside CDC director Robert Redfield) was not a success, either in terms of interagency coordination or in its ability to give clear and consistent public health messages.[12] This was in large part because Trump was reluctant to act on national security intelligence because of the perception that it would have downward pressure on the economy and because of his impatience for closure in the face of a virus with an unpredictable narrative. Wistfully, Trump sought a "burst of light" in spring 2020 that would put a swift end to what Fauci, speaking on Easter Sunday, called a "terrible affront to us as a nation, to our health and our well-being."[13] While Fauci was measured in his response, stressing what was known and unknown about the virus, Trump forayed into magical thinking.[14] He bragged about the speed with which stockpiles had been replenished, the slickness of the nation's testing capacity, and his ability to instruct state governors how to behave with respect to quarantine procedures and the temporary closing of public institutions. Ironically, eight White House staffers contracted the virus at a super-spreader Trump campaign rally in Tulsa in June 2020, where few face masks were in evidence. And despite the president's repeated promises about the imminence of a COVID-19 vaccine, the FDA did not approve a rollout for a vaccine until mid-December 2020, six weeks after Trump had lost the presidential election to Joe Biden.[15]

Public Health and Technological Imperatives

It was no surprise the federal government and medical leaders sought a biotech solution to the mounting infections and death toll via an immunization program after the initial plans to mitigate viral spread via contact tracing were, at best, only a partial success. Yet Trump and those in his close circle, such as advisor Peter Navarro and Secretary of State Mike Pompeo, stirred a cauldron of suggestion and misinformation about the cause, prevalence, and likely trajectory of the SARS-CoV-2 virus, inflamed by unfounded "deep state" conspiracy theories circulating on both mainstream and fringe media platforms that supported Trump's antigovernment policies.[16] Fauci was often criticized by Trump White House officials and the right-wing media for prioritizing public health over the economy and for his conviction that the virus originated from zoonotic transmission between animals and humans rather than from a laboratory experiment—a topic to which I turn in the next section.[17]

Yet within this crossfire of blame and conjecture, what has been called an "incoherent patchwork of interventions" emanating from Trump's White House played an oversized role in the reason that many citizens experienced uncertainty and social division during the first year of the pandemic, a topic Spike Lee's HBO series *NYC Epicenters* explores.[18] At its core, the erratic approach of Trump and some state officials contributed to a "post-truth" climate of contradictory messaging and "alternative facts," to use Trump counselor Kellyanne Conway's now-famous phrase of 2017. This not only mirrored the president's high-risk approach to international relations but placed public institutions under immense strain, so much so that it seemed to be eroding what Robert Bellah called the "exceptionally powerful institutional order" that binds together the nation and creates a bedrock of public trust.[19] Although the chair of the White House Coronavirus Task Force, Vice-President Mike Pence, defended a "whole-of-America approach, focusing on business innovation and state-based solutions" to counter an overmedicalized narrative of precautionary measures, Trump's seemingly cavalier attitude toward mitigating risk forced health care workers to improvise in order to save lives and stoked extreme emotions that led some Republicans to reject common sense regarding low-tech masking and high-tech vaccinations because of their belief that civil liberties should triumph over health security and their suspicion of Big Tech.[20]

It is in recognition of the chaos that engulfed Washington, DC, in 2020 that I open this final part of *Transformed States* by tracing how heroic premillennial biotech dreams foundered in the COVID-19 world emergency. In this discussion, I move outward from the focus on life stages and selfhood in chapters 5 and 6 to broader yet entangled questions of community and environment in this final part, by focusing on the urban transmissibility of viruses in this chapter and toxic threats to fragile coastal locations in chapter 8. In the following pages, I assess the holistic health effects of COVID-19 by analyzing its political, biomedical, and cultural intersections through a postmillennial lens of near misses of epidemics. I do so by focusing on the beginnings, ends, and uncertain middles of pandemics from the vantage point of two prescient pre-COVID texts: the disease-outbreak film *Contagion* (2011) and Ling Ma's 2018 pandemic novel *Severance*. As a route through the polarizing politics of immunization and vaccination, I then turn to Italian political theorist Roberto Esposito's influential theories of immunity to link Esposito's affirmatory biopolitics with Robert Bellah's call to rejuvenate citizenship. The chapter's final section develops this theme by returning to the biohacking theme in order to differentiate homeopathic and wellness techniques from the speculative health remedies emanating from Trump's White House during 2020.

Not only did the pandemic raise questions about national preparedness and technological efficacy, but also moral leadership and interagency coordination. Just as importantly, it revealed deep tensions between the rallying message that "we are all in this together" and the health vulnerabilities and inequalities differing communities and demographics experienced; older, Black, and Latinx Americans were at a disproportionately higher risk of contracting COVID-19 than younger white Americans.[21] These tensions were compounded by the racist abuse Asian Americans received in the wake of what Trump labeled the "China virus," while some LGBTQ+ community members were at a heightened risk of losing their jobs or experiencing domestic abuse or having hormone treatments disrupted during lockdown. As the editors of a special pandemic issue of *Perspectives on Politics* note, these economic, spatial, and racial disparities caused "unequal impacts" during the pandemic that illuminate "the central role of power and powerlessness in generating well-being and illness."[22]

Digital technologies played a vital role in connecting dispersed families, alongside telemedicine, which facilitated remote health care consultations and repeat prescriptions during the worst months of the pandemic. While Silicon Valley companies such as Mindstrong (est. 2014) were promising to revolutionize mental health care by tracking moods on smart phones and wearables, other technologies tended to reinforce health inequities rather than erase them as many workplaces became digitized and contact tracing and vaccine certification relied on mobile apps.[23] Families without broadband keenly felt digital inequalities, especially parents whose children faced periods of school closure and those living in isolated communities where internet coverage was patchy.[24] What historian Jeremy Greene sees as a technical problem of establishing physician-patient intimacy via remote technologies only exacerbated health challenges for some, while others struggled psychologically with lack of human contact during lockdown.[25] A July 2022 House hearing emphasized how the neurological and somatic symptoms of long COVID lingered after the vaccine rollout for an estimated 8.1 percent of working-age Americans in the form of depression, chronic muscle fatigue, ADHD, brain fog, sleep disturbance, and poor lung and pulmonary capacity, and, a year earlier, Surgeon General Vivek Murthy acknowledged that the pandemic was compounding the difficult mental health experiences many young Americans faced as he challenged tech companies to fight pandemic misinformation on social media.[26]

Had the Trump White House acted sooner—in January or early February rather than March 2020—and had the messages from the Coronavirus Task Force been consistent, it is likely that more American lives would have been saved. Shana Gadarian and colleagues portray "a decaying and politicized health care environment, economic and racial inequality, Trump himself, and, above all, partisan polarization" as a toxic mixture that created a kind of "time zero," which meant that the virus reproduced at a higher rate than it likely would have otherwise.[27] Yet while the pitch and consequences of the pandemic were acute in the United States, other nations that seemed to have relative success during phases of the pandemic in mitigating viral spread, such as New Zealand and China (two countries of contrasting sizes, demographics, political systems, and approaches to civil liberties), could not keep politics out of their zero COVID strategies and arguably only deferred a health crisis.[28]

It is easy to blame national governments in the face of sharp spikes in hospitalization and deaths, but cross-border alliances were also under strain, especially with respect to travel guidelines and vaccine production.[29] While WHO officials were trying to ensure that wealthy countries did not neglect vulnerable global regions when it came to vaccine availability, embodied by the COVAX (COVID-19 Vaccines Global Access) scheme, Trump was blaming officials for not detecting the virus early enough and for being soft on China. This was an obvious ploy to shift blame away from the White House onto the UN's health agency, despite efforts by the WHO in the 2010s to escalate its efforts to "keep the world safe, and serve the vulnerable," in order to make "a measurable difference in people's health at country level" by improving global cooperation.[30] Yet international institutions also stumbled in the world emergency, prompting the WHO to develop—arguably belatedly—an intergovernmental "prevention, preparedness and response" treaty committed to whole-of-government and whole-of-society approaches in the aftermath of the pandemic.[31]

It is clear from this account that the biopolitical implications of pandemic culture are far reaching and that questions of power, trust, and leadership go far beyond the White House and Congress. Writing in 1991, Robert Bellah argued that social institutions need to reaffirm their moral responsibility if they are to nurture a healthy society, recognizing that the "heritage of trust that has been the basis of our stable democracy is eroding" and that it is "much easier to destroy than renew."[32] Bellah was suspicious of laissez-faire politics, arguing that markets need realigning to promote "public aims," but he had nothing to say in specific terms about what management strategies would facilitate this or how pandemics impact institutional behavior when trust is in short supply and infrastructures face functional strain.[33] So although NIH leaders Francis Collins and Anthony Fauci bolstered trust by warning against the pernicious effects of the culture wars and by recommending that citizens observe public health guidelines, industry leaders continued to tout a heroic narrative of endeavor, particularly as the Pfizer and Moderna vaccines were available only ten months after the first reported American deaths in late February 2020.[34]

In the private sector, Jeremy Levin, Ovid Therapeutics CEO and chair of the Biotechnology Innovation Organization, writing in the first year of the pandemic, contrasted the "global dislocation" caused by the emergency with an optimistic vision of massive voluntary effort within the biomedical community "to confront and turn back the virus" by pitting "viral biology against human intellect and capability."[35] Levin's emphasis on companies swiftly making the collective moral decision to "step forward voluntarily" was a move to offset the criticism that Big Pharma benefited from the pandemic, given the need for national governments to quickly procure therapeutics.[36] His collaborative book with biopharmaceutical leaders, *Biotechnology in a Time of COVID-19*, argued that responsible biotech was "the frontline of defense against this grave threat, and we are doing so with good intentions for the benefit of humankind."[37]

Levin had little to say about government relations or procurements, although he blamed the media for giving the pandemic a political slant and some of his collaborators insisted that it was the responsibility of the Biomedical Advanced Research and Development Authority (formed in 2006 within the Department of Health and Human Services) to help companies innovate if the biotech industry was to help the country prepare for pandemic threats effectively.[38] Nonetheless, Levin's portrayal of a battle between heroic science and a deadly killer chimes with the rhetoric of warfare that marked a chain of White House health policies.[39] Trump's war against opioids in 2018–2019, when he promised the nation to "win the battle," pivoted in 2020 to a "fierce battle" of our "nation's scientific brilliance" against variants of an invisible, highly transmissible, and rapidly mutating coronavirus, which he believed "the most aggressive mobilization since the Second World War" would vanquish, as he told the UN General Assembly.[40] Even Mike Pence, one of the most overtly Christian vice-presidents, used combat metaphors to defend the administration's COVID response.[41] Neither leader acknowledged that the average life expectancy in the United States was already declining prior to the pandemic from a combination of opioid-related deaths, heart and liver disease, and a spike in suicides. This reveals how Trump's braggadocio deflected from a focus on the social codeterminants of health and threats to humans living healthier for longer, about which Robert Butler had warned the nation a decade earlier in *The Longevity Revolution*.[42]

This rhetorical war against an invisible enemy strained against two other modes of pandemic response: an intensification of practices of emergency care to treat vulnerable Americans suffering from a symptomatically complex disease, often in isolation from their families; and a culture of public-mindedness in which families, neighbors, and communities found ways to look out for one another—especially older Americans—despite the imperative of social distancing.[43] It was nonetheless difficult to move beyond metaphors of warfare, especially in the early months of the pandemic. This is in part because, as literary scholar Priscilla Wald recognized in 2008, viruses impart "a mythical case to their battle with human beings" in their invasion of host's body, a view that aligns with what anthropologist Elizabeth Povinelli describes as the virus erasing "the difference between nonlife and life . . . in order to extend itself."[44]

Writing over a decade later, during the intensity of COVID-19, Wald revisited her 2008 book *Contagious* by arguing that such warfare metaphors are a distraction from the lesson of the pandemic about how "we live with our microbes" via a combination of heightened personal awareness and an "integrative understanding of human-environment relationships" that goes beyond a pathological disease model.[45] These social and ecological lessons intersect with biomedical lessons about vaccine availability and health care capacity, prompting us to assess the relative stability or fragility of health environments that "intersect across multiple spatial and temporal scales."[46] As these final two chapters argue, an ecological approach to health can help us regain the lateral vision and somatic ethics that Paul Virilio and Nikolas Rose call for, pushing us to critically question the heroic narrative that biotechnical science is an "endless resource" (to revive the Clinton-era phrase from chapter 1) and think about health in a holistic way that sees biotechnology as heuristic rather than offering a grand solution. On this level, this fourth part of *Transformed States* takes up the challenge social historian Tim Cooper poses when he argues that "the question 'how did it come to this?' must be answered before we can meaningfully ask 'what is to be done?'"[47]

Beginnings, Ends, and Uncertain Middles

Obsession with how pandemics arise and what it takes to end them has a long history, going back before the Great Influenza of 1918–1919. The search for a primary viral cause is often frustrating but is typically overshadowed by an orientation toward pandemic endings, when a perilous narrative fades into the background of daily life at a threshold when population immunity is widespread. On this point, the protagonist Candace Chen of Ling Ma's pandemic novel *Severance* reflects that "The End begins before you are ever aware of it. It passes as ordinary."[48] In Candace's case, an eschatological version of "The End" resonates with her job at a Bible publisher and aligns with her retreat into personal rituals and commodity culture in the face of the fatal Shen virus. Reflecting also on middles, only later does Candace realize that one effect of the virus is to tilt individuals toward zombie-like rituals instead of helping them discern the colliding crises of late capitalism, of which health security is just one facet.

Set largely in New York City during the Obama years, Ling Ma's novel portrays a paradoxically fraying and insulated country in the middle of a pandemic that is far from President Obama's emphasis on hope and "confidence that we can ease suffering and make a difference," as he asserted in the 2014 speech at the NIH the chapter began with.[49] Instead of depicting the city as a laboratory in search of control of a virus, as it became in the worst months of COVID, urban spaces in *Severance* mask threats of transmissibility and immanent endings—at least until it is too late.[50] "Beginning of the end" was a common media phrase during the coronavirus vaccine rollout, even though there were risks that different viral strains would return in unpredictable ways. However, this phrase does not signal a simple concept, as Mike Chen explores in his 2020 novel *A Beginning at the End*, in which ends signify potentially apocalyptic repetitions rather than a return to pre-viral normality.[51]

I return to *Severance* later in this section, but it felt like a new dawn when a number of national health departments in the winter of 2022 affirmed the shift into an endemic phase of COVID-19, given the nearly three years of high mortality rates spanning over two hundred countries. In September 2022, UN director-general Tedros Adhanom Ghebreyesus announced that "we have never been in a better position to end the pandemic," although he warned that we were "not there yet" because the mutability of SARS-CoV-2 meant that its trajectory was hard to predict, especially given the lack of a single-dose vaccine that could offer long-term immunity.[52] Even after Ghebreyesus declared in May 2023 that the global threat of COVID had finally receded, he recognized the need to address comorbidities that make some individuals and global communities more vulnerable than others together with the persistent threat of resistant bacterial infections.

The scale and speed of COVID-19 transmission were unprecedented, but the biomedical concern that the virus had jumped between animals and humans inflected both the sense of uncertain endings and conspiracies about the origins of the novel coronavirus. Following the Wuhan Municipal Health Commission's announcement of December 2019 that twenty-seven cases of viral pneumonia had emerged from Wuhan's Huanan Seafood Wholesale Market, most epidemiologists at the time (including those at the NIH and the WHO) believed the virus emerged from the wet market, possibly from a bat or a raccoon dog.[53] This wet-market theory echoes the final montage of Steven Soderbergh's 2011 film

Contagion, which traces a SARS-like virus, MEV-1, that is transmitted by a colony of bats whose Hong Kong habitat has been disturbed by deforestation practices. Scriptwriter Scott Z. Burns consulted with WHO specialists to ensure that the film was epidemiologically accurate in its depiction of CDC and WHO officials collaborating in a race against the clock to find a life-saving vaccine.[54] A decade later, Burns recognized a stark contrast between the dedicated work of public health officials in *Contagion* and the precarious nature of trust in institutional integrity during the COVID pandemic, commenting that "I never thought in a million years that the scientists and public health people would be questioned and doubted and defunded and, in many cases, dismissed from their posts."[55]

During COVID lockdowns, *Contagion* enjoyed new interest among Anglophone audiences searching for cultural relevance on television. Its final montage sequence is especially resonant in its visual dramatization of events that lead a young pig to consume fruit excreted by a displaced bat, an event that in all likelihood creates a genetic mutation. We see three young pigs caged and transported to a Macao casino, before cutting to the casino's head chef preparing what we assume to be the infected pig for human consumption. The ceremonial photograph that marketing manager Beth Emhoff (Gwyneth Paltrow) poses for after shaking hands with the chef on what the film informs viewers is "Day 1" reveals how beginnings and ends intertwine in viral narratives, returning us to "Day 2" of the film's opening montage, in which travelers taking different routes home from Hong Kong show symptoms of fever, two days before Emhoff's gruesome death following a violent seizure. Film studies scholar Marco Grosoli describes this narrative loop as a "collective, dispersed, fragmented structure" in which characters are abandoned or appear late or disappear suddenly, arguing that this global disease pattern of disrupted life experiences is a metaphor for a crisis in late capitalism.[56] Thus, a narrative of food contamination morphs in the final montage into a critique of neoliberal exploitation. The process of deforestation enacted by Emhoff's company's bulldozers and the conspicuous consumption of a suckling pig in a casino is a deadly mix, as Emhoff travels 7,500 miles home to Minneapolis, where she unwittingly becomes patient zero.

Despite its circular and dispersed narrative, like the earlier patient-zero medical thriller *Outbreak* (1995), there is little that *Contagion* does not resolve in its emphasis on the identifiable origins of the virus, the contact points where the virus was transmitted, and the quest for a vaccine that could end the pandemic. In the time of COVID, this arc was reassuring but it did not mirror alternative accounts of viral origins or how long a succession of coronavirus variants continued to circuit through communities. That arc leads Sari Altschuler to argue that "the outbreak narrative's linear plot is directly harmful in a pandemic," suspending us "in a helpless position of expecting a cure that isn't coming."[57] Instead of ends and beginnings, COVID-19 was characterized by a prolonged and uncertain middle. A number of false dawns deepened the collective and individual psychological burden that compounded the primary respiratory danger, aligned with Altschuler's argument that "a midpandemic near future is unimaginable."[58]

The uncertainty stemmed in part from the mutability of the virus but also from misinformation and deliberate disinformation surrounding COVID that circulated on social media. This kind of "infodemic" (a term coined in 2003 during the SARS outbreak, three years before Twitter was launched) is illustrated in *Contagion* by blogger Alan Krumwiede (Jude Law), who falsely claims that he has cured himself with the homeopathic remedy forsythia. Justice is served when Krumwiede is arrested for fraud. But that does not stop him from peddling unfounded conspiracies about the WHO and the CDC, presaging the acceleration of social media activity in the late 2010s that during the pandemic amplified conspiracies about the origins of the novel coronavirus and the hidden intentions of public health institutions.[59]

Scientific studies reinforced the wet-market theory as the origin of SARS-CoV-2 because it aligned with causal explanations of the SARS and MERS viruses.[60] This biomedical consensus about natural viral origins did not prevent Kentucky senator and ophthalmologist Rand Paul from speculating that COVID-19 was created by "gain-of-function" biotech research at the Wuhan Institute of Virology laboratory sponsored by the NIH that made SARS-related viruses transmissible between bats and humans. This was not as extreme as Trump's messaging that the virus was a hoax concocted by Democrats and left-leaning media. Yet with the sketchiest of evidence and supported by right-wing media platforms that used First Amendment rights and disdain for Chinese communism to propel an anti-science agenda, Paul held Fauci responsible for using government funds to sponsor "high risk research that creates new potential pandemic pathogens that exist only in the lab not in nature" during a pause in federal funding for chimeric research that seeks to alter the molecular structure of viruses.[61]

In responding to these accusations by Paul at a July 2021 congressional hearing, Fauci (by then President Biden's chief medical advisor) dismissed the implication that NIH funding had been used for gain-of-function research, adding that it was "molecularly impossible" for such research to lead to the emergence of SARS-CoV-2 because the Wuhan research was genetically distinct. Acting NIH director Lawrence Tabak reiterated this point in early 2023, when the FBI and the Department of Energy revived the lab-leak theory, albeit without clear proof.[62] Paul accused Fauci of obscuring "responsibility for four million people from dying around the world from a pandemic," echoing Trump's accusations that the WHO had unleashed "the contagion around the world" and the first series of the German techno-thriller *Biohackers*, in which a rogue biologist releases a vivarium of deadly genetically modified mosquitos on a German train.[63] Fauci retorted that the senator was lying for partisan reasons, with Paul levelling his sights on the country's best-known public health official in an effort to accuse NIH of being the research wing of big government and a pivotal player in a global network of rogue science.

Sensing that he could realize his ambition to make what he calls "government bullies" accountable, Paul published on his website a July 2022 letter he had sent to the NIH's acting director, Lawrence Tabak (following Francis Collins' retirement the previous year), that claimed that the NIH might be "improperly withholding information from the public related to COVID-19 for political reasons."[64] Paul criticized the NIH for disregarding the Freedom of Information Act, for being slow to release details his team had requested, and for heavily redacting released material. He went further, accusing the NIH of deliberate censorship, quoting a court statement that the agency is "withholding portions of emails between employees because they 'could be used out of context and serve to amplify the already prevalent misinformation regarding the origins of the coronavirus pandemic.'"[65] That Paul attacked a government health agency rather than the biotech industry speaks to his libertarian politics, his belief in health freedom, and his efforts to loosen FDA regulation over market-sensitive pharmaceuticals, as evidenced in 2016, when he sponsored the Accelerating New Pharmaceutical Competition Act (a bill did that not reach the Senate floor). Notably, a month after Paul's July 2021 attack on Fauci, it came to light that in February 2020, his wife, Kelley Paul, had bought stock in Gilead Sciences, which manufactures the antiviral remdesivir, suggesting a gross double standard when it comes to transparency. This February purchase date was two months before Fauci announced that remdesivir was "quite good news" and nine months before the FDA approved it for COVID use, which implies that Kelley Paul had access to industry-sensitive information that was circulating in Congress (although the Pauls deny this).[66]

One of the effects of this political crossfire was that it distracted from the reality that the country was still facing a medical emergency in the summer of 2021, when infections, hospitalizations, and deaths from the Delta variant were on an upward curve and only 56 percent of the population had received one dose of the two-dose vaccine.[67] Paul's obsession with alternative accounts of the origins of the virus did not stem from an interest in epidemiology that could help biotech companies produce more effective vaccines or help the NIH prepare for future waves. Instead, he claimed in an online interview he was "kind of pro-vaccine, but also pro-freedom."[68] This was an expression of his "case against socialism," the title of his 2021 book that champions civil liberties over what he sees as a tyrannical surveillance state, and of his suspicion that the mRNA vaccine culture was a form of experimental gene therapy.[69] He was reckless about following quarantine measures when he contracted COVID-19 in March 2020, and he claimed that he did not need a vaccine as he had "natural immunity" only for a photograph to circulate on social media in August 2021 of him being inoculated.[70] As such, Paul's behavior is a manifestation of what the Carter administration advisor and communitarian thinker Amitai Etzioni calls radical individualism, which aims to paralyze public authorities and carries "grave human and moral consequences."[71]

Ignoring the federal oversight role played by the U.S. National Science Advisory Board for Biosecurity (est. 2005), Paul seemed more interested in conjuring alternative viral origins to indict the deep state than in establishing medical truth.[72] Paul's conspiratorial statements as a senator and a private citizen were part of the cloud of obfuscation that continued to envelop the domestic COVID narrative beyond Trump's term in the White House. Paul was not the only one to prolong this fog of uncertainty. For example, Florida governor Ron DeSantis sought to establish a state committee that consisted of vaccine skeptics and filed a petition with the Florida Supreme Court in December 2022 to investigate "any and all wrongdoing in Florida with respect to COVID-19 vaccines" in an effort to blame the NIH, the CDC, and vaccine manufacturers.[73] We might ignore such politics of outrage, as epitomized by the groundless statements about a "Fauci-funded China virus" from Colorado representative Lauren Boebert.[74] But the fact that House Republicans elevated the lab-leak theory to an official GOP platform in 2023 reveals the persistence of polarization about the issue of trust in public health officials.

Paul contributed to the zombie outbreak of disinformation and used his privileged position in the U.S. Senate to influence public opinion under the guise of freedom of speech, arguing that it is himself and others like him whose civil liberties were under assault by the deep state. He pictured his fear in an October 2019 congressional hearing he chaired for the Senate Homeland Security and Governmental Affairs Committee, where he proclaimed: "We are here the day before Halloween to talk about zombies. These are not the kind of zombies we see on *The Walking Dead.* . . . These zombies are far scarier. They are zombie government programs that have sometimes not been reauthorized for decades."[75] In this instance, Paul offered a "zombie cure" by arguing that federal programs should be reauthorized every four years.[76] This zombie discourse linked twenty-first-century pandemic culture to Cold War fears of enemies within and alien invasions, as evidenced by the 2007 post-apocalypse zombie film *I Am Legend*, adapted from Richard Matheson's early Cold War novel.

The concept of a zombie apocalypse was far from a new phenomenon as evidenced by a succession of science fiction and horror stories since the late 1960s. However, many media commentators noted how apposite it was in the early months of COVID.[77] A more immediate horizon was established by Max Brooks in his books *Zombie Survival Guide* (2003) and *World War Z* (2006), published during the George W. Bush administration, when bioterrorism was a national security priority. The books envisage an outbreak of the fictional Solanum virus, which transforms humans into zombies whose lives can never end. Within twenty-four hours of infection, the virus undermines bodily functions, then mutates into "a completely new organ," while the brain stays "alive but dormant," untethered from the body.[78] Biotechnology proves useless in this world. There are no vaccinations that can prevent infection, and when a former UN medical investigator finds a twelve-year-old patient zero in Dachang, China, at the beginning of *World War Z*, the boy is depicted as being possessed by violent, almost bestial movements, as if his humanity has been extinguished.[79]

World War Z is an apocalyptic global narrative in which essential services and social structures collapse, but it is also a geopolitical story about the United States. The federal government does not take the threat seriously at first, but then it ramps up to a full-scale battle against mass zombie attacks that lasts for three years. The U.S. president is removed from office following a nervous breakdown and the new government retreats from Washington, DC to Honolulu, while many Americans try to flee to Canada, only to perish without the survival skills they need to thrive in a colder climate. *World War Z* is far fetched, especially its Hollywood film adaptation of 2013. Nonetheless, the novel dramatizes how the virus exposes frailty in the social fabric and, as Brooks commented in July 2020, the "gap between the American people and those who protect them" when civil order breaks down and public institutions cease to function.[80]

Brooks argues that the "wholeness of nation" approach to border security eroded in the post–Cold War era, partly because conflicting notions of truth and social media distractions meant that the nation was less prepared for biothreats, at least compared to the civilian preparedness campaign of the early Cold War years. This is perhaps the reason why the Department of Defense developed a zombie defense training exercise and the CDC released a blog in 2011 called "Preparedness 101: Zombie Apocalypse," arguing that if Americans were prepared for such a mythical invasion then they would also be ready for other public health emergencies.[81] Within this alarmist framework, Ling Ma's *Severance* both evokes and moves on from Cold War invasion narratives by presenting a quieter apocalypse—one in which its casualties are zombified by the fatal Shen virus, which travels via spores carried on trade routes from the manufacturing hub of Shenzhen, China, to rapidly spread undetected across the United States. Avoiding

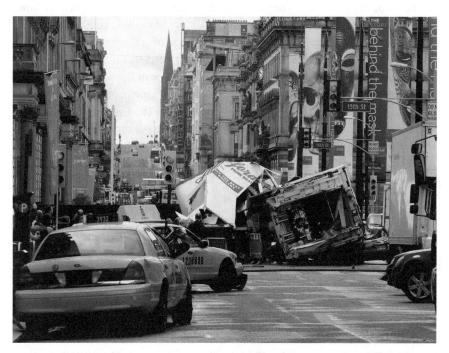

Figure 7.1. Social order collapses in New York City in the wake of a rapidly transmissible virus. *World War Z* (2013), filmed in Glasgow, Scotland. Say Cheese/Alamy Photo.

the horror genre of the long-running Netflix zombie apocalypse series *Z Nation* (2014–2018), *Severance* more subtly explores what happens when social cohesion crumbles in the face of a pandemic and questions how robust common culture is when it is fueled by late capitalist consumerism. Ling Ma's protagonist Candace, who is immune from the fictional Shen fever (perhaps because of her genetics as a second-generation Chinese American), reflects that New York City "lulled you into thinking that there were so many options, but most of the options had to do with buying things."[82] It is tempting to read *Severance* as an allegory of late capitalism as a zombie system, but journalist Jiayang Fan argues that the novel resists a straight allegorical reading and is better approached for its "pervasive mood—anxious and bleak."[83]

Set in 2011, *Severance* intertwines present and past into a meditation on a country that is almost silently consumed by a virus that pushes its casualties into mindless routines as their bodies enter a state of decrepitude. This trait is framed within the zombie genre as one of Candace's friends and erstwhile group leader Bob reflects that zombie horror narratives are not about "a specific villain" in the way that vampire stories often are, because "one zombie can be easily killed, but a hundred zombies is another issue. Only amassed do they really pose a threat. This narrative, then, is not about any individual entity, per se, but about an abstract force . . . [which] strikes at any time, whenever, wherever, like a natural disaster, a hurricane, an earthquake."[84] Candace initially does not think the zombie paradigm is applicable to Shen fever ("The fevered aren't zombies. They don't attack us or try to eat us. They don't do anything to us") only to realize later, when Bob starts to reveal zombie-like behavior, that the numb mindlessness of the zombie life is an unquestioning acceptance of a force seemingly beyond control.[85] In the early pages, the still-human Bob describes it as a "mob mentality" that often arises in the early phase of pandemics in the form of erratic and compulsive behavior, panic buying, hoarding, or marking out territory (an example from real life would be the spike in gun sales in the United States in 2020–2021). It is also difficult to counter such self-serving yet paranoid behavior if public leaders and social institutions do not act responsibly—within what Bellah calls a moral ecology—to ensure that both self-care and care of others are consistently high on the national agenda.

Significantly, politicians, public health officials, and the mainstream media do not feature heavily in *Severance*, aside from news reports about travel bans and airport closures. Instead, Candace depends on a company FAQ handout and Google to find out about Shen fever, with the recognition that communication networks will not last long as infrastructures start to crumble and the looting of abandoned facilities becomes rife.[86] The FAQ handout determines that the virus is hard to detect on transmission but that there is the likelihood of early "memory lapses, headaches, disorientations, shortness of breath, and fatigue," then within one to four weeks "malnourishment, lapse of hygiene, bruising on the skin, and impaired motor coordination," and finally "fatal loss of consciousness."[87] What the handout does not initially include is advice on prevention. When the FAQ handout is revised halfway through the novel, more detail is given about the origins of the virus and about the recommendations of the CDC that people avoid dusty environments and wear an N95 respirator so as not to inhale the microscopic spores.[88] Yet at no point does the handout discuss behavioral adjustments or safeguarding wellness, as if human life is expendable as long as capitalist wheels keep turning.

The fact that Candace learns about the virus in a piecemeal way that is arguably too late for many of her fellow citizens is one of the novel's lessons. So too is the intertwining of different kinds of narratives about viruses that tend to dominate the uncertain middle of pandemics. The subdued, possibly depressed Candace has her own blog, NY Ghost, on which she documents changes in her increasingly abandoned city. She reflects, "Who knew what was true. The sheer density of information and misinformation at the End, encapsulated in news articles and message-board theories and clickbait traps that had propagated hysterically through retweets and shares, had effectively rendered us more ignorant, more helpless."[89] Such an insight about the viral consequences of what Alison Bashford calls "the touch of words" is especially relevant for the COVID-19 pandemic.[90]

On this theme, Yoram Lass, the former director of Israel's Ministry of Health, declared COVID-19 "the first epidemic in history which is accompanied by another epidemic—the virus of social networks. These new media have brainwashed entire populations. What you get is fear and anxiety, and an inability to look at real data . . . all the ingredients for monstrous hysteria."[91] This observation was echoed in 2022 by Anthony Fauci's comment that Twitter is a "cesspool of interaction."[92] Such views overlook the benefits of social media for helping dispersed families and friendship groups remain in touch and access information. Yet Lass's comments also highlight how the psychological aspect of pandemics overlaps with threats to physical health. (Twitter and Facebook responded to this dynamic in 2020–2022 by including label warnings on misleading COVID-19 information, and YouTube temporarily suspended Rand Paul for making bogus claims about masking.) As such, *Severance* has a tighter focus on holistic health than *Contagion*, prompting a return in the next section to the role of biotech during pandemics, framed by questions of natural versus induced immunity.

The Vaccine Calculus and Long COVID

Despite the erratic messaging of Trump's White House and the strain placed on health care systems over a sequence of viral surges, the race to find a SARS-CoV-2 vaccine via collaboration between industry and public institutions was a success story. Compared with the lengthy searches to discover a polio vaccine and effective therapeutics for HIV/AIDS and Alzheimer's, three biotech companies, Pfizer-BioNTech and Moderna in the United States and Oxford-AstraZeneca in Europe, between them produced "the fastest vaccine in history."[93] Although Operation Warp Speed, the federal initiative to "maximally expedite a safe effective vaccine," envisioned an October launch—a deadline Vice-President Pence reiterated in the summer of 2020, when Phase 3 trials were just starting—all three vaccines were rolled out at the turn of 2021, starting with frontline workers and vulnerable groups. By the end of 2022, at least 80 percent of the U.S. population had received at least one dose of a vaccine, a public health initiative that was judged to have helped prevent 18 million hospitalizations and to have saved 3 million lives.[94]

The apparent success of the COVID vaccine is an example of what Al Gore at the beginning of the 1990s called the "complex ethical calculus" of responsible biotechnology in the face of a world emergency.[95] Although the speed of the development of SARS-CoV-2 vaccines was undoubtedly aided by research on SARS and MERS (Middle Eastern respiratory syndrome coronavirus), Pfizer and Moderna innovated by using adaptable mRNA technology that can stimulate an immune response in patients from the protein's genetic code. These DNA vaccines were judged to be a "fast and flexible platform," although two doses were required because a single vaccine shot offered only "limited immunogenicity," especially because multiple variants and subvariants were circulating in overlapping waves.[96] The FDA and the WHO were cautious about gene mutations that mRNA vaccines might cause, but the agencies deemed that the risks of heart inflammation, arrhythmia, embolism, thrombosis, kidney damage, and pneumonia-like illnesses were greater in unvaccinated individuals.[97]

The short-term effects of the vaccine were varied, ranging from headaches, blurred vision, and nausea to fever, fatigue, and flu symptoms through to no adverse effects at all. The Pfizer, Moderna, and AstraZeneca vaccines were all modeled on two doses. Only Johnson & Johnson manufactured a one-dose vaccine, which it released in February 2021, although the CDC noted that it posed pulmonary and neurological health risks to some. The two-dose vaccine experience meant that some patients suffered mild versions of COVID more than once, especially when booster shots were administered in the winters of 2021 and 2022 to counteract new variants. For many, this was, of course, preferable to the high risk of a life-threating illness among those over fifty and those with weak immune systems; the chance of death was estimated to be fourteen times higher among unvaccinated Americans than among those who had received two doses of a vaccine.[98] This did not prevent anti-vaxxers, both conservative and liberal, from arguing that vaccines contain unhealthy chemicals, might trigger allergies and autism, or can heighten the risk of stroke, based on some reports about possible side effects of the Pfizer vaccine.[99] Some viewed vaccines and antivirals like Paxlovid (which the FDA granted emergency-use authorization in December 2021) as agents of a medical-industrial complex designed to turn citizens into zombies, as one Illinois woman told the *Washington Post*, citing the film *I Am Legend*, in which a botched virology experiment creates a deadly disease (although she changed her mind about vaccines after talking to a health professional).[100]

Discourses of immunity in the post-9/11 years raised questions of autoimmunity on somatic and state levels in the face of geopolitical instability, which both revived and moved on from Cold War fears of invasion and assaults on democratic values. Biothreats became headline news when a number of letters sent to members of Congress and media outlets tested positive for anthrax in the weeks following 9/11, leading to five deaths, wild conspiracy theories, and what has been called the "largest biodefense program in American history."[101] This anthrax spore wave normalized the fear that bioweapons would likely be used against the United States. Making a playbook post–Cold War move, President George W. Bush's rhetoric cast the danger to American health and prosperity as an outside threat on the part of bad actors in Afghanistan and Iraq, providing a road map for Trump's attacks on China and the WHO during the early months of COVID-19.

Domestic tensions between Washington, DC, and individual states were palpable. Trump's son-in-law, Jared Kushner, sought federal control over the national stockpile of therapeutics while Trump sought to blame state governors, especially those in blue states. New York governor Andrew Cuomo, who appeared heroic in the first year of COVID, helped fuel these accusations with a sexual misconduct scandal and opaque statistics about the rate of infections in nursing homes.[102] In contrast, California governor Gavin Newsom escaped Trump's ire, perhaps because he was affirmative about the federal response, but that did not mean that he escaped criticism from other Republicans. The numbers of cases and hospitalizations fluctuated widely across California in 2020–2021 and some commentators claimed that greater vaccine availability and vaccine take-up might have saved the lives of some of the 100,000 Californians who died at the start of 2023. In the wake of a recall election in the summer of 2021 during which the electorate questioned the efficacy of state restrictions and stay-at-home orders, Newsom unveiled a statewide SMARTER plan that put equity and investment at the core of public health.[103] The pressures Newsom faced—in one of the bluest states—showed that any governance move, no matter how well considered, was liable to tilt opinion polls, either because it strained the capacity of the health care system or because some argued that it curtailed civil liberties.

Aside from the regional specificities of these cases, it is important to recognize (following sociologist Nik Brown) that immunization is "rife with acute tensions between participation within, and also withdrawal from, necessarily mutual vaccination programmes."[104] To address these tensions, it is helpful to reflect on Italian theorist Roberto Esposito's landmark trilogy, *Communitas* (1998), *Immunitas* (2002), and *Bios* (2004), which opens up a space for biopolitics as an ethic of mutual care. Developing a responsive and responsible bioethics is no easy task, especially in the midst of health crises, when biomedicine "takes centre stage in tensions between the community and the individual."[105] Esposito recognized this in a June 2020 interview conducted during a period of prolonged isolation at home in Naples, Italy. In this lockdown interview he argued that immunization collapses life and death, building on his early argument that health is inseparable "from the mortal risk that runs through it" in overthrowing and re-creating "rules for life."[106] Vaccines may seem like a solution for restabilizing health ecologies and lowering transmission rates, but Esposito contends that administering the patient a nonlethal dose of a virus creates an "immunitary paradigm" that works in reactive mode by hindering "another force from coming into being."[107] Because the vaccine interlinks health and illness, it gives resonance to Esposito's phrase "the enemy is now life's propulsive force" and anchors abstract questions about natural versus induced immunity in the context of the patchwork of decisions individuals and families must make when neither total compliance nor an individualistic response seem wholly appropriate.[108]

Esposito reflected on the relevance of his ideas in the midst of a pandemic when sadness and anxiety were his overriding feelings during an anxious time for Italy. Realizing that immunization was now central to everyday life, Esposito argued that not only was medicine politicized but politics was medicalized, "treating the citizen as a patient in need of perpetual care and turning social deviance into an epidemic disruption to be treated or suppressed."[109] He did not dwell on anti-vaxxers or faith-based objectionists, yet the protocol around public health compliance was precisely why Trump, Paul, and alt-right Christian groups were suspicious of overmedicalization. Herd immunity is unpalatable for its implicit sacrifice of life, but Esposito also realized the economic and psychological dangers of lockdown. Balancing faith in immunization with a recognition of lockdown "desocialization," he cautioned against extremes, arguing that the immune system destroys itself if it crosses "a certain threshold," whereas prolonged isolation creates a "total rupture of social bonds."[110]

In this interview, Esposito tempered his earlier view that "there is no community without some kind of immunity apparatus" with a recognition that extreme immunization erodes community by sealing individuals against one another.[111] He used the immunity metaphor of building barriers against outside forces, but he recognized its dangers because it forces life "into a sort of cage where not only our freedom gets lost but also the very meaning of our existence."[112] Because of this, he argued, immunity has a "bivalent character," both "positive and negative, protective and destructive."[113] Esposito's solution to this entrapment was, first, to recognize the dialectic relationship between community and immunity; and second, to enact a "radical ecological reform" of the capitalist system to deepen commitment to the common good.[114] He sees in this ecological vision a recognition that health and illness intersect and an expansive view of life that affirms the interdependence of personal and social health.

Esposito conceives this vision of an affirmative bioethics as a rejuvenated philosophy of life, arguing in *Terms of the Political* (2008) that "there is never a moment in which the individual can be enclosed in himself or be blocked in a closed system, and so removed from the movement that binds him to his own biological matrix."[115] In this way, he moves beyond both Giorgio Agamben's notion of bare life and Michel Foucault's concept of biopower as the subjection of human bodies to the body politic. For Esposito, the "dual, interlinking process" between medicine and politics is an aspect of the modern state, but he argues that bodies can be the site of resistance rather than just the locus of exploitation.[116] Despite their theoretical differences, Esposito and Foucault each emphasized the theme of care—self-care for Foucault, a caring community for Esposito—which undergirds a somatic ethics that can navigate the subjugating forces of governmentality, including public health governance.

Esposito sees this affirmatory vision as coterminous with a more intense form of community that "constitutes us without belonging to us" in which biopolitics is the continuum "of life" rather than a force "over life."[117] He identifies such a vision in democratic—as opposed to authoritarian—societies as "a point of intersection and tension" rather than a coherent political philosophy, gesturing toward the "common good" (a term he prefers over "public life") that can nurture the "potentiality of life's becoming."[118] Esposito's lack of specific examples is frustrating. Nonetheless, he sees the fulfilment of this potential as resting on the responsibility of caring public institutions to stimulate a communal recognition that individual and collective lives are part of the same ecology.

It is possible to read Esposito's recommendation as a form of health citizenship that hinges not on obedience to a body politic but on voluntary cooperation and mutual care, recognizing that one's own life and health are bound to others. We can see examples of this in the WHO's emphasis on bottom-up approaches to health literacy and health access and in Robert Bellah's vision of citizenship as a deeper communal language inspired by what he calls a "politics of imagination" that recognizes the variegated health landscape beyond the horizon of one's own subject position. Just as Esposito sees an affirmative biopolitics as always open to "more than one feature" of life, so Bellah discerns a combination of "local participation" and "national dialogue" that is aware of multiple scales of communal existence.[119] Although Bellah does not use the term biopolitics, this vision of "active citizen involvement and discussion," characterized by a long-term perspective and "common moral grounding," opens up a middle ground between the extremes of radical individualism on the one side and the unapproachable apparatus of state on the other, creating "spaces for reflection, participation, and the transformation of our institutions."[120]

We can credit Esposito and Bellah with uncoupling Leon Kass's idea of a rich public bioethics from his conservative politics. But there are some limitations. In Bellah's case, the exceptionalist discourse of a good society that "takes social inclusion and participation as a key theme" does not interrogate exclusions, whether due to illness, disability, imprisonment, or other forms of marginalization, while Esposito's focus on physical and community health arguably neglects psychological aspects that can go undetected or are not perceived as readily as what is physically visible.[121] So, although Esposito's affirmative biopolitics seek to go beyond Agamben's conception of bare life, COVID stripped life down to raw existence for many global citizens. This is not the apocalyptic scenario of the zombie noncommunity in Ling Ma's *Severance*, yet the world emergency hinged on threats to physical health on a mass scale, compounded by the anxiety and stress of living in the midst of a prolonged pandemic, leading some researchers to posit the emergence of "COVID stress syndrome."[122]

I have already mentioned some symptoms that lingered long beyond a viral infection and even after vaccination, but as a bridge to the next section on pandemic well-being, I turn to the implications of long COVID—or post-acute sequelae of COVID-19, to use its scientific name—for thinking through the relationship between immunization and biotechnology. Esposito sees immunization as the start rather than an endpoint because if immunity is taken too far it undermines the possibility of community. He was also wary of an overemphasis on medicine or on what he calls the "technicization of life" because reliance on biotechnological solutions brings back into play the negative (or Foucauldian) version of biopower.[123] This backsliding prompted Esposito to write in 2013 that "devices of control and subjugation lead to a corresponding decrease in individual and collective freedoms." Although Rand Paul would jump on this comment to denounce the apparatus of the bioscientific establishment, Esposito meant that when we rely too heavily on technological apparatuses to stay alive and keep in touch with one another, the concept of community becomes thinner and is more precariously circumscribed by the politico-medical force of immunization.[124]

In this climate of precarity, the reinforcement of the message that "we are all in it together" becomes a call for compliance rather than a recognition that some communities and demographics will need more care than others. In describing this thinning of community and diminishment of "vital power," Esposito focuses on bodies over minds, commenting that "no longer content merely to besiege us from the outside, technique has now taken up residence in our very limbs."[125] However, whether it was from infection with the virus, the side effects of vaccination, or the mere endurance of lockdown, when alcohol use, depression, suicide, and domestic violence were all on the rise, minds were also under siege at a time when health care services were at capacity saving bodies.[126] The U.S. Census Bureau calculated that 42 percent of Americans in December 2020 were suffering from depression compared to around 11 percent the previous year, but many mental health challenges overlapped with physical symptoms and proved tricky to treat at a time when health care institutions were operating at full stretch in their attempts to save lives. Given the global spread of COVID, these challenges have arcs that span different generations and communities, but the aftereffects of the pandemic spilled into "a mass disabling event": an estimated 18 million Americans had long COVID at the end of 2022, a condition without a technological fix nearly three years after the first deaths in the pandemic.

While the biotech race for an effective and safe vaccine propelled the national pandemic story, a less coherent and often submerged set of smaller narratives resonated with Americans experiencing isolation behind closed doors at a distance from one another and health care workers—what Bruno Latour called a "carapace of consequences" that he learned "to drag around" during the "ground zero" of lockdown.[127] In such a state, it is difficult to maintain peripheral vision when the Zoom or telehealth screen becomes the primary medium of communication. Rather than a "catastrophic rupture," this reality approximates to what Elizabeth Povinelli calls the "ordinary exhaustion" of life under prolonged lockdown when most experiences became "quasi events."[128] But instead of Latour's and Povinelli's encaged yet dislocated reality undermining Esposito's search for an affirmative biopolitics, it injects more urgency into ensuring the common good is not lost by retreating into isolation, relying too heavily on digitized data, or putting supreme faith in technofixes. As I discuss in the final section, just staying well in a time of COVID was challenging, especially when there was so much contention about lifestyle choice and therapeutics. Yet the possibility of emergent practices and interconnected communities meant that not all life was bare.

Keeping Well in a Time of COVID

When Trump emerged from Walter Reed National Military Medical Center on October 5, 2020, following treatment for coronavirus, he used the occasion as a public relations stunt. Following an initial White House announcement four days earlier that the president had tested positive for SARS-CoV-2, the official medical report implied that there was one concerning moment when his oxygen levels had dipped, but the *New York Times* later reported that his oxygen level had been precarious and that he had had pulmonary infiltrates, although he had not been put on a ventilator.[129] The official announcements were crafted to ensure that the president did not look weak or overly reliant on medicine. Nonetheless, it was the combination of therapeutics he received at Walter Reed that seemingly helped the seventy-four-year-old president recover enough to leave after three days. Trump was reported to have received remdesivir, the steroid dexamethasone, Pepcid for heartburn, and an infusion of polyclonal antibodies. The biotech company Regeneron Pharmaceuticals had announced its preliminary findings just a few days earlier that the Regn-CoV2 antibody cocktail showed signs of reducing the viral load after a Phase 3 trial for nonhospitalized patients whose immune systems appeared unresponsive to other treatments.[130] However, because Regeneron had not yet opened discussions with the FDA about the use of this new treatment on hospitalized patients at risk of a severe case of COVID-19, Trump received an experimental infusion that would not have been administered to most other Americans at that stage.

Just eight days after being released from Walter Reed, Trump returned to the reelection campaign trail. Speaking unmasked at a rally in Johnstown, Pennsylvania, he claimed that he "felt like Superman" and promised his Republican followers that "the vaccines are coming soon, the therapeutics, and frankly the cure. All I know is I took something—whatever the hell it was, I felt good very quickly."[131] Not only was the president quick to show the public he was strong enough to be elected, but he both praised his medical team ("what great talented people") and trivialized medicine, again attacking the WHO, obscuring the treatment he received ("I don't know what it was, antibodies, antibodies, I don't know"), and claiming that he could have been back on the campaign trail five days earlier. More dangerously, and without evidence, he asserted he was now immune from SARS-CoV-2 and "could come down and start kissing everybody," before pivoting to his rival, Joe Biden, who masked assiduously in public: "Biden would terminate our recovery, delay the vaccine, prolong the pandemic, and annihilate the economy with draconian unscientific lockdowns."[132] In this statement, not only did Trump claim that science was on his side, but he returned to one of his 2016 campaign themes that he alone could fix the whole system.

Trump's phrase "I alone can fix it" when he accepted the Republican nomination in July 2016 took on ominous proportions four years later as he stoked tribal loyalties instead of seeking to balance public health integrity, fiscal prudence, civil rights, and social cohesion, alongside an honest conversation with medical and scientific experts about strategy, capacity, and messaging. We have already seen how the tensions within the Trump White House Coronavirus Response Team led to mixed messaging, but the president's opinions on therapeutics hovered between dangerous and ludicrous. At a press briefing on April 23, 2020, Trump told Deborah Birx, his coronavirus response coordinator, that health officials should research whether "powerful light brought inside the body" or injecting "disinfectant" into the lungs could help patients fight COVID. Two profound problems were that Trump did not attend briefings and was not well informed on science. The president also liked to ad lib, so when the acting homeland security under-secretary for science and technology William Bryan said that "bleach will kill the virus" on external surfaces "in five minutes" Trump misunderstood Bryan to mean that this can be used on the human body.[133]

Arguably, this bleach incident was the moment the White House lost control over the pandemic narrative, but there were other instances of dangerous public health advice. Even as he was keen to grant FDA approval to Gilead Sciences for administering remdesivir to hospitalized patients, Trump continued to pitch the anti-malaria drug hydroxychloroquine, saying without any scientific evidence, "What do you have to lose? Take it."[134] Although hydroxychloroquine had undergone a small-scale French trial, social media figures such as Elon Musk and pundits on Fox News seemed to be Trump's chief influencers rather than NIH scientists, given that Fauci repeatedly warned against its experimental use.[135] Trump habitually defended himself by claiming that he was floating hydroxychloroquine as one choice among others alongside the anti-bacterial antibiotic Zithromax to reduce the risks of patients with COVID infections being hospitalized and being put on ventilators.[136] But behind the scenes he was pressurizing Indian prime minister Narendra Modi to release hydroxychloroquine supplies, and the Department of Health and Human Services received a whistleblower complaint that the federal government was risking scientific credibility by pushing "technologies that lack merit."[137] These incidents show how casual remarks about health freedom linked to shadow White House policies that were in tension with medical science.

Groups like the People's CDC Movement believed that state public health messaging was too lax and that questions needed to be asked about the efficacy and integrity of the CDC.[138] The antiscience grip on the White House tightened in August 2020, when the president chose to add neuroradiologist Scott Atlas to the Coronavirus Task Force. With the relationship between Trump and Fauci ever more strained, Atlas became the president's medical advisor. He shared Trump's skepticism about mask mandates and school closures and his disdain for the

Affordable Care Act. Atlas had advised previous Republican leaders, but it seems that Trump chose him because of his Fox News appearances and his status as an outsider in the medical community, as evidenced by a letter a group of immunologists and microbiologists published denouncing "the falsehoods and misrepresentations of science recently fostered by Dr. Scott Atlas" soon after his appointment to the White House team.[139] These Stanford University infectious disease experts believed that Atlas was undermining "the credible science that guides effective public health policy," especially his implication that herd immunity was an answer to COVID, as he told Fox News just before joining the president's team.[140] Atlas stated that he was following science, but he blamed left-leaning media for vilifying hydroxychloroquine. He claimed that it was a "super safe" drug (he could not have known its efficacy for SARS-CoV-2 when he said that) and he possibly fed the president "parallel data" prior to his role on the coronavirus task force that may have fueled Trump's early comments.[141] Dogged by controversy, Atlas resigned from the task force after Trump's election defeat in November, but his is appointment was a symbol of how ideologically distorted public health claims often hide behind the mask of science.

As well as dramatizing chaotic governance at a time of national crisis and the president's unwillingness to listen to the scientific community, the tumultuous months of 2020 also revealed a deeper structural issue related to the oversight of mainstream (allopathic) and alternative (homeopathic) drugs. Although rumors abounded about Trump's medication regime and the lax protocols followed by the medical team in the Trump White House, there is no evidence that he believed in homeopathic remedies (his presidential medical reports reputedly listed all the drugs he was taking).[142] Yet his opinions on hydroxychloroquine approximated to the homeopathic principle that like cures like, and his comments on sunlight and disinfectant might be framed as alternatives to allopathic medicine. These views also chimed with Trump's resistance to the federal system—in this case, the resistance of the FDA to approving homeopathic remedies. The FDA's regulatory framework does not extend to homeopathic remedies beyond listing them as dietary supplements, as codified by the Dietary Supplement Health and Education Act of 1994. However, FDA officials held a hearing in April 2015 to take into account public opinion on the issue, a consultation that led in 2019 to FDA withdrawing a long-standing Compliance Policy Guide on the premise that it had "encountered multiple situations in which homeopathic drug products posed a significant risk to patients," and in 2022 to final guidance on homeopathic products and safety.[143]

This FDA process began prior to COVID-19 but may have been sharpened by misinformation about pandemic origins and trajectories and by a recognition that the homeopathic market had grown significantly since it had established its policy guide in 1988, especially as between 2007 and 2012 the proportion of U.S. adults who used homeopathic medicine increase by an estimated 15 percent. The revised FDA guidelines were the opposite of what some alternative medicine and health freedom advocates desired when they lobbied the White House in the early 1990s, a time President Clinton was aiming for a major reform of health care. Homeopathic practitioners were unhappy that Clinton's Task Force on National Health Care Reform did not include alternative remedies in its health insurance bracket. The White House received a number of letters in 1993 from concerned individuals, one of whom wrote passionately that health freedom is enshrined in the Constitution and that the FDA was "viciously suppressing . . . truthful information about natural/alternative health benefits, supplements and herbs."[144]

Despite the activism of the National Health Federation, a group that defends consumer rights to use dietary supplements, there was no evidence then that the FDA was suppressing information about homeopathy, especially given that Clinton established a Commission on Complementary and Alternative Health Policy within the Department of Health and Human Services in his final year as president to consider health and wellness from pluralistic perspectives.[145] However, in 2019, the FDA began to differentiate responsible homeopathy from dubious marketing practices, issuing warnings to companies for violating good manufacturing regulations in a number of cases because the products were falsely marketed as containing only sterile ingredients.[146] Seductive marketing during a pandemic is particularly dangerous when consumers feel more vulnerable about their own or their family's health and when health services are stretched because they are dealing with infections and hospitalizations. An illustrative case in point is the forsythia fruit remedy promoted by blogger Alan Krumwiede in *Contagion*, a substance that is typically used in Chinese medicine either orally to treat conditions including tonsillitis, heart disease, vomiting, fever, and muscle soreness or intravenously in combination for treating bronchiolitis. Although forsythia may have antiviral or antibacterial properties, no clinical trials have corroborated its benefits or determined what dosage is effective or safe, except that it should not be taken during pregnancy.[147] The case of Krumwiede is less about whether forsythia counteracts viral infection and more about the fact that he fakes his infection (claiming on his blog Truth Serum Now "If I'm here tomorrow, you'll know it works") in order to dupe his followers into buying the remedy from him while simultaneously resisting the state-sponsored MEV-1 vaccine.

In *Contagion*, Krumwiede is a lone operator who seeks celebrity and profit with no regard for the health of others and exploits the media channels available to him. A decade later, in the midst of the COVID-19 pandemic, the volume and scope of digital information had grown exponentially.[148] Social media can also be a bewildering space of opinion rather than reliable health advice, and there was little in 2020 that could help Americans navigate the over two hundred symptoms of long COVID, including brain fog and extreme fatigue.[149] Medical evidence and more responsible congressional oversight in 2021–2022 improved recognition of long COVID, yet there was no authentic medical test for it and it went underreported in communities of color and among poorer Americans who could rarely afford time away from work.[150] Media outlets speculated that brain fog was an immune reaction, was caused by brain inflammation, or was due to microstrokes. This confusion heightened the scariness and unpredictability of the health expe-

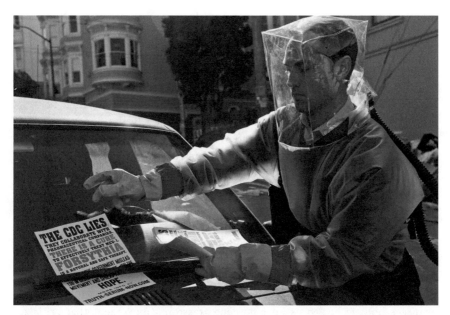

Figure 7.2. Alan Krumwiede (Jude Law) posting anti-CDC propaganda. *Contagion* (2011). Moviestore Collection Ltd/Alamy Photo.

riences. "Everything in my brain was white static" said a thirty-one-year-old female lawyer, while a sixty-year-old Californian male described wandering around a grocery store "like a zombie" after he thought he had recovered.[151] These *New York Times* interviews, published the day of an altercation between Rand Paul and Anthony Fauci in the Senate chamber, emphasized that brain fog could hit all ages in bewildering ways, leading to an inability to work and a sharp erosion of quality of life, but the report offered no therapeutic trajectory that might alleviate brain fog, aside from community support via a Survivor Corps network.

At the time of writing there is no definitive allopathic treatment for long COVID brain fog. However, by late 2022 reports had begun to appear about the potential effectiveness of a combination of guanfacine (typically used to treat ADHD) and N-acetylcysteine (used for traumatic brain injury), although the small patient sample of a Yale Medical School trial means that controlled trials that include a placebo under the auspices of the NIH's RECOVER Initiative (Researching COVID to Enhance Recovery) and a new federal Office of Long Covid Research and Practice within the Biden administration will be needed to gauge efficacy.[152]

Other pharmaceuticals such as naltrexone (which is typically prescribed for addiction) have shown some benefits for brain fog, while memory-enhancing supplements such as magnesium, vitamin D, and spirulina may alleviate chronic stress, although without clinical trials it is hard to know to what extent these supplements target the complex symptoms of long COVID. The growing interest of the biohacking community in ancestral medicine and the homeopathic use of fungi and tree bark like lion's mane mushrooms and ginkgo biloba may also have short-term benefits for mental health while boosting immunity. Some biohackers look beyond mood and cognition, such as Canadian nutritionist Brittany Ford (see chapter 5). In focusing on optimizing mitochondrial health by taking vitamin B12 and on microdosing with the cannabinoid THCV and the psychedelic fungi psilocybin, Ford echoes Dave Asprey's emphasis on a healthy gut to promote well-being, to protect against the accrual of zombie cells that hasten senescence, and to prevent the buildup of toxins such as mercury, lead, and mold.[153]

It is clear that long COVID has accelerated interest in specific therapeutics the FDA has approved for treating SARS-CoV-2 and within the biohacking community in a more holistic awareness of health, ranging from exercise and yoga to red light therapy and vagus nerve stimulation to NAD+ supplements and DIY microdosing. However, given the significant increase in antidepressants prescribed by physicians in response to widespread reports of anxiety, depression, and ADHD symptoms in 2020–2022, there is a danger that the COVID acceleration merely intensified drug dependency.[154] In response, the biohacking community sees holistic health as an emergent grassroots movement that criticizes public health for being an institutional system of top-down interventions and warnings—an impetus that leads Asprey to uphold biological autonomy while declaring "back off central tracking!" in his critique of what he believes are forms of government overreach.[155]

The libertarian wing of the biohacking movement that propels a quest for alternatives to modern medicine might be seen as empowering at both the individual and group level. Yet it can also lead to a trial-and-error approach to health. This DIWO (doing it with others) ethos is a far cry from Trump's antiscience speculations about potential cures for SARS-CoV-2. Nonetheless, the biohacker space shares a quest to evade the state apparatus of public health by yoking ancestral practices to a piecemeal embrace of technology. Rather than embracing an accessible and inclusive middle space for wellness, DIY biohacking, in its emphasis on health freedom, may exacerbate health risks while simultaneously ignoring health inequities inflected by race, class, gender, and sexuality. Ultimately, during the COVID years, biohacker wariness of Big Tech and the move toward deep state conspiracy theories were in direct tension with the intensified democratic community that Roberto Esposito believes is needed to nurture affirmatory bioethics and ecologically attuned public health.

8   *Invisible Toxicities*

ENVIRONMENTAL HEALTH AND

THE LIMITS OF BIOTECHNOLOGY

In June 2001, management consultant Darryl Vernon Poole, founder of the Cambridge Institute for Applied Research think tank, briefed George W. Bush's Domestic Policy Council about potential improvements in health care and environmental policy. Although Bush had been in the White House for only six months, the briefing was clear that health care issues would be central to the 2004 election, spanning Medicaid to fund car seats for children to "what the public regards as Environmental Affairs: Water & Air Pollution & Contamination."[1] National economic productivity in a "new Industrial Age" was the chief driver behind these recommendations, rather than the global ecological implications of the Anthropocene, a now-familiar term Dutch meteorologist Paul Crutzen had coined the previous year to demarcate an era in which the health of the environment and animals is circumscribed by human activity.[2] In an exclamatory mood, Poole stressed that "it's not the Environment, it's HEALTH!," adding that "the real issue to most Americans is Health. In terms of Environment that means whatever may impact personal Health <u>First</u>, and quality of life <u>Second</u>."

In his briefing, Poole coupled policy areas that are often held at arm's length in government, even though he was not a specialist in human health or environmental health. The periodic coupling and uncoupling of these two aspects of health is a major theme of this final chapter and in this particular instance, it raises two key points.[3] The first is the ways that environmental health is typically delimited by instrumental concerns about human health; the second is how both health and the environment are often reduced at the government level to talking points that can give an electoral advantage to a candidate or party. Think tanks are often persuasive voices that offer practical pathways for government officials, yet in chasing voting trends they are not necessarily philosophically consistent or robust in their definitions, especially on complex topics like health. This variability is acute for environmental health because, as Jennifer Thomson argues in *The Wild and the Toxic* (2019), "fundamental questions about the meaning of health, to whom it applies, and how it should be measured and protected remain unasked."[4] I return to Thomson's insights to extend the discussion of ecological health from chapter 7 as a route to forging perspective and praxis in an age of biotech. But it is important to note that White House briefings do not always sway federal technology policy, although they can have an indirect influence. While Bush clearly did not heed Poole's advice to shift from carbon to hydrogen to meet the demands of the "New Industrial Age," in the summer of 2001 he claimed that he was taking climate change "very seriously," including controlling diesel emissions and developing biomonitoring techniques to assess the effects of climate change on human health.[5]

Pivotal for understanding early-century planetary politics was the Bush administration's view that the Kyoto Protocol of 1997 was "fatally flawed" in its efforts to push governments to reduce greenhouse gas emissions, mainly because it posed an economic risk to the United States.[6] This did not mean that the Bush administration eschewed all environmental policies. For example, in his June 2001 speech on climate change, Bush affirmed his commitment to international cooperation and a "science-based response to the issue of global warming" drawn from "a wide spectrum of views."[7] Such views included the Arizona-based conservative nonprofit Doctors for Disaster Preparedness, the head of which wrote to the White House to state that "the scientific evidence is decisively *against* the prospect of any severe anthropogenic climate changes now or in the foreseeable future" and to tout the benefits of carbon dioxide emission.[8] In his public speeches, Bush sidestepped denial of global warming while recognizing the responsibility of the United States to reduce greenhouse gas emissions (although reports have suggested that Vice-President Cheney led a covert disinformation campaign to obscure the pace of climate change).[9] However, Bush believed that the Kyoto targets were unrealistic and that China and India should play their roles in the global effort without the exemptions the Kyoto Protocol offered them. Bush announced national climate change initiatives that sought to devise creative technological solutions and resolve uncertainties, but because of his administration's commitment to big business and free enterprise, nature was seen as an exploitable resource.[10] For this reason, although Bush began this 2001 speech by stating that he cherished "Earth's well-being," his administration's emphasis on "economic growth and prosperity" failed to recognize that complex ecosystems were facing profound threats at the dawn of the twenty-first century that might intensify health risks for both human and nonhuman populations.[11]

We might be tempted to look toward recent Democratic administrations for more progressive responses to climate change. However, although Clinton, Obama, and Biden occasionally acknowledged the fragile health of the planet, political topics relating to environmental health typically skewed toward anthropocentric concerns during their political careers. For example, in the spring of 2007, Illinois senator Obama gave an impassioned speech about the need to cut energy dependence, even evoking President Nixon in his argument that "for the sake of our security, our economy, our jobs and our planet, the age of oil must end in our time."[12] Obama continued the planet-in-peril theme into his presidency. This included a commitment to reducing carbon emissions and efforts to bring federal government departments into closer dialogue with the Environmental Protection Agency (EPA) and the National Center for Environmental Health of the Centers for Disease Control and Prevention (CDC) in order to tackle the physical health vulnerabilities of climate change, leading him to focus his remarks at an April 2015 event at Howard University on health care training, the rising rates of asthma and malaria, and a progressive attitude toward open data.[13] This tendency to frame planetary issues in humanistic terms was epitomized by a White House summit two months later that emphasized empowering local communities, a direct response to reports about poor air quality, food scarcity, and a potential mass animal extinction due to ecosystem degradation.[14]

The environmental health pendulum swung sharply from planetary management to denial of the climate crisis when Donald Trump entered the White House in January 2017. Trump not only amplified the skepticism of many congressional Republicans about the scientific consensus that global warming is long term and created by humans, he also sought a divergent path to the United Nations Framework Convention on Climate Change and the World Health Organization (WHO), a foreshadowing of his criticisms of international health governance during the COVID-19 pandemic (see chapter 7).

In contrast to Trump's tendency to reduce the health consequences of extreme weather events to legalistic approaches to land management, President Joe Biden featured the pandemic and global warming as two of the four colliding crises he outlined in his campaign speeches of 2020, approximating to Bruno Latour's view that COVID-19 revealed how we are all "entangled, ensnared, enmired" with the Earth.[15] Breathing a sigh of relief at the outcome of the presidential election with respect to "taking climate seriously," the editors of *Time* magazine declared that Biden's climate policy will "shape the 21st century geopolitical and economic landscape and help determine whether the world can stave off the worst effects of catastrophic climate change."[16] By recognizing that Earth's inhabitants are already in what Latour calls the "critical zone," an early sign of this eco-promise was Biden's marking of the EPA's fifty-year anniversary in December 2020.[17] At that event, Biden promised "bold, progressive action" on the climate crisis, echoing the emphasis of his presidential envoy for climate, John Kerry, on the vital importance of maintaining healthy oceans and lowering pollutants, although this perspective was also an ecologically palatable way of mitigating national security threats and promoting a "clean-tech revolution."[18]

Between Ecoskepticism and Climate Activism

It is not just to the executive branch we should turn to assess why a balanced understanding of environmental health is such a rarity. Impediments are also visible in an increasingly polarized U.S. Congress, in which recognition of the links between climate change and public health emerge only occasionally. Even when catastrophic events are discussed in Congress, the discourse tends to be delimited. A case in point is a Senate hearing on the health impacts of global warming held in October 2007. Democrats had retaken control of Congress that January after a six-year wait and were eager to discuss how federal mobilization in response to Hurricane Katrina might have been improved. Michael McCally, director of Physicians for Social Responsibility, called the Gulf Coast disaster a shameful event in which vulnerable Louisianans received "inadequate or no health care at all."[19] But the hearing focused squarely on the devastating impact to human health instead of considering the long-term damage to marine and coastal ecosystems which, as I discuss below, came into sharp focus after the spill from BP's Deepwater Horizon oil rig in the Gulf three years later.

At the time of writing, few national governments have placed the health of the environment over the drive for economic prosperity: Denmark may be the exception, although health questions might be asked about its territory of Greenland, as the final section of this chapter explores. Bioethical concerns that conservationist Rachel Carson brought to the attention of the federal government and industry in the 1960s and 1970s have since become deeply divisive, and the relatively neutral term "climate change" is now frequently replaced by the potentially apocalyptic "climate crisis" as the earth's temperature climbs and extreme weather events increase in frequency.[20] As earlier chapters have shown, there are questions to be asked about how much science political leaders understand. Questions need also to be asked about rival truth claims that are charged when it comes to climate science. The speculative claims of pressure groups such as the Doctors for Disaster Preparedness have undermined trust in public institutions by "employing (often quite marginal) counter-scientific claims" that discourage meaningful participation in climate issues at community level.[21]

In particular, questions about the sustainability of food sources has intensified the manufacture of genetically modified foods in the search for "improvements to the quality and quantity of our Nation's food supply," as George W. Bush said when he launched National Biotechnology Week in May 2001, which was linked to the search for hardier crop varieties and vegetables with longer cycles of edibility.[22] Working within a coordinated framework, the U.S. Department of Agriculture, the EPA, and the FDA have developed a science-based approach to agricultural biotechnology, balancing a commitment to innovation and productivity with a careful assessment of the biosafety of genetically modified organisms and the risks they pose to human health.[23] The interagency view is that genetically modified crops can offer incremental improvements to food chain supplies and the reduction of waste.

However, the Department of Agriculture has done little to allay the health concerns of environmental activists about the biotechnologies big agrochemical corporations such as Monsanto use. The controversy regarding Monsanto has centered on its use of herbicides and pesticides in an effort to cultivate hardier crops, but which had a disproportionate health impact upon Black communities, notably in Anniston, Alabama, where a Monsanto plant produced polychlorinated biphenyl (PCB) for nearly five decades.[24] The temptation is to go big when dealing with environmental toxicity, as Paolo Bacigalupi does in his 2009 novel *The Windup Girl*, about the exploitative agricultural corporation Agri-Gen, which releases branded genetically modified products in order to prevent the future world from tipping into mass starvation. But links between local and national reflections are equally important. For example, the environmentally aware novelist Ruth Ozeki dramatizes the conflicting world views of corporations and activists in her Idaho novel *All Over Creation* (2013), and ecoactivist singer Neil Young castigates Monsanto's use of "poison-ready" crops in the title track of his 2015 album *The Monsanto Years* and in his short Alabama-based film *Seeding Fear*, about the corporation's efforts to destroy the viability of small-scale farming.[25] Just as important for spotlighting national health and safety risks, mainstream media outlets occasionally react to Monsanto's "harvest of fear," as *Vanity Fair* called it, despite the company's efforts to discredit journalists who disagree with its claims. Going further, independent researchers have challenged Monsanto about the safety of its herbicides, contesting its marketing assertions that transgenic crop biotechnologies will safely produce food surpluses—some researchers have gone so far as to suggest a conspiratorial pact between the EPA and Monsanto.[26]

The rise of climate activism at both the local and global levels in the 2010s has heightened consumer awareness of so-called Frankenfoods and has prevented government officials and big business leaders from monopolizing discourses of sustainability.[27] But the danger is that deeply polarized views about the reality, provenance, and speed of global warming do not facilitate the kind of reasoned middle ground in which both behavioral and technological transformations can coexist. Robert Butler called for such an intermediary space in *The Longevity Revolution* (2008), not only emphasizing the perilous state of the ozone layer, the quality of water, and the temperature of the earth's surface, but the increased prevalence of a range of diseases that do not stop at national borders, including malaria, cholera, the return of tuberculosis, and a heightened risk of cancer.[28] Butler's vision of longevity turns in the final section of his book to heightened risks of "shortevity" as a physical and existential threat not just for countries with developing economies but also for vulnerable American communities.[29] Butler is mindful of the important role of environmental consciousness raising, but the middle ground he seeks consists of a "constructive alliance between nature and economic development, ensuring mutual adaptability."[30]

In contrast to federal policy that sometimes shirks tough confrontations with big business (such as requiring that genetically modified foods be labeled), environmental activists are keen to level blame at politicians and corporations and raise questions about tech solutions. Some activists eschew technology, while others advocate its responsible deployment. For the international Ecomodernist Project, this entails the recognition that "the modernization processes that have increasingly liberated humanity from nature" are "double-edged, since they have also degraded the natural environment," as expressed in its 2015 manifesto.[31] This emphasis on responsible tech chimes with the commitment to renewable biosolutions of the World Economic Forum and the Organisation for Economic Co-operation and Development. Yet British activist George Monbiot is critical of the Ecomodernist Project for privileging urban over rural life and ignoring the benefits of small-scale farming, while the group's push "to leave nature behind" conflicts with the argument of Canadian ecoactivist Bill McKibben that it is important to mobilize local environmental engagement for a "durable future."[32]

McKibben began his writing career in 1989 by warning against the "end of nature," a year prior to George H. W. Bush proclaiming that "today science and technology are assuming a broader and more interrelated role in human life than ever before," especially with an increase in the use of biotechnologies for food production.[33] *The End of Nature* closes with a pessimistic account of how inertia undermines the possibility of a collective environmentalist effort, but McKibben's 2003 book *Enough: Staying Human in an Engineered Age* develops a more nuanced picture of early twenty-first century humanity. While George H. W. Bush was celebrating the "eye of technology" for "etching the idea of freedom on the psyche of humanity," McKibben argued in *The End of Nature* that western societies already have enough sophisticated technologies to make their lives comfortable.[34] McKibben believes that any more technology will not only create instability in the infrastructure but will further destabilize global and regional ecosystems already under siege from the extraction of unsustainable energy sources. In contrast to his enthusiastic advocacy of the "deep economy" that he discerns in local activism is his growing despair about the future of the planet, given the sluggish response of the world's largest countries to climate change. This pessimistic turn leads McKibben to argue in both *The End of Nature* and *Enough* that "human meaning dangles by a far thinner thread than we had thought" and that a collective "we"—community, nation, species—might vanish forever. This vision is even more apocalyptic than the face in the sand washed away by the tide that Michel Foucault evoked nearly forty years earlier, as discussed in the introduction.[35]

McKibben has developed this view further in *Eaarth* (2011) and *Falter* (2019) and in his work for the grassroots organization 350.org (est. 2008). He argues that the planet has become a radically different place in the twenty-first century and that this transformative shift demands that human communities adopt an intensified approach to environmental care and justice.[36] Jennifer Thomson reads McKibben as an environmental conservative with a focus on "lifestyle curation" and "scientific management" rather than a figure who embraces biocentrism as a "radical more-than-human democracy open to interruptions."[37] Although Thomson's reading is persuasive, McKibben does not avoid critiquing administrations. In addition to agreeing with progressive Vermont senator Bernie Sanders (and many others) that the Trump administration was a clear and present danger to the climate crisis, he called Obama "the carbon president" in 2011, wrote an open letter to Hillary Clinton during her presidential run in 2015 that judged her climate crisis rhetoric to be "correct but eye-glazing," and made swipes at Congress while noting promise in the Biden administration and President Biden's stand against the oil industry.[38]

More helpfully, McKibben's stance might be positioned at the convergence of environmental ideas and energies that enable him to speak meaningfully in both scientific and political registers. One task of this middle ground is to maintain—or regain—a sense of proportion, especially because the immensity of climate change can lead to what Timothy Clark terms "derangements of scale" that slide across perspectives on person, place, and planet for delineating the zonal impact of climate change.[39] In exploring what Latour calls the "implications, folds, overlaps, entanglements" of human and environmental health, this chapter returns to these interrelations between person, place, and planet in tandem with the ecological view that degradation of one aspect of an ecosystem causes direct and indirect stresses throughout the biosphere, from microbiomes to apex predators.[40]

In focusing primarily on the 2010s, this chapter explores the contested yet pivotal place of health within environmental politics. It focuses particularly on human-generated toxins that cause physical and psychological harm to planetary life. Emphasizing the importance of a holistic approach to health in appraising the damage and potentiality of climate technologies, the next section deploys literary critic Heather Houser's concept of ecosickness to explore conflicting government and ecoactivist responses to degraded environments and the health consequences for their human and nonhuman populations in hot and cold places. I contrast the technique of bioremediation for cleaning up toxic spills in the Gulf of Mexico and in Florida with the ecoactivist writer Jeff VanderMeer's imaginative response to contaminated wilderness in his 2014 Southern Reach trilogy and his 2017 speculative biotech novel *Borne*, then move in the final section to discuss toxic legacies in the contrasting perilous spaces of subarctic Alaska and arctic Greenland. Focusing on the potential for an ecological reimagining as a responsible and revitalizing path through the complex health landscapes of the early twenty-first century, these final two sections assess the overlap between rewilding techniques and extinction revival, or "de-extinction," a controversial biotechnology for reviving fragile ecosystems.

Eco-Anxiety and Invisible Toxicities

It is open to debate whether genetically modified foods make consumers sick, but there is no doubt that environmental anxieties relating to food insecurity, pollutants, and global warming have deleterious effects on the body and the mind.[41] When people assess climate change and toxicity, physical health is regularly prioritized over mental health, as evidenced by the dearth of comprehensive psychiatric and sociological studies of climate change anxiety at the time of writing. Nonetheless, surveys revealing different forms of eco-anxiety and emerging concepts such as "solastalgia" and "ecological grief" point to the intensifying health impacts of environmental strain and global warming—for example, in a forum run by the UK's Mental Health Foundation charity at the 2021 UN Climate Change Conference at Glasgow (COP26) and a WHO study of vulnerable children and extreme weather events.[42]

It is often difficult to separate science from rumor when the consequences of toxicity for holistic health are discussed. Take, for example, the Republican suspicions that fluoride in national water supplies during the early Cold War was not an aid to dental health but a brainwashing agent, a conspiracy theory that the National Health Federation, a natural medicine lobbying group, was still circulating in the 1990s.[43] Pathological metaphors have long been deployed to amplify environmental threats, but the truth is that climate anxiety and ecosickness have become more pervasive in the postgenomic period, despite warnings such as Rachel Carson's landmark book *Silent Spring* (1962) about the effects of pollution on coastal ecosystems and the consciousness raising of the ecoactivist groups Friends of the Earth and Greenpeace USA in the 1970s and 1980s. The palpable and impalpable collide in the term ecosickness, with small symptoms hiding large toxic dangers that are neither reported nor easily detectable, accompanied by uncertainty about both cause and cure. Heather Houser argues that the difference between effect and affect is indistinct because the line between toxic environments and human disease is difficult to trace for scientists, physicians, and patients alike. In Houser's view, this is because climate anxiety "can excite different affects in different people, and sometimes affect has no specifiable catalyst," even though it is felt physically, cognitively, and emotionally.[44]

Houser opens her 2014 book *Ecosickness in Contemporary U.S. Fiction* with the example of the fictional Los Angeles housewife Carol White, played by Julianne Moore in Todd Haynes's 1995 film *Safe*, who experiences "asthma attacks, headaches, stinging red eyes, hive outbreaks, and seizures" that are lumped together under the wastebasket diagnosis of "multiple chemical sensitivity" because no other diagnosis fits.[45] Carol's intolerance of chemicals in *Safe* seems to be caused by external toxins rather than electromagnetic sensitivity, but it also stems from her barely articulated experiences of depression, headaches, panic attacks, and sleeplessness that exacerbate feelings of paranoia. In her analysis of millennial fictions, Houser shows how ecosickness is a "powerful organizing concept" that interconnects organisms and environments.[46] Yet if we are to regain bioethically attuned lateral vision, we need to keep both cultural affects and scientific etiologies in the frame.

One guide to this double vision is weird science writer Jeff VanderMeer, to whom I turn at key points in this chapter for his demarcation of a critical space for ecological health. For example, in VanderMeer's 2017 novel *Borne*, the half-animal, half-human eponymous figure who possesses a heightened environmental sensibility says "I see it, I taste it. All the contamination. The low-level radiation, the storage sites, the runoff. Every place is sick—there's sick everywhere."[47] This vision of ecosickness as sensed by an outsider figure points to the importance of combating what a 1997 Environmental Defense Fund report calls "toxic ignorance" about chemicals that might pose health hazards, despite the development of the EPA's Toxics Release Inventory since the mid-1980s.[48] We might think of toxins as triggering skin rashes and respiratory problems, but there is evidence to show that air and water pollutants are associated with an increased risk of psychiatric disorders, which might explain Carol White's form of ecosickness.[49] A key facet of consumer advice in the *Toxic Ignorance* report is to retain proportion, especially because ecosickness skews stable frames of reference. Just as chapter 7 showed that it is important that citizens not passively absorb public health warnings issued in the national interest, this Environmental

Defense Fund report is useful in helping consumers retain critical insights while guiding them away from apocalyptic imaginings about a reckless biomedical-industrial complex.

In this section, I use Susan Prescott's and Jeffrey Bland's argument of 2020 that discourses of planetary health often blur scales of person, place, and planet in order to work through concepts of clarity and opacity that characterize the relationship between toxicity and environmental health.[50] I do so by extending the frame of public health to consider fauna and flora in different habitats—southern in this section, northern in the next—that are often overlooked in discourses that focus on the preservation of human lives. I initially focus on two southern localities in an effort to rescue perspective and praxis from these complex bioethical debates. The first is the Gulf Coast, the site of Hurricane Katrina in 2005 and the Deepwater Horizon petrochemical disaster in 2010. The second is the fragile ecosystem of the Everglades in south Florida as a conservation concern for both environmentalists and politicians. These two southern case studies enable me to assess different scales of toxicity and degradation in relation to the health of human and nonhuman life, illustrated by a reading of VanderMeer's Southern Reach trilogy of 2014, which explores the health consequences and existential triggers of the enigmatic and potentially dangerous Area X.

The unprecedented oil spill fifty miles from the Louisiana coast caused by a blowout on the BP Deepwater Horizon drilling platform on April 20, 2010, was a catastrophic threat to a marine and coastal ecosystem still recovering from the toxic floodwaters and traumatic impact of Hurricane Katrina. Exacerbating the health threats of an eighty-five-mile stretch between Baton Rouge and New Orleans that had long been called "cancer alley" due to the high concentration of industrial facilities and lingering toxicity of PCBs, the fifteen-foot waters precipitated by Katrina flooded largely low-income coastal communities, submerging countless cars and houses and leading to the release of gasoline, antifreeze, lead, and asbestos into the Gulf of Mexico and domestic water supplies.[51] Less than five years later, the Deepwater Horizon explosion released 200 to 350 million gallons of crude oil over eighty-seven days, further testing the resilience of vulnerable coastal communities and posing profound health threats to marine and coastal fauna.[52]

Oil prospecting in the Gulf developed rapidly after World War II, but the idea that offshore drilling could be seen as environmentally responsible because it protects "natural resource," as George H. W. Bush argued in 1992, was not borne out by the environmental consequences of oil spills.[53] When the Republicans adopted the campaign slogan "Drill, baby, drill!" at their 2008 national convention, seventy years after the first offshore well was established in the Louisiana wetlands, it was clear that profits were more important than health or environmentalism. The Deepwater Horizon oil spill echoed an incident two decades earlier, when the *Exxon Valdez* oil tanker ran aground on Alaska's southern coast, contaminating one thousand miles of shoreline. Even though the cleanup in 2010, which was coordinated by the National Oceanic and Atmospheric Administration, was much larger, it was more efficient than the sluggish response of the

Exxon Corporation in 1989, in part due to more sophisticated bioremediation techniques that used bacteria to absorb hydrocarbon molecules in the natural gas and the construction of boom barriers to protect the coastline. Bioremediation was more effective on the light crude oil of Deepwater Horizon than on the heavy crude spill of the *Exxon Valdez*, in part because by 2010, the EPA had developed more robust decontamination standards, even though microbes were ineffective for preventing the formation of heavy tar-like substances. Less successful, though, was the attempt to degrade the BP oil spill by using the chemical dispersant Corexit 9500, which created oil plumes on the ocean floor.[54]

We might be tempted to consider the six months of the Deepwater Horizon cleanup a relative success story, as President Obama summarized in his review of his administration's work in 2010, through the mobilization of the U.S. Coast Guard and the EPA.[55] Nonetheless, along with the eleven deaths and seventeen injuries among oil rig workers, Obama recognized the profound consequences of the oil spill on marine and coastal habitats along coastal regions of Louisiana, Mississippi, Alabama, and the Florida Panhandle. He went further by expressing solidarity with "the anger and frustration felt by our neighbors in the Gulf" and demanding that BP and allied oil companies be held responsible for such disasters, particularly as BP had a patchy health and safety record.[56] The federal response was a six-month ban on deepwater drilling and a five-year restriction on BP collaborating with the federal government, but this did little to allay health vulnerabilities along the Gulf. Contaminated food and water were obvious threats to the food chain, but ecosickness manifested itself in anxieties about toxicity and fears of infertility that exacerbated eye, lung, and skin problems cleanup workers and coastal communities faced, prompting a congressional hearing that focused on "human exposure and environmental fate."[57]

While the disaster was on Obama's mind through 2010 and he was keen to ensure that BP paid compensation, the deleterious impact on wildlife was beneath his radar, beyond the effects on Gulf Coast fishing as a way of life.[58] The fact that it took nearly three months for BP to contain the oil spill was evidence of how little bioremediation actually helped accelerate the cleanup process. The Alabama-based disaster relief organization Mobile Baykeeper estimated that more than 8,300 species were affected, including fish, birds, crabs, dolphins, and sea turtles, and that the impacts on organ health and fertility are still discernible in some species a decade later.[59] In *A Million Fragile Bones*, a 2017 novel exploring the health consequences of the BP oil spill, Connie May Fowler contrasts the myopia of politicians and corporations with what she calls her "edge of the world" home at Alligator Point, separated from the Florida Panhandle by the Ochlockonee Bay and an open harbor.

She depicts Alligator Point as a complex and fragile "living human body," a fragility that is emphasized by the fate of up to 200,000 Gulf of Mexico sea turtles that died in the spill or that laid eggs but could not return to the nest to hatch.[60] Although the spill did not drift as far east as Alligator Point, Fowler shares novelist Paolo Bacigalupi's view that BP "couldn't see that the step-by-step actions were gonna cascade into something much bigger than themselves," with diverse story-lines veering off in directions that no one can control.[61] These unintended directions do not mitigate responsibility. Fowler's account followed Jane Fulton Alt's 2010 photographic collection *Crude Awakening*, which featured beach visitors smeared to resemble the oil slick, and the documentaries *The Big Fix* (2011) and *Pretty Slick* (2015) that comment on health aspects of the spill. Fowler does not just blame corporate greed in *A Million Fragile Bones*, but she highlights BP's use of Corexit, which transformed "the oil into droplets so small, they permeate—thus poisoning—the membranes of the living" and ensured "a dead zone" on the ocean floor.[62] The use of what the EPA had flagged as a controversial oil dispersant did not just raise health risks for cleanup workers (Fowler calls it "cancer-inducing"), but in making a visible spectacle invisible the dispersant exacerbated the toxic threats to marine and coastal creatures and their habitats.[63]

The environmental threat to the Everglades—what novelist Zane Grey called "this last and wildest region" in 1924—is of a very different nature from the threat the Deepwater Horizon spill posed.[64] We might call this the slow violence of long-term degradation (to appropriate Rob Nixon's term), that has been ongoing since the construction of the Tamiami Trail in 1928.[65] The fragility of the Everglades intensified following the greenhouse summer of 1988, four decades after Harry Truman remarked on how the subtropical marshland region is "tranquil in its quiet beauty" during his dedication of the Everglades National Park as a means of preserving "an irreplaceable primitive area."[66] Often a shorthand for unspoiled nature in a tourist-friendly state, the Everglades featured in Bill Clinton's speeches of the late 1990s to signal the commitment of his administration—and a bipartisan Congress—to protecting the region through environmental restoration and responsible water resource management.[67] We might conclude that the motive of the federal government was to protect the "economic structure of American agriculture," despite Clinton's reminder to the public of the therapeutic benefits of walking in unspoiled landscapes, echoing Truman's view that "conservation of the human spirit" is linked to stewardship of biodiversity.[68] As the Everglades National Park approached its fiftieth year, the inaugural White House Conference on Climate Change in 1997 offered a unique forum for both global warming believers and deniers to "talk with each other rather than past each other." Clinton used this phrase in his opening remarks with the goal of ensuring "the continued vitality of our planet and expanding economic growth and opportunity for our people."[69]

Clinton and Gore emphasized their pledge to environmental stewardship throughout the second term of their administration. One of the clearest manifestations of this commitment is the multidecade Comprehensive Everglades Restoration Plan, which the U.S. Army Corps of Engineers drafted and Congress approved in 2000 as part of the Water Resources Development Act. Beyond legislation, Clinton and Gore recognized the need for citizens and communities to be involved in restoration projects, but they rarely discussed the public and environmental health aspects of climate change in detail, aside from warning that viruses are likely to increase in subtropical regions, where mosquitos thrive in seasonally warmer climates.[70] For Clinton, environmental stewardship was not explicitly about stabilizing ecosystems, mitigating risk, and protecting endangered species such as the Florida panther. Instead, he cast it in business terms as an effort to improve quality of life by "protecting farmlands, parklands, and other green spaces, rewarding consumers who buy cars and houses that reduce greenhouse gas pollution, controlling polluted runoff to lakes and streams, and improving the quality of the air we breathe."[71]

Al Gore visited the Everglades as vice-president in December 1997 to mark fifty years since President Truman dedicated the national park, and George W. Bush visited as president in the summer of 2001 to emphasize his administration's endeavors in advancing the Comprehensive Everglades Restoration Plan and to underscore his commitment to the National Parks Legacy Project.[72] In the presence of his brother, Florida governor Jeb Bush (one of the architects of the plan), President Bush highlighted the need for the care of, attention to, and protection of the ecosystem and the more than forty endangered species that inhabit the Everglades.[73] Bush's speech of June 4, 2001 is as rhetorically powerful as Clinton's in its emphasis on stewardship, but Bush went further by recognizing "nature's prior claims" to the region and that "the demands of growth" should not harm "the very things that give Florida and the Everglades their beauty."[74]

Despite the rhetoric, in the post-Clinton years the most extensive restoration project ever fell behind schedule, largely because of a reduced budget but also because of resistance within the executive branch and a Republican-controlled Congress (that included former Florida governor Rick Scott) to taking the Kyoto Protocol and global warming seriously. The result was the heightened vulnerability of charismatic mammals and thirty-eight other threatened and endangered native Florida species. These native inhabitants experienced a number of threats: new invasive species like the Burmese python, the Nile monitor, and the bromeliad beetle; arboviruses carried by mosquitos; a degradation of biodiversity down to the microbial level; and the bioaccumulation of mercury, phosphorus, and nitrates linked to increases in hurricanes, floods, and periodic drought.[75] Extreme weather brings its own risks. For example, experts believe that in 1992 Hurricane Andrew brought pythons to the Everglades when it destroyed a local breeding facility, and that in 2017 Hurricane Irma caused gaps in almost half the forest canopy.[76] While high levels of mercury in fish and increases in toxic blue-green algae blooms are hazards to human health caused by agricultural pollution, saltwater intrusion from rising sea waters threaten creatures living in Everglades marshes despite efforts at the state level to accelerate plans for a reservoir south of Lake Okeechobee to restore freshwater flow and a CDC study of cyanotoxins in the air and health advice about how to avoid blooms. In addition, the Biden administration has allocated $2 billion for accelerating Everglades restoration, a decade after a congressional hearing on the topic, and Obama and Biden visited in 2012 and 2015, respectively, to highlight awareness of the impact of global warming and to pledge federal support for Everglades restoration.[77]

The history of the Everglades restoration project swings between optimism and concern that the pace of change is too slow or the environmental challenge too immense. As Heather Houser notes, hope tends to be a form of techno-optimism, for example with regard to technologies that test changes in bioaccumulation and the use of computer modeling to increase understanding of ecosystem needs and resilience.[78] However, there are environmental and existential questions to ask about the restoration project itself, as the EPA acknowledged in a 2007 report. Significantly, the EPA authors used the language of health to express deep concern about water quality: "If nothing is done, the health of the Everglades will continue to decline, water quality will degrade further, water shortages for urban and agriculture users will become more frequent, and the ability to protect people and their property from flooding will be compromised."[79]

These concerns persist into the present day, despite a system of levees and canals that are designed to transform the subtropical wetlands into a controlled hydrological space. For activists, this managed environment has done little to protect the slow-moving marshy water system of the Everglades from air, water, and soil pollutants from suburban developments to the north and east.[80] The non-profit Miami-based Friends of the Everglades, in particular, recognizes that the restoration project will be successful only if federal and state governments take seriously efforts to reduce pollution and mitigate the environmental and human health risks of global warming. This includes a measured view of what growth in tourism, biotech, and pharmaceuticals in Palm Beach and Broward Counties both brings and degrades and a more collaborative approach to cleaning up toxic spills, with evidence suggesting that community activism is currently a deterrent to EPA-funded remediation.[81]

When Friends of the Everglades staged a "clean water conversation" with Tallahassee resident Jeff VanderMeer in the spring of 2022, its goals were first to highlight the "systemic pillaging of Florida" and second to protest suburban over-development and the lobbying power of wealthy special-interest groups that ignore vulnerable communities. Echoing his anger after the Deepwater Horizon oil spill twelve years earlier, VanderMeer took a holistic perspective of environmental health and degradation that aligns with the views of activists eager to develop biodiverse wildlife corridors. VanderMeer concludes that despite the steady stream of government leaders making the right noises about conservation, Florida is experiencing "ecocide" because he believes "state leaders and developers have chosen a cruel, unsustainable legacy involving the nonstop slaughter of wildlife and the destruction of habitat."[82]

Area X: Contamination beyond Bioknowledge

Preceding his "Annihilation of Florida" essay by eight years, Jeff VanderMeer's Southern Reach trilogy is a major cultural assessment of the fragility of environmental health in the early twenty-first century. The weird science trilogy *Annihilation*, *Authority*, and *Acceptance*, published over an eight-month period in 2014, defies generic conventions, blending empirical science, science fiction, horror, magic realism, fantasy, and speculative fiction in its exploration of the mysterious fictional Area X, located in a southern coastal region.[83] Area X is reminiscent of St. Marks National Wildlife Refuge, forty-three miles of coastal wilderness in Apalachee Bay, a thirty-minute drive south of VanderMeer's Tallahassee home. Although Deepwater Horizon did not directly contaminate the wildlife refuge, VanderMeer says that the trilogy was inspired by the oil spill, which morphed in his mind from "a dark, horrible spiral" as he lay in bed with bronchitis and "came back out of me in unexpected ways," just as "at the microscopic level the oil was still infiltrating and contaminating the environment." In his feverish state, the "spiral of oil" spilled through his mind to become an imagined encounter with a "tower sunk into the ground" with "living words" made out of moss and fungi on its walls.[84]

The link between the spillage and the "strange matter" of Area X remains allusive, deliberately so, it seems, because VanderMeer evokes the eco-philosopher Timothy Morton's theory of "hyperobjects" that are too immense to perceive clearly but nonetheless have a "threatening proximity."[85] Morton's focus on this uncanny dyad of visibility and invisibility is especially resonant for VanderMeer because "association, correlation, and probability are the only thing we have to go on, for now," although both Morton and VanderMeer explore the psychological and visceral stickiness of hyperobjects.[86] The BP oil spill epitomizes this viscosity for Morton ("non-humans and humans alike were coated with a layer of oil, inside and outside their bodies") and raises questions of scale and duration that align with VanderMeer's almost-unimaginable sense that the disaster might keep "unfolding for twenty years."[87] The trilogy enables VanderMeer to work through two intertwined themes that emerge from the vision he had while he was sick. First, the theme of transformation pushes him to explore the health consequences of invisible contaminants for human and nonhuman life, linking to the concept of an as-yet-unknown pathogen that the WHO calls Disease X (see chapter 7). Second, the theme of illegibility shows how mass-scale environmental disasters exceed any scientific, corporate, or political frame that is typically superimposed on them.

Area X initially seems to conform to what sociologist Steve Lerner calls a "sacrifice zone," given VanderMeer's statement that the BP oil spill "created Area X" and that for many Panhandle residents it was for years "gushing in our minds . . . haunting us day and night."[88] Lerner offers a range of examples of poor communities exposed to chemical toxicity such as charcoal and dioxin contamination in Florida cities as diverse as Ocala and Pensacola (the latter was affected by the Deepwater Horizon spill) that compounds other contamination events in the Gulf, such as a collision of three vessels carrying oil and jet fuel near Tampa Bay in 1993 that blackened fourteen miles of beaches. The sacrifice zone concept may not be directly applicable to Area X given its remote location, surrounded by military security and "possibly even government-trained colonies of apex predators and genetically modified poison berries."[89] However, the concept is problem-atized in the trilogy, given the twin contexts of the Deepwater Horizon spill and divergent views about Everglades restoration, plus the fact that Area X is an elastic zone with a toxic health risk on lands that were formerly home to the Apalachee Indigenous group.[90] Now the land provokes "vagueness and confu-sion" in the public as "a dark fairy tale" shrouded in conspiratorial mystery. Rumors are fueled by a local Séance and Science Brigade that claims to have detected paranormal activity and by nonspecific official statements that "secret government experiments" have degraded the terrain, possibly leading to a "human-made ecological disaster area."[91] Compounding this uncertainty are the unclear motives of the Southern Reach agency, which seems to be operating in a protectionist rather than an investigative mode, though we are told in *Authority* that "no one seemed to care much" about the "dormant secret" anymore.[92]

Area X is much more than a potential contamination zone in its embodiment of the dialectic of clarity and opacity. VanderMeer calls it a "strange pristine wil-derness" that is difficult to clearly map scientifically or conceptualize philosophi-cally yet has a transformative effect on those who enter it.[93] Echoing contamination fictions such as Michael Crichton's *The Andromeda Strain* of 1969, *Annihilation* is not a conventional invasion story or a solvable environmental mystery. In fact, Area X might be an antidote to contamination, a radically animate wilderness that is "more what it had always been without human interference: less contami-nated, less compromised."[94] Given this ambiguity, Area X is untranslatable in its eccentricity. Nonetheless, the region leaves open the possibility that topo-graphical receptivity may help us navigate empirical and existential aspects of climate change, revealing itself in "unexpected ways" in the "breath or thickness of molecules."[95]

VanderMeer's understanding of weird science provides one clue to the trajec-tory of the Southern Reach trilogy. As a version of Southern Gothic, he sees its task to be a subverting of "romanticized ideas about place found in traditional fantasy."[96] He does not see weird science as "overtly political," though the hybrid genre is "acutely aware of the modern world" and carries political freight in exposing what is covered over. These themes of invisibility and legibility are most evident in the first volume, *Annihilation*, and in Alex Garland's substantially revised film adaptation of 2018. In both versions, the human world is brought into focus through the biologist who struggles to interpret the nonhuman world via observation and cellular testing, as evidenced in an iconic image from the film in which Natalie Portman's character stares into a void in the earth. The biologist is one of four female explorers (alongside the anthropologist, the psychologist, and the surveyor) who are known only by their abstract professional titles in the nov-els, their real names having been stripped from them in training "to make condi-tioning and hypnosis more effective."[97] (The film retains first names and gives them biomedical professions.) The four, who are not emotionally close, become aware that their maps and epistemologies are inadequate to the task.

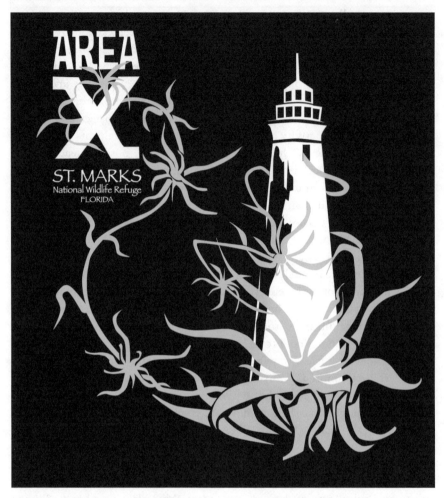

Figure 8.1. Area X logo. Artist Rita LaBlanc. Image courtesy of Friends of St. Marks Wildlife Refuge, Florida.

As well as invoking what Timothy Clark calls the uselessness of maps "when it comes to relating [climate threats] to daily questions," this epistemological redundancy is exemplified in a scene in which the biologist encounters a large starfish that "bled a dark gold color into the still water as if it were on fire."[98] At close range, the starfish is incomprehensible, especially when in her mind it grows to fill the tidal pool and then the whole world.[99] This experience makes her realize that she knows "nothing at all—about nature, about ecosystems," and the beholding prompts her to muse that "I knew less than nothing about myself as well."[100] In this moment, the biologist feels dislocated and can no longer distinguish between sky and sea as she experiences a derangement of scale. This incident intensifies an earlier feeling, after the anthropologist's death, when the biologist begins to doubt the validity of her empirical method in the face of what she experiences as a "brightness" spreading within her, a toxic contaminant from a cluster of spores that affects body and mind. Instead of spore contamination constituting a zombifying pandemic threat (as it does in the 2023 HBO ecoapocalyptic series *The Last of Us*), nature starts to speak to and through her via indecipherable moss-like letters on the walls of a tower that she discovers.

It is notable that the four members of this twelfth expedition into Area X rely on private journals rather than technologies or an interdisciplinary master document to record their observations. That the biologist's observations are not as detailed as they first appear might be attributed to the trauma she recently experienced when she lost her husband to the eleventh Area X expedition: he returned as "a shell, an automaton going through the motions" before he and his estranged expedition companions all died of cancer.[101] The biologist appears to possess strong self-awareness, at least initially, recognizing in the wilderness that "things were not quite what they seemed," and she has to "fight the sensation before it could overwhelm [her] scientific objectivity."[102] Yet her retrospective account makes us question her sagacity and doubt the reliability of place and perception. Through a series of textual dislocations, VanderMeer answers the Mortonian question "How might ontology think nonlocality?" in the "mid-Collapse" of the Anthropocene.[103] Endangered health and identity disintegration hang over the biologist, leading her to a tower previous scientists have recorded and then to a lighthouse that contains traces of previous expeditions. The location of these sites, which are inspired by the complex history of St. Marks Lighthouse at the tip of the wildlife refuge (including numerous rebuilds in slightly different locations), seems deliberately unclear in the trilogy, leading the Southern Reach director to later ask the biologist about "topographical anomalies"—as illustrated in artist Rita La Blanc's striking yet entangled design for that incorporates VanderMeer's Area X in the logo for St. Marks Wildlife Refuge.[104]

Midway through *Annihilation*, the biologist stumbles across the body of the missing psychologist, whom she discovers in the lighthouse half-consumed by a "fibrous green-gold fuzziness," and later she finds the anthropologist covered in a "carpet of hand-shaped parasites that lived among the words on the wall."[105] The fate of the anthropologist and the psychologist seem to be attributable to more than nature just reclaiming its domain. Lurking in the wild habitat are perilous forces—not just contaminants that might induce cancer but something potentially monstrous. Instead of the lighthouse illuminating the region's secrets, a brightness growing within the biologist draws her back into the darkness. She struggles to make legible the "massively distributed, sentient being" that spreads through Area X and feels compelled to anthropomorphize its central energy force as "the Crawler," despite her initial reluctance to superimpose human qualities on nonhuman creatures.[106]

VanderMeer's uncanny story can read as a double metaphor. First, the inadequacy of knowledge at "the edges of something unprecedented" alludes to the ways that nature evades human conceptualizations and the technologies humans use to control it.[107] On this figurative level, the trilogy both represents and fails to represent the consequences of environmental and public health disasters by

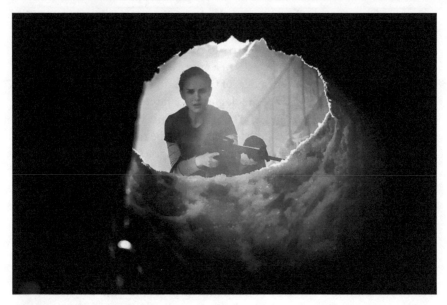

Figure 8.2. The biologist (Natalie Portman) encounters a void in *Annihilation*. Paramount Pictures, 2018. Pictorial Press Ltd/Alamy Photo.

revealing an invisible plenum that can only be glimpsed rather than recorded. VanderMeer's recognition of inaccessibility is especially relevant for assessing an oil economy as "an omnipresent, but slippery force" that "is both beyond human cognition and everywhere."[108] In this way, the trilogy can be read as a "textual manifestation of the spill" as we work through layers of textual suggestion and evidence without ever seeing the whole picture.[109] Second, the brightness that invades the biologist is a metaphor for the ways invisible toxins from multiple sources and with manifold effects pathologize human and nonhuman life. The biologist wonders if the natural world "had become a kind of camouflage" for an experiment gone wrong and for which there are only traces, such as a glimpse of a dolphin with a human eye (possibly her husband's) that unnerves because it evokes the possibility of transgenic experiments.[110]

The disintegration of the biologist's stable viewpoint means we can never be sure of the cause or degree of contamination. We see only these half-glimpses and the effect of brightness as a "refracted phosphorescence" that heightens her senses yet induces a state of delirium as the bioluminescence mirrors the lettering she first saw in the tower.[111] The biologist chooses to remain in Area X after all her companions have died, not just so she can continue the quest for her presumed-dead husband, but also because she is experiencing an ecological merging of self and environment as she is consumed by a "cone of energy" that rises from the tower.[112] It seems that no matter how many decades of journals the biologist uncovers from previous expeditions into Area X, none will hold the key to understanding its provenance or its evolving trajectory. This is emphasized by the imagery of the documents, which VanderMeer describes as "torn pages, crushed pages, journal covers warped and damp" that merge with the environment as mold infiltrates the books.[113]

Adding to the epistemological confusion of Area X is the emergence of existential doubles that link to the environmental haunting of the BP oil spill and the Anthropocene at large. By the end of *Annihilation*, the biologist undergoes a form of psychic splitting in which a doppelgänger called Ghost Bird emerges to leave Area X, while the brightness within the biologist herself compels her to remain, as she adds her journal to the decomposing pile she earlier discovered. This doubling continues through volumes two and three. In the second volume, *Authority*, the new Southern Reach director, John "Control" Rodriguez, sees himself as the dark counterpart of the bright Ghost Bird, who responds tersely to his questions about the expedition. When she does speak, her phrases are detached with "undercurrents and hidden references" that Control fears he will never understand.[114]

Not only are the biologist and Ghost Bird versions of each other (they are described as "haunted twins"), but we also encounter zombie versions of the surveyor, the anthropologist, and the missing psychologist, who reemerges in the final volume historically in her human form and transgenically when the biologist detects the psychologist's resemblance in the face of a moaning creature as a "mask of utter uncomprehending anguish."[115] The biologist's husband also reappears, it seems, in the form of an owl, prompting her to conclude that the "lines between the eccentricities of wildlife and the awareness imposed by Area X are difficult to separate at times."[116] Area X seems to have a double life as a contaminated region that the government and Big Science seek to contain and as an untamed energy force that shifts the boundaries between life and death and collapses human time. This theme of radical doubling taps into a history of Southern Gothic writing that gestures on the one hand toward environmental and existential dangers and on the other to a wilderness that defies management strategies, yet in moments of "silence and solitude" reveals "a sense of invisible things stitching through."[117]

The intertwining of biodiversity and toxicity is allusive in the Southern Reach trilogy and it is difficult to locate hope, even as VanderMeer injects radical uncertainty into all kinds of master discourses and practices. Although biotechnology is not the central focus of the trilogy, it exists on its edges through the biologist's glimpses of what appears at times to be a contaminated wilderness, as well as the seemingly haphazard experiments of Southern Reach: for example, the decision of its science division in the mid-1990s to release two thousand white rabbits fifty feet from Area X to see if they can overwhelm its border protection, only for most to completely disappear and others to attack the scientists.[118] But just as he illuminates links between the Deepwater Horizon spill and the experiments of the Southern Reach agency, it is clear from VanderMeer's nonfiction writings and his 2017 novel *Borne* that he targets the intersection of biotechnology and climate change as a "witness-bearer, chronicler, storyteller, truthsayer," in the words of Connie May Fowler, with an activist consciousness that seeks to unearth deep truths about the environment, both present and future.[119]

These multiple roles come together in what Beatriz da Costa and Kavita Philip call "tactical biopolitics" via VanderMeer's interrogation of what "governs scientific statements, their thinkability."[120] These tactical biopolitics are evident in his critique of biotechnology, and his concern about the mistreatment of animals (such as Southern Reach's ethical disregard for the white rabbits) becomes a dominant theme in *Borne*. This is illustrated both through the transformation of Borne as a radically evolving transgenic creature, with a voice, intelligence, and a capacity for empathy, and partly through the narrator Rachel's partner, Wick, who worked on a human-fish interspecies project for his previous employer. The plans for this experiment have disintegrated over the years, making them illegible "dark clouds of scribbles," but Rachel discovers that Wick has revisited these "monstrous visions of projects never completed," albeit only in his imagination.[121] Although we see Borne evolving from plant to animal to a distinct personality, Rachel's empathic connection to him makes him far from the "monstrous vision" of Margaret Atwood's *Oryx and Crake*. Although VanderMeer echoes Atwood's portrayal of a chaotic biosphere full of transgenic boundary crossing, as discussed in chapter 1, *Borne* centers on the enigmatic unknowability of nature and human responsibility toward creatures born via genetic manipulation.[122]

Borne is VanderMeer's most compelling statement to date about the well-being of transgenic creatures, but his tactical biopolitics are also on display in a speculative 2019 op-ed for the *New York Times* in which he imagines that humans have bioengineered their own extinction by 2071 because leaders have avoided pressing bioethical questions and because the needs of nonhuman life are typically ignored in the drive to progress technologically. This bleak future is not merely one where biotechnology is dominant but where it turns against humans after decades of slack regulation.[123] I switch to another aspect of VanderMeer's tactical biopolitics in the final section via his practice of rewilding, but in the speculative future of this op-ed he pictures humans as abject beings who are facing ecosickness and are contaminated by the consequences of their transgenic experiments.

Ecological Reimagining: De-Extinction as/versus Rewilding

In April 2006, the cover of *Time* magazine featured a lone and seemingly bewildered polar bear on a small float of Arctic ice, set against the apocalyptic header "Worried. Be Very Worried." This cover coincided with fears of a sixth mass extinction and the concerns of the International Union for the Conservation of Nature (IUCN) about the well-being of the polar bear. The IUCN upgraded its threatened species classification to vulnerable that year, following its adherence to the long-standing international accord on the conservation of polar bears that the United States joined in 1977. This 2006 issue of *Time* appeared a fortnight before the twenty-sixth Earth Day turned the focus of the magazine to the subject of science and faith. In that discussion, a distrust of materialism and a commitment to environmental stewardship offered a bridge between seemingly conflictual world views. Yet the April headline was less concerned about restoring the polar bear's habitat and more concerned about "how it affects you, your kids, and their kids as well." The article associated with the headline illustrates this by switching the geographic focus to the catastrophic damage to human health and habitat caused by Hurricane Katrina the previous year.[124]

This was not the first time that polar bears featured on a cover of *Time*. Six years earlier, a stranded male had looked down from a tower of ice to the headline "Arctic Meltdown," followed by the message that "the polar bear's in danger, and so are you" because the sea ice that helps control global temperatures was 40 percent thinner than it had been twenty years earlier.[125] Given the prediction that the polar bear population could decrease to near extinction by 2100, over these six years the creature became the "most recognizable image of climate change."[126] The Arctic meltdown prediction was a feature of consciousness raising by grassroots activists and prominent celebrities such as Daryl Hannah and Leonardo DiCaprio; DiCaprio appeared on a cover of *Vanity Fair* in a photograph by Annie Leibovitz standing next to a digital image of a polar bear cub.[127] Coinciding with Earth Day 2007, this cover image was resonant at the start of a warm summer in the Arctic during which the melting of the ice cap had accelerated dramatically. However, even though the polar bear became a recognizable "poster child" for environmentalism—including a World Wildlife Fund animated film of a melting polar bear that coincided with the 2021 COP26 summit in Glasgow—these discourses teetered between calls to save animals from extinction and discussions of how global warming primarily impacts human life.

Polar bear politics on the fulcrum between biocentric and anthropocentric world views are exemplified by Al Gore's 2006 documentary and accompanying book *An Inconvenient Truth*.[128] Gore's rhetorical strategy of interlinking the personal and the planetary is embodied in a short yet poignant animated sequence of a solitary polar bear failing to find an ice float stable enough to take its weight. In his lecture presentation that structures the film, Gore cites a 2005 study that revealed that some polar bears swim sixty miles to find stable ice, a scenario that has since worsened, as emphasized by the follow-up film *An Inconvenient Sequel* of 2017.[129] He steers away from polar bears in this more pessimistic sequel, but that same year the online version of *National Geographic* featured video footage of a starving polar bear (taken by SeaLegacy biologist Paul Nicklin) with the tagline "this is what climate change looks like."[130] The animated sequence of *An Inconvenient Truth* and the SeaLegacy video are open to charges of exploiting polar bears to illustrate the thinning of the arctic ice cap. Conversely, we might decide that both accounts are honest in their efforts to demonstrate how the cumulative effects of global warming are a matter of "accretion rather than accident" within a project that seeks to stimulate citizen science.[131] These accounts couple science and symbolism to drive home to the public the growing threat to endangered species and to fragile ecosystems that support all planetary life.

Just as Bill McKibben argues that global warning has "broken the Arctic," it is no accident that Gore focuses on arctic and subarctic regions.[132] As a senator, he decried the *Exxon Valdez* oil spill, demanding that Exxon Corporation intensify

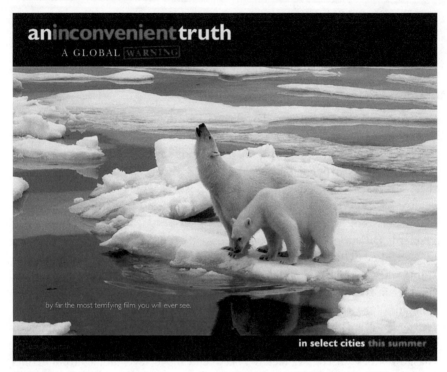

Figure 8.3. Polar bears movie poster for *An Inconvenient Truth* (2006). AJ Pics/Alamy Photo.

its cleanup efforts. The spill not only endangered fish, coastal birds, and marine animals but also posed threats to the health of Alaskan native communities living near Prince William Sound, including rashes from exposure to oil, accidental ingestion of oil, mental health challenges, and drug and alcohol use.[133] This interest in Alaska inflected Gore's warning about the rise of greenhouse gasses during his terms as a Tennessee senator and as vice-president, but the backlash he faced shows just how polarizing environmental politics are and how "derangements of scale" play out politically (to recall Timothy Clark's concept). High-profile Republican climate change deniers such as former Alaska governor Sarah Palin have pushed back on Gore's claims, alongside other less prominent figures like Fairbanks sculptor Stephen Dean, who created the first of an annual series of Al Gore ice sculptures in January 2009 for the Compeau's powersports firm.[134] The owners of Compeau's blew exhaust fumes through the mouth of the 2010 version of "Frozen Gore" to a soundtrack of excerpts of Gore's UN Climate Change Conference speech of that year, creating political theater to illustrate the relatively low emission of Ford trucks compared to those of the Lear jet Gore used to fly to the Copenhagen conference.[135]

There is some truth that Gore's engaged yet pragmatic approach to global warming tips into alarmism, using the image of "the edge" to direct eyes north and to shape public opinion that time is running short to act. Take his environmentalist stance in his 2007 book *The Future*: "We have been slow to recognize the extreme danger we are creating" because governments typically focus on short-term horizons and tech solutions based on a single strategy such as carbon capture or nuclear energy.[136] Here he interweaves dramatic language and autobiographical reflection to spur readers to engage with a "collective global conscience" and to navigate "persistent confusion" about the sources of fear.[137] However, Gore's fearmongering is open to criticism that he is pitting humans against the natural world as a collision of interests, superimposing a political and cultural lens on environmental diversity and fragility.[138]

Gore is not in search of a technofix, but his faith in restoring balance through tech solutions is arguably at the expense of sensitivity to human-animal relationships and communications. This rhetoric of restoring balance stems from his 1992 book *Earth in the Balance* and inflects the depiction of an ailing planet in his Nobel Lecture of December 2007: "The earth has a fever. The fever is rising. The experts have told us it is not a passing affliction that will heal by itself."[139] It also shapes the rhetorical and visual strategy of *An Inconvenient Truth*, which mixes scientific analysis of environmental threats with fearmongering about human disregard for fragile ecosystems as he strives to make the larger point that the fates of animals and humans intertwine. Despite Gore's interest in cold and warm habitats (the Everglades feature in *An Inconvenient Sequel*), he sometimes projects an imagined Arctic onto an inhabited space and overlooks communities that are living symbiotically with their environment and do not typically seek technological answers.

We can bring Gore's neglect of diverse communities into focus if we zoom in from a global perspective to consider the subsistence lifestyle of Inuit, their close interaction with polar bears, and the melting habitat that is making Artic communities more isolated.[140] From this perspective, instead of romanticizing polar bears via emotive imagery, Subhankar Banerjee reminds us that the "intertwined tragic fates of the bears and the Inuit underscore the differential nature of accountability and vulnerability in cases of environmental violence and challenge the universalizing tendency of the Anthropocene narrative."[141] As Steve Lerner documents with respect to St. Lawrence Island off the northwest coast of Alaska, arctic lands are increasingly vulnerable in the face of global warming and because of the "toxic legacy" of military bases (that were operational on St. Lawrence Island during World War II and the Cold War) that spilled contaminants or dumped them on otherwise pristine lands, where they entered the food chain for decades after demobilization, leaving what anthropologist Jocelyn Cassady (quoting an Iñupiaq elder) calls a "tundra of sickness" in mainland northern Alaska.[142] The health consequences on St. Lawrence Island were manifold: contaminated drinking water, elevated cancer rates in the local community, high levels of PCBs in the bloodstreams of community residents, dead coastal birds, and seals turning yellow from diesel fuel.[143]

Sheila Watt-Cloutier, former chair of the Inuit Circumpolar Council and a Nobel Peace Prize nominee in 2007, echoes Lerner's view that disease clusters derive from multiple sources of environmental stress. In recognizing that the front line of climate change spans diverse species, Watt-Cloutier is careful to avoid focusing on "haunting images of polar bears struggling to find ice" at the expense of other arctic creatures that tug less "at the heartstrings of 'Southerners.'"[144] She is also wary about the fact that political and public attention is usually on charismatic animals and shows how the erosion of habitat has profound health consequences for all inhabitants of the Artic. This is a major aspect of her 2015 book *The Right to Be Cold*, published the year the Obama administration added an Arctic theme to its Climate Data Initiative in order to better assess climate change risks for northern communities, a few days after President Obama met with Alaska Native leaders and attended a "Global Leadership in the Artic" conference in Anchorage.[145] The key issues are as much existential as they are about leadership. On the one hand, polar bears facing exhaustion or irregular cycles of diet and fasting are likely to experience distress because they typically lose weight during their time on land and because modified mating patterns mean fewer births. On the other hand, the Inuit communities of northern Canada and Greenland are experiencing one of the highest suicide rates globally as well as multiple health risks, including heart and liver problems, psychosocial challenges, and growing instances of skin cancer and cataracts due to the thinning ozone layer.[146] Vulnerability to suicide is especially acute for young Inuit, many of whom feel insecure and disempowered in the face of intractable global processes yet have few health care resources in a context in which national governments and WHO are not intervening.[147]

Watt-Cloutier is concerned that climate change is making persistent organic pollutants, including PCBs, pesticides, herbicides, and manufacturing effluents, an imminent health threat to both Inuit and marine animals as warmer winds carry these toxins farther to arctic and subarctic regions.[148] These pollutants are often invisible, and it is easier to document physical symptoms than it is to document the anxiety that sustained habitat changes can trigger, especially among communities for whom health facilities are scarce. Animals are also likely to experience chronic distress in a rapidly changing habitat that may prevent them from maintaining normal species behavior based on regular sources of food, shelter, and kinship bonds. Discourses of mental health hinge on philosophical precepts about the relative levels of consciousness of different genera and species, and it is debatable whether it is advisable to demarcate the physical and mental health of animals, following research in the 2010s that focused primarily on the welfare of farm, zoo, and companion animals.[149] However, epidemiological evidence suggests that polar bears kept in captivity reveal distress through repetitive and unpurposeful behavior that approximates to obsessive-compulsive disorder, while practices of administering Prozac to polar bears at Calgary Zoo in the 1990s to control erratic moods and preserve their appeal for the public elicited criticism from conservation groups.[150]

Climate change deniers who care enough might argue that oil spills can be cleaned up with bioremediation and biodegradation and that animals will adapt to changes in seasons or can be given supplementary food sources. On the first point there is inconclusive evidence that microbiotic agents used for cleaning up the Gulf of Mexico would also work for oil spills in Arctic waters.[151] There are hints of demographic and genetic evidence on the second point. For example, a survey conducted in the 2010s revealed a polar bear subpopulation living in fjords in southeastern Greenland that is less reliant on sea ice than other arctic populations.[152] Nevertheless, the lead scientist, Kristin Laidre at University of Washington's Polar Science Center, argues that identifying genetic diversity within a species and the adaptive patterns of some subpopulations is only a partial story, despite mitochondrial and genomic studies that show how polar bears can regulate energy production differently, depending on climate and habitat.[153] For Laidre, this evidence links to a recognition that loss of sea ice affects all Arctic animals and habitats.

Alongside pharmacological research on treating compulsive behavior among animals held in captivity and seeking solutions for microbial resistance to antibiotics by commercializing the biological resources of the Arctic, the most prominent response from the biotech community to threatened species has been to focus on postgenomic efforts to reverse the extinction cycle.[154] The terrain of de-extinction echoes my discussion of longevity in chapter 5, spanning a spectrum of viewpoints, from the scientifically valid to the seemingly fanciful, all of which can be considered strategies for surviving "climatological disaster" by providing scientific and public reassurance that previous extinction events "have already been anticipated, remediated, survived."[155] The rise of extinction recovery projects in the 2010s pits the genetically possible practices of back breeding (with the aim of restoring ancestral genetic traits) and cloning (using somatic cell nuclear transfer or Crispr techniques) against the implausible idea of resurrecting long-extinct species like the woolly mammoth, the quagga zebra, and the Tasmanian tiger. This breadth of ambition and practice led the IUCN's Special Survival Commission to promote de-extinction guidelines in an effort to establish clarity and regulation that can steer responsible bioethical practice.[156]

Just as the millennial imagination was stirred by the real cloning of a domestic sheep and the imaginative de-extinction of dinosaurs in Michael Crichton's *Jurassic Park* (visualized on the screen by Stephen Spielberg in 1993), so the biotech turn to the Arctic in the early twenty-first century has at least the potential to help preserve the ice cap and slow global warming. A wave of de-extinction projects using genetic engineering to rescue lost species followed a high-profile TEDx DeExtinction event held at the National Geographic Headquarters in Washington, DC, in the spring of 2013. The event, which was run by the newly formed California-based nonprofit biotech company Revive & Restore, was accompanied by a *National Geographic* cover that posed the question "Reviving Extinct Species: We Can, But Should We?"[157] The de-extinction gaze is often fixed on reviving magnificent creatures that Britt Wray calls "charismatic necrofauna" because these are more likely to stir public interest than keystone animals, plants, and microorganisms that create stability in the ecosystem.[158] Some de-extinction advocates are wary of overhyping a complex science and allowing media doom-sayers to turn to apocalyptic discourses. They counter extremes by offering what Beth Shapiro calls "solutions, success stories, reintroductions," in part to dilute worries about the future by showing how the past can be reinvented.[159] Yet de-extinction projects place faith in the inherent value of postgenomic practices to re-create discrete species from the past instead of muddying bioethical waters by editing an animal's genes to improve their chances of survival or producing hybrid interspecies or even contemplating the promethean task of resurrecting long-extinct Neanderthals using ancient DNA samples.[160]

This is not to say there is no biodiversity justification for de-extinction proj-ects, especially because large mammals at the top of the food pyramid are often influential in regulating ecosystems.[161] Apex predators are not always the focus, however. For example, according to geneticist George Church, the lead researcher of the AI company Hypergiant, a number of woolly mammoth de-extinction projects in the United States, Japan, and Russia are efforts to ensure that carbon gasses remain trapped in the ice by means of restored mammoth herds grazing on and maintaining the steppe grassland ecosystem.[162] Church believes that de-extinction will revitalize the conservation movement by injecting "new hope and new technologies," and he envisions a new age of "panspermia" that mixes ancient and futurist ideas.[163] More terrestrially, Church has founded a number of start-ups that face the biotech future, including Colossal Biosciences (est. 2021), through which tech entrepreneur Ben Lamm and he are collaborating with a University of Melbourne research team to revive the iconic Tasmanian tiger, which became extinct in the 1930s.[164] The cloning of the Arctic wolf in autumn 2022 by the Beijing pet-cloning company Sinogene Biotechnology is a more mod-est yet no less significant effort to address species threat, although its focus is on using somatic cell nuclear transfer to maintain the genetic diversity of Arctic wolves kept in captivity rather than on repopulating endangered species in the polar north.[165]

The debate is inconclusive about whether de-extinction practices can restore a preindustrial balance of ecosystems by reversing extinction threats or whether they simply ignore the degrading effects of toxins by attending to spectacular projects that can be commercialized. Critics of what geographer Juanita Sund-berg calls "capitalocentrism" argue that teleological narratives of de-extinction always contain the seeds of creative destruction, revealing what literary critic Ashley Dawson describes as the "leading edge of contemporary capitalism's con-tradictions."[166] Instead of perpetuating a war between neoliberal technocracy and grassroots eco-resistance, Sundberg promotes research projects rooted in local communities that can bring equal health benefits to people, places, and the planet. Yet it is reasonable to ask if this mode of health citizenship underpinned by culturally congruent research is liable to have unintended consequences that might be based on competing power interests, conflictual histories, and diver-gent belief systems.

For environmentalists, rewilding is a more palatable praxis than de-extinction, largely because it is less interventionist and embraces a more holistic sense of environment. As a form of wilderness restoration, rewilding also often embodies an anticapitalist ethos of living non-extractively and of letting nature restore itself. This practice is embodied in the efforts of Jeff VanderMeer to rewild his Tallahassee yard with the aim of restoring biodiversity on a modest budget without herbicides or pesticides, thereby helping stimulate "a chain reaction of behavioral change," in the words of environmentalist Michael Pollan.[167] It is easy to view de-extinction and rewilding as divergent philosophies—the first high-tech and spectacular, the second low-tech and holistic immanent—but that perspective ignores the increasing inexpensiveness of genomic sequencing and current projects that blend the two philosophies. In his 2019 novel *Hummingbird Salamander*, which was released the year that scientists were calling for a "Global Deal for Nature" to protect biodiversity in the face of climate change, VanderMeer upholds the need to respect animals despite his skepticism about whether the collapsing biosphere can now be fixed at all.[168] Yet two examples of arguably respectful rewilding de-extinction projects are American and Scandinavian research teams seeking to rewild the Arctic with reindeer (to protect tundra and prevent the release of carbon gases) and a collaboration between Revive & Restore and the U.S. Fish and Wildlife Service to clone the endangered black-footed ferret from historic DNA samples in order to restore genetic diversity and increase the number of the only indigenous North American ferrets living in the wild.[169]

If we shift away from seeing rewilding as a technique and more as a life philosophy predicted on care, then we can identify an epistemological and ontological gap between grand adventurist biotech projects and the more immanent biohacking practices I trace through the second half of this book.[170] There are some warnings here. First, if genomic sequencing moves out of the laboratory, it will increase the risk of rogue interspecies research that may damage ecosystems more than regulated de-extinction projects. This possibility leads Britt Wray to remind her readers that American citizens can "genetically modify an organism and release it on [their] own land" just as long as it is not endangered. Sinogene has already used a beagle to mother the cloned Arctic wolf and a Dubai research team has experimented with injecting germ cells from a chicken into duck eggs in order to produce chicken sperm. In this open biohacking terrain, a regulatory framework is vital at a global level to reinforce national research protocols. Second, although top-down biotechnology and bottom-up biohacking can be equally individualistic, the sharing of rewilding knowledge can help foster a revival of ancestral practices that can strengthen ecosystems and promote "nature-integrated lives" in human communities, to quote nutritionist Daniel Vitalis.[171]

Essentially, emergent practices that put wellness and care at their core may help us understand how better to reimagine ecosystems by tackling often-invisible toxins and may also deter us from viewing mental health as either the sole domain of human beings or an anthropocentric lens superimposed upon animals. Aligned with what environmental ethicist Ben Minteer calls "pragmatic preservationism," post-anthropocentric wellness practices respect nonhuman health experiences and ecologies as coequal in status to human health.[172] This perspective does not repudiate biotechnology in favor of spiritual rewilding. Instead, it embodies a version of Nikolas Rose's somatic ethics in a shared terrain that avoids beguiling projections of anthropomorphism and recognizes environmental health on its own terms.

Conclusion

MENTAL HEALTH AND
BIOTECHNOLOGY BEYOND 2030

When President Biden signed an executive order on September 12, 2022 to launch a new National Biotechnology and Biomanufacturing Initiative, he echoed a sequence of White House policies that looked toward technology to stimulate the economy, which included a National Bioeconomy Blueprint of ten years earlier when he was vice-president.[1] This whole-of-government initiative sought to release the "potential of biology" to "make almost anything that we use in our day-to-day lives, from medicines to fuels to plastics" in an effort to "drive U.S. innovation into economic and societal success."[2] Speaking at a historic White House summit on September 14th, the director of the Office of Science and Technology Policy, Alondra Nelson—whose scholarly work highlights structural and technological inequalities—called 2022 a "momentous summer" for science innovation, as the federal initiative had the potential to benefit diverse communities through $2 billion of new government investment.

It is unsurprising to see such technological optimism, wedded to goals of "equity, ethics, safety, and security," in the aftermath of the COVID-19 emergency. Yet the emphasis on productivity not only echoes the priorities of previous post–Cold War presidents, it also subordinates health care to national security, biosafety, and market opportunity.[3] Seeking to avoid reviving the Cold War in light of Russia's recent invasion of Ukraine while championing American technology in a multipolar world, Biden's executive order was more progressive than Trump's overtly aggressive efforts to reduce biotech regulations as a means to stimulate a favorable competitive trading climate for the United States.[4] The Biden administration took a further step by establishing a National Bioeconomy Board in spring 2024 that linked to its Investing in America infrastructural agenda by seeking to "advance societal well-being, national security, sustainability, economic productivity, and competitiveness."[5] Nonetheless, had the Biotechnology and Biomanufacturing Initiative been led by an agency other than the National Security Council, and had it made strengthening health care via public and private biotech partnerships its central focus, it most likely would have struck a more resonant chord for a post-pandemic nation.

Transformed States has shown how American biotechnology and health care periodically couple and uncouple in the post–Cold War period, with the promise of technofixes often a rallying call for more government investment in the biomedical quest to deepen preventive health care and cure major diseases. However, the economy or security invariably continue to take precedence over improving care. The Biden executive order affirms this coupling by emphasizing the importance of "life-saving diagnostics, therapeutics, and vaccines" as elements of a broader ambition to jump-start the bioeconomy. It is not that the components of this multipronged initiative are wrongheaded, but more that fiscal and national security concerns take priority over tackling ill health and health inequities.

The executive order was cautious about setting concrete objectives beyond the first-term Biden administration except for the goal of carbon net zero by 2050, a goal aligned with United Nation ambitions. This caution is understandable given that new administrations often unpick signature initiatives of their predecessors and that Biden's internationalist values were in tension with Trump's isolationist America First ideology that still held sway among a vocal group of congressional Republicans. Although Biden may have felt that too much emphasis on health care would fuel his political opponents' caricature of a socialist president, it might nevertheless have been more effective if the initiative had placed health and well-being front and center.

Had it done so, it would have aligned with the long-running Healthy People federal initiative, inaugurated by a landmark report of 1979 by President Carter's surgeon general, Julius B. Richmond, which initially sought to reduce health disparities and more recently eliminate them.[6] Healthy People followed on from Richmond's recommendations of the late 1960s (when he was working in the Office of Economic Opportunity for the Johnson administration) to forge new synergies between institutions and practices of health care through an interagency approach to addressing systemic health disparities.[7] It is disappointing, if not unexpected, that Biden's executive order four decades later did not align itself more closely with the fifth iteration of Healthy People, which set health goals toward 2030. Perhaps the emphasis Biden chose was designed to mask the fact that the country was unhealthier in 2022 than it was at the millennium due to rising deaths from opioid use, COVID infections, and a spike in homicides and suicides. Perhaps the evasion was also intended to deflect from the fact that the health of Americans had worsened in some priority areas, including obesity, depression among young people, and deaths from injury. On other fronts, Biden sought to protect Medicare and Medicaid entitlements, to restore faith in Obamacare, to reduce prescription drug costs, and to stimulate a national strategy for mental health in tandem with his surgeon general, Vivek Murthy, who was looking to renewed social connectedness to combat "our epidemic of loneliness and isolation" rather than to biotechnological solutions or digital health care.[8] As a corrective to the disregard of the Trump presidency, Biden's executive order might have usefully integrated agendas and echoed the emphasis of Healthy People 2030 on health literacy and well-being from a lifespan perspective with the aim of creating "a thriving, equitable society" through collective responsibility.[9]

Biden's secretary of the Department of Health and Human Services, Xavier Becerra, had a seat at the table at the 2022 biotechnology summit, but his felt like a secondary voice following the excitement of the opening speakers about scaling up bioproduction and tech innovation. Becerra affirmed the prominence of biotech in the health space, but he said that the primary role of Health and Human Services was to collaborate with the National Institutes of Health in steering biopharmaceutical innovations, expanding developments in synthetic biology, and addressing international biosafety concerns, especially given the escalation of the COVID-19 lab-leak theory.[10] While the executive order—and the subsequent action plan—recognized that biotechnology spans an ecosystem of research, development, application, and user access, the role of Health and Human Services was at arm's length from the challenges Healthy People had tackled since the early 1980s, now with heightened intensity given that by 2030 the proportion of population over sixty-five will be double that of 2000 and mental ill health will by then likely be the leading cause of morbidity globally.[11]

In fact, there was nothing specific in the September 2022 biotechnology initiative to address mental health challenges, which is surprising given that President Biden had spoken about mental health as a key aspect of his "unity agenda for the Nation" in his State of the Union Address six months earlier.[12] Biden's State of the Union remarks focused on protecting young Americans from the encroachment of digital technologies on well-being, technologies that novelist Jennifer Egan thinks will have completely eroded privacy by the 2030s.[13] But the president's brief comments brushed over the broader recognition by the White House and Health and Human Services that strengthening system capacity, increasing access to health care, and creating healthy environments are vital for decreasing the nation's mental health burden.[14] This whole-of-society perspective shares the intent of the World Health Organization to produce finely granulated health data beneath national statistics. But the biomanufacturing emphasis of Biden's executive order and the targets of Healthy People that focus on macro data missed key World Health Organization sustainable development goals with respect to gender equality and planetary protection that a more ecological approach might achieve, given that nearly 60 percent of the global mental health burden is borne by inhabitants of low- and middle-income countries.[15]

That said, the gap between federal tech initiatives and the equity commitments of Healthy People is narrower than it first looks if we take into account the audacious assertions of biotech adventurists such as Gregory Stock, Peter Thiel, and George Church, who seek to take a high-tech path through "the many forks in the road ahead . . . to its logical extreme."[16] However, as the biohacking thread running through the second half of *Transformed States* shows, this high-tech path is far from inevitable and low-tech and ancestral medical practices still have a place in the health care ecosystem. Yet, as the introduction discusses, when adventurists consider bioethical issues, proactionary rhetoric usually overshadows the precautionary principle by conjuring alluring visions of what enhancement technologies will bring to the world. On this proactionary front, we might recall the "endless resource" of science evoked by the federal Office of Science and Technology Policy in the 1990s (rhetoric Alondra Nelson echoed at the 2022 White House biotechnology summit), but for President Clinton science was pivotal to securing a democratic future, guided by bioethical commissions to ensure that the biosciences do not run amok. As early chapters discussed, the rich public bioethics of Leon Kass during the first term of the George W. Bush administration need not necessarily be undergirded by conservative technoskepticism or unwarranted suspicion of the deep state, but can instead be an affirmatory and bipartisan guide through the evolving landscape of red biotechnology.[17]

The Healthy People initiative is also in tension with the trajectory of industry influencers that capitalize on the growing global market for biotechnology, which is estimated to increase at an annual rate of 13 to 18 percent through the 2020s. These influencers include the long-established Japanese public relations company Dentsu, which looks to a super high-tech future that will soon put the economic and health challenges of COVID-19 pandemic in the rearview mirror. Dentsu foresee four key trends that will be realized by 2030 within what they call "the Age of Inclusive Intelligence."[18] After consulting with futurists, business strategists, and specialists (including two science fiction writers), Dentsu charted four consumer trends. First, "universal activism" that goes beyond established subject positions, particularly in respect to climate change and data use; second, "a widespread embrace of synthetic enhancements and virtual experiences that improve our health"; third, the deepening of brand loyalty, especially with respect to personal health; and, fourth, "the human dividend" in which "the traits and capabilities that make us human" will intensify to offset the tech acceleration. Realizing that many predictions about biotech upgrades are likely to be socially divisive, yet not considering low-tech alternatives, Dentsu sees the 2020s as a time of "progress and peril." The company's primary aim is to help industry and consumers retain their agency in an augmented future, but it is significant that physical and mental health bind all four themes within a vision of upgraded lives that avoids the extremes of utopian technophilia and knee-jerk technophobia.[19]

The Dentsu report portrays the 2020s as a decade when humanist and posthuman rhetoric will finally align. However, it focuses on tech companies adapting to consumer demand, and there is nothing in it about downturns in biotech investment or the role of the state and public services, aside from as regulators of social media misinformation. Undoubtedly, the early 2020s are a more complex and contested time than the report acknowledges, including widespread suspicions of Big Tech; risks of unregulated genomic and AI experiments; probes into the integrity of state-sponsored science around the emergence, mitigation, and treatment of SARS-CoV-2; and fiercely divided views on reproductive technologies, access to gender-affirming care, and the depth of environmental degradation.[20] Despite collaborative biotech landmarks—such as a pangenome map that accounts for global genetic variation and potential breakthroughs for neurodegenerative conditions—it is unlikely these conflicts across so many fronts will settle down anytime soon.[21] The Organization for Economic Co-operation and Development sensed this when, in 2009, it sketched two visions of 2030, either as the culmination of rapid biotechnological change or a continued period of "muddling through" premised on a "dysfunctional set of systems" that "cannot envisage a different future."[22] The OECD report recognized the risks of rapid tech development but pictured the alternative muddling-through scenario as one in which the state continues to have a piecemeal relationship with biotech industries, focusing on hotspots that influence elections, putting the brakes on some accelerations, and leaving the market to shape others.

In contrast to this vision of bifurcating paths, an issue-specific attention of federal and state government to biotech debates and efforts to ensure that institutions act ethically might actually be seen as a basic building block for working through Robert Bellah's conception of "the good society" in terms of improving quality of life by tackling major diseases, protecting health data, democratizing digital communications, and facilitating health citizenship via a significant change in the ethics of organizational behavior. However, as this book has shown, technology has a limited place in Bellah's vision of a good society. Instead of seeing science as an endless resource, Bellah prioritized a "politics of imagination" that encourages citizens to look beyond their own subject positions and their locality to acquire lateral vision and to deepen values rooted in "social inclusion and participation."[23]

For Bellah, the politics of imagination is as much a place of reflection as it is of participation, a vantage point as well as a method of envisaging new democratic vistas. Although this strategy is insufficient for eliminating racism, sexism, and homophobia at the structural level, it nonetheless opens up a crucial space for creative and reflective accounts of the technological consequences this book has traced through a range of cultural texts.[24] It also puts Bellah at odds with the centrality of agency in Richard Rorty's vision of "achieving our country" through a regalvanized leftist politics.[25] As the introduction discusses, in affirming democracy as a "form of moral and social faith," Rorty prioritizes John Dewey's model of progressive pragmatism over Martin Heidegger's cultural pessimism.[26] Rorty thinks that a pragmatist can "play along" with Heidegger's efforts to put "technology in its proper place" but that ultimately Heidegger's gloomy outlook is at odds with the contingency that underpins Dewey's faith in pragmatism.[27] Nonetheless, Rorty misses a trick in not following Heidegger's gaze back to expansive ancient science as a lost resource that can ensure that imaginative poiesis is given the same importance as instrumental modern science.

If the arc of history is moving to a better day, to recall Barack Obama's campaign speeches of 2008, then a patchwork approach to congressional oversight that puts economics before health is unlikely to realize a good society by encouraging institutions to act responsibly over the long term. It is not just progressive politics that are at stake here, despite the risks to stable health care governance that will be shaped by the balance of power in Washington, DC during the second half of the 2020s. Regardless of who is in the White House, this patchwork approach is unlikely to facilitate the bioethical oversight needed to recalibrate social order, given Francis Fukuyama's argument that the "rate of technological change" often exceeds "the rate of social adjustment," as he wrote in his 1999 book *The Great Disruption*.[28] In 2007, fueled by conservative anxieties about a radically transformed future and in an effort to break institutional deadlock, Fukuyama called for an independent commission that is accountable, responsible, "technically competent," and "morally credible."[29] Such a commission is welcome if it prevents sharp fluctuations between congressional terms. However, history shows that an independent commission is unlikely to be free of partisan politics in terms of safeguarding long-term federal appropriations or swaying deeply held beliefs about reproductive technologies.

Writing in the same year that Fukuyama set out his "proposal for modernizing the regulation of human technologies," Nikolas Rose offered a different approach by envisaging the future as one that "will emerge from the intersection of a number of contingent pathways that, as they intertwine, might create something new."[30] Elements of contingency and disruption are features of Rose's perspective, suggesting that not all natural processes are translatable into technological instrumentalism. Rose also suspects that triumphant visions of a post-human future of "radical transformation" are a mirage and that "bioeconomic predictions" will likely turn out to be "wildly optimistic."[31] Arguing that advanced economies will continue to find themselves in the midst of change, Rose thinks that when the future comes we might not even notice it, stating that "biotechnological change will be gradual rather than revolutionary, incremental rather than epochal."[32] This view is predicated on the multiple trajectories *Transformed States* has charted through biotech practices that span the biomedical imaginary. It also recognizes the deeper embeddedness of technologies in our everyday lives, which may "soon become so integral to our ways of seeing, thinking, and acting that it will be hard to recognize their novelty."[33]

Despite this technoskeptical lens, Rose is optimistic about emergent possibility, not only in developing a somatic ethics but in health practices that operate from the bottom up, despite the dynamics of state and market biopower. Co-writing with philosopher Paul Rabinow, Rose argued that in the case of the biopolitics of mental health, we might witness a deeper recognition that quality of life matters more than radical transformations, a quality of life that is shaped more by local and global movements than by state interventions, even well-meaning ones like the September 2022 White House biotechnology summit with its emphasis on biosecurity over bioethics. Rabinow and Rose think that this potential shift might reconfigure the "knowledge, power, and expertise" that pathologize diagnoses and experiences of mental ill health by "reshaping the ways in which individuals themselves think about, judge, and act upon themselves in the name of mental health."[34]

Rose develops his thoughts on mental health in *Our Psychiatric Future* (2019), where he envisions an alternative mode of biopolitics that, first, pays as much attention to the social sciences as the life sciences and, second, takes an ecological approach to health within lived environments.[35] This ecological process aligns with the arguments of *Transformed States* in seeking a dynamic middle path between top-down and bottom-up energies as a way of embedding and rejuvenating bioethics at personal, community, and environmental levels while recognizing contingency and uncertainty. Lived experience is not a return to the identity politics that Bellah warns would delimit a politics of imagination in favor of group self-interest, but it is a key aspect of an inclusive form of health citizenship and what Rose calls "neuroecosociality" that sidesteps industrial models of the biosciences to take a more holistic approach to health that recognizes the interconnectedness of planetary life.[36]

This ecological perspective was not entirely absent at the 2022 biotechnology summit. Notably, Gilda Barabino, president of the American Association for the Advancement of Science, emphasized the role of communities in co-creating tech solutions, an increasingly diverse workforce in terms of race and gender, and the equal centrality of technical training, bioliteracy, and cultural understanding. There is democratic potential here. However, the integrated solutions typically sought in the biotech sphere place future hope in models of growth and productivity rather than in shared values, participation, and an emergent yet affirmative bioethics that recognizes the intertwined futures of all planetary life as a driving force for shaping health toward and beyond 2030.

Acknowledgments

Transformed States, the final instalment of a project I began fifteen years ago, has been a long time coming. This is in part due to other projects distracting me and in part due to the COVID-19 pandemic that, among its many more profound disruptions, prevented me visiting archives for over two years. Yet in truth, the book needed longer to gestate than I had anticipated. Despite feeling the weight of a trilogy-shaped albatross for longer than intended, there have been major gains. First, my decision to take a historical step back to 1990, offering a decade overlap with the second volume, *Voices of Mental Health*, gave me a post–Cold War perspective on biotechnology, with world events in the early years of the Biden administration exposing jagged lines between nation-state and global community that seemed to align at the millennium. Second, I refocused the book's final part in the light of planetary trends emerging in the late 2010s but that could not be fully gauged until my final and most intensive phase of writing in 2021–2023. Third, the longer-than-expected writing period gave me a stronger conceptual sense of what I wanted the book to achieve, especially in pursuing holistic and ecological views of health, in which the demarcation between mental health and physical health is deliberately less sharp than in my first two volumes.

The extra time it took to complete the book raised other issues, in which the bad and good sometimes interrupted each other. A lack of momentum and the interruption of COVID-19 fell on the negative side. But a relocation from Leicester to Manchester is very much on the positive. There, Kristen and Ignatius have transformed my life, and I owe them so much love and thanks—for everything large and small. Since moving to the Northwest, I have also gained immensely from being a visiting fellow in the School of Arts, Languages and Cultures at the University of Manchester in 2020–2023. Thank you to Jerome de Groot and Ian Scott for facilitating this fellowship. In addition, I had the honor of being a visiting research scholar in the Center for Health and Wellbeing at Princeton University in 2022–2023, where I presented a version of chapter 5 at the Princeton School of Public and International Affairs. My thanks here go to Janet Currie, Kate Ho, Heather Howard, Debra Pino Betancourt, and Justine Conoline for being so helpful and welcoming during my New Jersey visits.

Even though the COVID years were among my most taxing professionally, the University of Leicester, both materially and intellectually, continues to support my research in consequential ways. This book could not have been written without the professional and personal support of colleagues in the Centre for American Studies—Nick Everett, Zalfa Feghali, Andrew Johnstone, George Lewis, Catherine Morley, and Alex Waddan—as well as colleagues in the School of Arts: David Christopher, Gowan Dawson, Lucy Evans, and Mark Rawlinson. I was working on this book during my involvement in an international project that straddled the COVID years between the universities of Leicester and Guyana focusing on mental health in Guyana's prison system. This was such a valuable interdisciplinary collaboration and I must thank, particularly, Clare Anderson, Tammy Ayres, Queenela Cameron, Melissa Ifill, Dylan Kerrigan, Kevin Pilgrim, and Kristy Warren.

In addition, my thanks go to Sari Altschuler, Sara Alzahrani, Jonathan Bell, Caitlin Hawke, Paul Hegarty, Brian Jarvis, Zuzanna Ladyga, Danny Lutz, Andy Mousley, Joel Rasmussen, Joe Street, Casey Wallace, Brian Ward, and Alex Zagaria for offering valuable suggestions that helped in developing this project. I am grateful to Nicholas Manning for his American Literature and Therapeutic Cultures initiative (including a June 2023 conference at Université Grenoble Alpes, where I presented a version of chapter 2) and for giving me the opportunity to reflect upon my research over the last quarter century for *Revue francaise d'études américaines* 170, no. 1 (2022). I also want to thank Sophie Jones, my coeditor for the *Edinburgh Companion to the Politics of American Health*, the research for which intersected with elements of this book. Published in 2022, this thirty-five-essay volume includes some fantastic authors whose work assisted me in thinking through aspects of *Transformed States*.

I am very grateful for the assistance of librarians and archivists throughout this project, especially those at the William J. Clinton Presidential Library, Little Rock, Arkansas; the George H. W. Bush Presidential Library, College Station, Texas; the George W. Bush Presidential Library, Dallas, Texas (including assistance processing Freedom of Information Act requests at both Bush libraries on redacted documents relating to the Decade of the Brain initiative, bioethics, stem cell research, and partial-birth abortion); the Arthur H. Aufses, Jr., MD Archives Icahn School of Medicine at Mount Sinai, New York City; the Robert N. Butler Columbia Aging Center Archives at the Mailman School of Public Health, Columbia University, New York City; the Elmer E. Rasmuson Library, University of Alaska Fairbanks; the Strozier Library, Florida State University, Tallahassee; the William Madison Randall Library, University of North Carolina Wilmington; the Harvey S. Firestone Memorial Library, Princeton University, Princeton, New Jersey; the University of South Florida Tampa Library; the Cecil H. Green Library, Stanford University, Stanford, California; the National Library of Medicine, Bethesda, Maryland; the Library of Congress, Washington, DC; and the Wellcome Collection Library, London.

Thank you to Antony Gormley who kindly provided permission to use a photograph I took on my 50th birthday on Crosby Beach, Merseyside, depicting a fragment of his *Another Place* installation of 1997. Photographed during the worst COVID year in the UK, the cover image is resonant of the ecological health theme of this book and offers a wonderful riposte to Michel Foucault's famous image of "a face drawn in sand at the edge of the sea" being washed away by the tide, as discussed in the introduction. I am grateful to all the copyright holders who granted permission to use the images in *Transformed States,* especially to Rita La Blanc and Jeff VanderMeer for their permission to reprint the Area X logo of St. Marks Wildlife Refuge, Florida in chapter 8. Thank you, too, to Peter Mickulas, my editor at Rutgers, who has been a long-term supporter of this endeavor, and to Kate Babbitt, Catherine Denning, and Angela Piliouras for their valuable editorial assistance. As ever, my thanks go to my family, especially my mum, dad, and brother, for putting up with my randomness for so many years—and for always being there.

Finally, I want to dedicate this book to two southern gentlemen who were central figures for much of my adult life and positive energies through these three volumes. One was born in Tennessee, the other in the District of Columbia. One was my PhD supervisor and so much more; the other was my Capitol Hill landlord who became a dear friend and companion, especially in his later years. Their personalities differed, but both thought capaciously and historically, made me think, made me laugh, did irony, and had powerful presences—although they would no doubt deny this. They never knew each other, but both studied at the University of Virginia and they may have shared a ride on the Washington, DC metro in the 1970s. On many fronts, they helped me keep my life together and I miss them both greatly. For these reasons, I dedicate this book to Richard H. King (1941–2022) and Carl B. Nelson (1946–2021).

Notes

NOTES TO PREFACE

1. Thomas L. Friedman, *Thank You for Being Late: An Optimist's Guide to Thriving in the Age of Accelerations* (New York: Farrar, Straus and Giroux, 2016), 22, 201, 298; "Investment in Biopharma Is Reaching an Inflection Point," Biospace, September 21, 2021, accessed February 1, 2023, https://www.biospace.com/article/investment-in-biopharma-is-reaching-an-inflection-point-.

2. The White House, National Bioeconomy Blueprint, April 2012, https://obamawhitehouse.archives.gov/administration/eop/ostp/library/bioeconomy. For the colors used to characterize different branches of biotechnology see Paweł Kafarski, "Rainbow Code of Biotechnology," *Chemik* 66, no. 8 (2012): 811–816.

3. John P. Holdren, Howard Shelanski, Darci Vetter, and Christy Goldfuss, "Improving Transparency and Ensuring Continued Safety in Biotechnology," July 2, 2015, accessed November 21, 2021, https://obamawhitehouse.archives.gov/blog/2015/07/02/improving-transparency-and-ensuring-continued-safety-biotechnology; President's Council of Advisors on Science and Technology to President Obama, November 2016, accessed November 21, 2021, https://obamawhitehouse.archives.gov/sites/default/files/microsites/ostp/PCAST/pcast_biodefense_letter_report_final.pdf. See also Paul Virilio and Sylvère Lotringer, *Crepuscular Dawn*, trans. Mike Taormina (Cambridge, MA: MIT Press, 2002); and Paul Virilio, *The Administration of Fear* (New York: Semiotext(e), 2012).

4. Achille Mbembe, *Necropolitics* (Durham, NC: Duke University Press, 2019), 14.

5. John Tomlinson, *The Culture of Speed: The Coming of Immediacy* (London: Sage, 2007), 10.

6. See John Pat Leary, "Innovation and the Neoliberal Idioms of Development," *boundary2*, August 2018, accessed November 30, 2021, https://www.boundary2.org/2018/08/leary.

7. Sherry Turkle, *Alone Together: Why We Expect More from Technology and Less from Each Other* (New York: Basic Books, 2011), 242–243.

8. Virilio, *Administration of Fear*, 37.

9. American Psychiatric Association, *Diagnostic and Statistical Manual of Mental Disorders*, 4th ed. (Washington, DC: American Psychiatric Association, 1994), #300.02.

10. Substance Abuse and Mental Health Services Administration, *Impact of the DSM-IV to DSM-5 Changes on the National Survey on Drug Use and Health* (Rockville, MD: Substance Abuse and Mental Health Services Administration, 2016), Table 3.15, accessed October 15, 2021, https://www.ncbi.nlm.nih.gov/books/NBK519704/table/ch3.t15. See

also Gavin Andrews, Megan J. Hobbs, Thomas D. Borkovec, Katja Beesdo, Michelle G. Craske, Richard G. Heimberg, Ronald M. Rapee, et al., "Generalized Worry Disorder: A Review of DSM-IV Generalized Anxiety Disorder and Options for DSM-V," *Depression and Anxiety* 27, no. 2 (2010): 134–147; Allan V. Horwitz and Jerome C. Wakefield, *All We Have to Fear: Psychiatry's Transformation of Natural Anxieties into Mental Disorders* (New York: Oxford University Press, 2012), 72.

11. See Mark J. Brosnan, *Technophobia: The Psychological Impact of Information Technology* (London: Routledge, 1998); Mark J. Brosnan and Susan J. Thorpe, "An Evaluation of Two Clinically-Derived Treatments for Technophobia," *Computers in Human Behavior* 22, no. 6 (2006): 1080–1095; Richard T. LeBeau, Daniel Glenn, Betty Liao, Hans-Ulrich Wittchen, Katja Beesdo-Baum, Thomas Ollendick, and Michelle G. Craske, "Specific Phobia: A Review of DSM-IV Specific Phobia and Preliminary Recommendations for DSM-V," *Depression and Anxiety* 27, no. 2 (2010): 148–167; Susan J. Thorpe and M. J. Brosnan, "Does Computer Anxiety Reach Levels which Conform to DSM-IV Criteria for Specific Phobia?," *Computers in Human Behavior* 23, no. 3 (2007): 1258–1272. See also Jonathan Haidt, *The Anxious Generation: How the Great Rewiring of Childhood is Causing an Epidemic of Mental Illness* (New York: Allen Lane, 2024).

12. Virilio, *Administration of Fear*, 15. On phobic responses, see Douglas Kellner, "Virilio, War and Technology: Some Critical Reflections," *Theory, Culture & Society* 16, no. 5/6 (1999): 103–125; and Paul E. Brodwin, ed., *Biotechnology and Culture: Bodies, Anxieties, Ethics* (Bloomington: Indiana University Press, 2000), 5.

13. Neil Postman, *Technopoly: The Surrender of Culture to Technology* (London: Vintage, 1993), 20.

14. Donna Haraway, *When Species Meet* (Minneapolis: University of Minnesota Press, 2007), 15.

15. See Douglas Eklund and Ian Alteveer, *Everything Is Connected: Art and Conspiracy* (New York: Metropolitan Museum of Art, 2018).

16. Matthew N. Hannah, "A Conspiracy of Data: QAnon, Social Media, and Information Visualization," *Social Media and Society* 7, no. 3 (2021), https://doi.org/10.1177/20563051211036064.

INTRODUCTION

1. "Decade of the Brain, 1990–1999," Proclamation 6158, July 17, 1990, 55 Fed. Reg. 140 (July 20, 1990), 29553.

2. Joint Resolution to Designate the Decade beginning January 1, 1990, as the "Decade of the Brain," Pub. L. 101–58, 103 Stat. 152 (July 25, 1989), https://www.congress.gov/101/statute/STATUTE-103/STATUTE-103-Pg152.pdf. For the initiatives of the National Advisory Neurological and Communicative Disorders and Stroke Council in the Bush era, see National Advisory Neurological and Communicative Disorders and Stroke Council, *Decade of the Brain: Answers through Scientific Research* (Bethesda, MD: U.S. Dept. of Health and Human Services, Public Health Service, National Institutes of Health,

1989). For National Institute of Mental Health initiatives, see Sandy Rovner, "Probing the Most Common Mental Disorder, High Anxiety," *Washington Post*, May 22, 1990.

3. George H. W. Bush, "Remarks to the National Academy of Sciences," April 23, 1990, in *Public Papers of the Presidents of the United States: George H. W. Bush, 1990*, Book 1, *January 1 to June 30, 1990* (Washington, DC: Government Printing Office, 1991), 547.

4. Carnegie Commission on Science, Technology, and Government, *A Science and Technology Agenda for the Nation: Recommendations for the President and Congress* (December 1992), 23, https://www.ccstg.org/pdfs/AgendaNation1292.pdf.

5. Murray Goldstein, "Decade of the Brain: An Agenda for the Nineties," *Western Journal of Medicine* 161 (September 1994): 239–241.

6. Richard Himelfarb and Rosanna Perotti, *Principle over Politics? The Domestic Policy of the George H. W. Bush Presidency* (Westport, CT: Praeger, 2004), 359.

7. George Bush, "Remarks at the Swearing-In Ceremony for Bernadine Healy as Director of the National Institutes for Health in Bethesda, Maryland," June 24, 1991, in *Public Papers of the Presidents of the United States: George H. W. Bush, 1991*, Book 1, *January 1 to June 30, 1991* (Washington, DC: Government Printing Office, 1992), 713–714.

8. President's Council on Competitiveness, *Report on National Biotechnology Policy* (February 1991), 4; Office of Science and Technology Policy, *U.S. Technology Policy* (September 26, 1990), 11; "Science and Technology (1990) (Bromley) [1]," Box 98, John Sununu Files, White House Office of Chief of Staff, George H. W. Bush Presidential Records, George H. W. Bush Presidential Library, College Station, Texas.

9. "Appendix 1: The Role of Technology in Bush Administration Policies," 4, "Science and Technology (Bromley) (1991) [1]," Box 99, John Sununu Files, White House Office of Chief of Staff.

10. See Susan Thaul and Dana Hotra, eds., *An Assessment of the NIH Women's Health Initiative* (Washington, DC: National Academies Press, 1993), 20. Bernadine Healy argued to Congress that "discrimination based on genotype must be prohibited as a matter of basic civil rights": US Congress, House of Representatives, Committee on Government Operations, Subcommittee on Government Information, Justice, and Agriculture, *Domestic and International Data Protection Issues: Possible Uses and Misuses of Genetic Information: Public Hearing* (Washington, DC: Government Printing Office, 1991). Notably, as president of the American Heart Association (1988–1989), Healy profiled the health consequences of heart disease for American women.

11. George H. W. Bush, "Remarks to the United States Chamber of Commerce National Action Rally," February 24, 1992, in *Public Papers of the Presidents: George H. W. Bush, 1992*, Book 1, *January 1 to July 31, 1992* (Washington, DC: Government Printing Office, 1993), 298.

12. George Bush, "Remarks to Stryker Corporation Employees in Kalamazoo, Michigan," March 13, 1992, in *Public Papers of the Presidents: George H. W. Bush, 1992*, Book 1, 441.

13. William J. Clinton, "Remarks on Signing Memorandums on Medical Research and Reproductive Health and an Exchange with Reporters," January 22, 1993, *Public*

Papers of the Presidents of the United States: William J. Clinton, 1993, Book 1, January 20 to July 31, 1993 (Washington, DC: Government Printing Office, 1994), 7. Clinton's speech redressed Bush's anti-abortion ethos by emphasizing women's and minority health.

14. See, for example, George Bush, "Question-and-Answer Session with Students at John F. Kennedy High School in Denver, Colorado," December 8, 1989, in *Public Papers of the Presidents of the United States: George H. W. Bush, 1989*, Book 2, *July 1 to December 31, 1989* (Washington, DC: Government Printing Office, 1990), 1671.

15. See Nicolas Rasmussen, *Gene Jockeys: Life Science and the Rise of the Biotech Enterprise* (Baltimore, MD: Johns Hopkins University Press, 2014), 160–182; Malcolm Gladwell, "For Genentech, Success Comes with High Price," *Washington Post*, May 15, 1988; Barry Stavro, "Gene Warfare," *Los Angeles Times*, December 4, 1988.

16. Cort Wrotnowski, *Biotechnology in the 1990s: Taking Stock* (Norwalk, CT: Business Communications, 1992), 1.

17. US Congress, Office of Technology Assessment, *Biotechnology in a Global Economy* (Washington, DC: Government Printing Office, October 1991), http://ota.fas.org/reports/9110.pdf. See also Office of Technology Assessment, *New Developments in Biotechnology* (Washington, DC: Government Printing Office, 1988).

18. Wrotnowski, *Biotechnology in the 1990s*, 8.

19. Echoing the 1947 Nuremberg Code, Clinton released a "Memorandum on Research Involving Human Subjects," February 17, 1994, in *Public Papers of the Presidents of the United States: William J. Clinton, 1994*, Book 1, *January 1 to July 31, 1994* (Washington, DC: Government Printing Office, 1995), 281; and a "Statement on Protections for Human Subjects of Classified Research," March 28, 1997, in *Public Papers of the Presidents of the United States: William J. Clinton, 1997*, Book 1, *January 1 to June 30, 1997* (Washington, DC: Government Printing Office, 1998), 359.

20. Elias A. Zerhouni, "US Biomedical Research: Basic, Translational, and Clinical Sciences," *JAMA* 294 (September 21, 2005): 1357; Elias A. Zerhouni, "Translational and Clinical Science—Time for a New Vision," *New England Journal of Medicine* 353 (October 2005): 1621–1623.

21. See Martin Kenney, *Biotechnology: The University-Industrial Complex* (New Haven, CT: Yale University Press, 1986); Albert Sasson, *Medical Biotechnology: Achievements, Prospects and Perceptions* (Tokyo: United Nations University Press, 2005); Junfu Zhang and Nikesh Patel, *The Dynamics of California's Biotechnology Industry* (San Francisco: Public Policy Institute of California, 2005); Kaushik Sunder Rajan, ed., *Lively Capital: Biotechnologies, Ethics, and Governance in Global Markets* (Durham, NC: Duke University Press, 2012).

22. See Chong-Moon Lee, *The Silicon Valley Edge: A Habitat for Innovation and Entrepreneurship* (Stanford, CA: Stanford University Press, 2000); Doogab Yi, *The Recombinant University: Genetic Engineering and the Emergence of Stanford Biotechnology* (Chicago: University of Chicago Press, 2015).

23. Maya Kosoff, "Peter Thiel Wants to Inject Himself with Young People's Blood," *Vanity Fair*, August 1, 2016.

24. Erin Griffith and Dan Primack, "The Age of Unicorns," *Fortune*, January 22, 2015; Adam Lashinsky, "The Age of Unicorns Wanes," *Fortune*, January 21, 2016.

25. "Vice President Biden Visits Bay Area Company That Could Soon Revolutionize Healthcare," CBS News, July 23, 2015, https://www.cbsnews.com/sanfrancisco/news/vice-president-joe-biden-theranos-elizabeth-holmes-newark-lab-test. Joe Biden's remarks are quoted in John Carreyrou, *Bad Blood: Secrets and Lies in a Silicon Valley Startup* (New York: Knopf, 2018), 265.

26. Dave Eggers, *The Circle* (New York: Knopf, 2013); David Sergeant, *The Near Future in 21st Century Fiction* (Cambridge: Cambridge University Press, 2022), 89.

27. On socio-regressive critiques, see Martin Paul Eve and Joe Street, "The Silicon Valley Novel," *Literature and History* 27 (May 2018): 81–97. On surveillance capitalism, see Critical Art Ensemble, *Flesh Machine: Cyborgs, Designer Babies, and New Eugenic Consciousness* (Brooklyn, NY: Autonomedia, 1998); and Richard Bingham, "The Disabled Body under Surveillance Capitalism: Tony Tulathimutte's *Private Citizens*," *C21 Literature: Journal of 21st-Century Writings* 8, no. 1 (2020): 1–28. On skepticism about venture capitalist biotechnology, see Arielle Emmett, "Biotech Start-Ups," *The Scientist*, June 2000, https://www.the-scientist.com/news/biotech-start-ups-55895.

28. Jemimah Steinfield, "Nonsense and Sensibility: An Interview with Dave Eggers," *Index on Censorship* 49 (September 2020): 60; Susan Squier, *Liminal Lives: Imagining the Human and the Frontiers of Biomedicine* (Durham, NC: Duke University Press, 2004), 17.

29. See Bernard D. Davis, ed., *The Genetic Revolution: Scientific Prospects and Human Perceptions* (Baltimore, MD: Johns Hopkins University Press, 1992).

30. Nikolas Rose and Joelle M. Abi-Rached, *Neuro: The New Brain Sciences and the Management of the Mind* (Princeton, NJ: Princeton University Press, 2013), 3–5.

31. Michel Foucault, *The Order of Things: An Archaeology of the Human Sciences* (1966; repr., New York: Routledge, 2005), 422.

32. Joseph Masco, "Atomic Health, or How the Bomb Altered American Notions of Death," in *Against Health: How Health Became the New Morality*, ed. Jonathan M. Metzl and Anna Kirkland (New York: New York University Press, 2010), 133.

33. Michael Mulkay, *The Embryo Research Debate: Science and the Politics of Reproduction* (Cambridge: Cambridge University Press, 1997), 117.

34. Boris Johnson, "PM Speech to the UN General Assembly: 24 September 2019," Gov.UK, https://www.gov.uk/government/speeches/pm-speech-to-the-un-general-assembly-24-september-2019.

35. Tina Stevens and Stuart Newman, *Biotech Juggernaut: Hope, Hype, and Hidden Agendas of Entrepreneurial Bioscience* (New York: Routledge, 2019); Gina Kolata, "Building a Better Human with Science? The Public Says, No Thanks," *New York Times*, July 26, 2016.

36. Stevens and Newman, *Biotech Juggernaut*, xi. See also US Department of Health and Human Services, *Healthy People 2000: National Health Promotion and Disease Prevention Objectives* (Washington, DC: Government Printing Office, 1990).

37. Nikolas Rose, *The Politics of Life Itself: Biomedicine, Power, and Subjectivity in the Twenty-First Century* (Princeton, NJ: Princeton University Press, 2007), 1; Sheryl Gay Stolberg, "A Genetic Future Both Tantalizing and Disturbing," *New York Times*, January 1, 2000.

38. William J. Clinton, "Remarks at the California Institute of Technology in Pasadena, California," January 21, 2000, in *Public Papers of the Presidents of the United States: William J. Clinton, 2000*, Book 1, *January 1 to June 30* (Washington, DC: Government Printing Office, 2001), 95.

39. See Philip Ball, *How to Grow a Human: Adventures in Who We Are and How We Are Made* (London: HarperCollins, 2019), vii–viii.

40. Giorgio Agamben, *Language and Death: The Place of Negativity*, trans. Karen E. Pinkus with Michael Hardt (1982; repr., Minneapolis: University of Minnesota Press, 1992), 56–57; Paul Virilio, "Ground Zero" (2002), in *The Paul Virilio Reader*, ed. Steve Redhead (New York: Columbia University Press, 2004), 251.

41. N. Katherine Hayles, *Unthought: The Power of the Cognitive Nonconscious* (Chicago: University of Chicago Press, 2017), 170. See also Bradley B. Onishi, "Information, Bodies, and Heidegger: Tracing Visions of the Posthuman," *Sophia* 50 (April 2011): 101–112.

42. Eugene Thacker, *Biomedia* (Minneapolis: University of Minnesota Press, 2004), 2.

43. William J. Clinton, "Statement on Signing Biotechnology Process Patent Legislation," November 1, 1995, in *Public Papers of the Presidents of the United States: William J. Clinton, 1995*, Book 2, *July 1 to December 31, 1995* (Washington, DC: Government Printing Office, 1996), 1704.

44. George W. Bush, "Remarks to the American Association of Community Colleges Convention in Minneapolis, Minnesota," April 26, 2004, in *Public Papers of the Presidents of the United States: George W. Bush, 2004*, Book 1, *January 1 to June 30, 2004* (Washington, DC: Government Printing Office, 2005), 676. Bush championed job growth in "high-skilled fields like health care and biotechnology" in his January 20, 2004, State of the Union Address.

45. Clinton, "Statement on Steps to Enhance the Safety of Clinical Trials," in *Public Papers of the Presidents of the United States: William J. Clinton, 2000*, Book 1, *January 1 to June 30* (Washington, DC: Government Printing Office, 2001), 1008. See also Harriet A. Washington, *Deadly Monopolies: The Shocking Corporate Takeover of Life Itself* (New York: Anchor, 2013).

46. Klaus Schwab, *The Fourth Industrial Revolution* (New York: Crown Business, 2016), 9, 98.

47. For this phrase, see Armand Doucet, Jelmer Evers, Elisa Guerra, Nadia Lopez, Michael Soskil, and Koen Timmers, *Teaching in the Fourth Industrial Revolution: Standing at the Precipice* (London: Routledge, 2018); and Rose, *The Politics of Life Itself*, 5.

48. Don DeLillo, *Zero K* (New York: Scribner, 2016), 245.

49. On tech progress narratives, see George Estreich, *Fables and Futures: Biotechnology, Disability, and the Stories We Tell Ourselves* (Cambridge, MA: MIT Press, 2019), xiv–xv.

50. Donna Haraway, *When Species Meet* (Minneapolis: University of Minnesota Press, 2007), 136.

51. Bruno Latour, *We Have Never Been Modern*, trans. Catherine Porter (Cambridge, MA: Harvard University Press, 1993); Bruno Latour "Can We Get Our Materialism Back, Please?," *Isis* 98 (2007): 138–142. Latour is critical of Heidegger in this essay.

52. On "bringing forth," see Martin Heidegger, "The Question Concerning Technology" (1962), in *Basic Writings*, rev. ed. (New York: Harper, 2008), 317–318.

53. Heidegger, "The Question Concerning Technology," 338.

54. Heidegger, "The Question Concerning Technology," 311–312.

55. Kevin Aho, ed., *Existential Medicine: Essays on Health and Illness* (Lanham, MD: Rowman and Littlefield, 2018).

56. See Kendall and Michel, "Thinking the Unthought," 145–146.

57. Heidegger, "Letter on Humanism" (1946), in *Basic Writings*, rev. ed. (New York: Harper, 2008), 265.

58. Martin Heidegger, "Science and Reflection" (1954), in *The Question Concerning Technology and Other Essays*, trans. William Lovitt (New York: Harper & Row, 1977), 155.

59. George H. W. Bush, "Remarks at the Swearing-In Ceremony for Bernadine Healy," June 24, 1991, in *Public Papers of the Presidents of the United States: George H. W. Bush, 1991, Book 1, January 1 to June 30, 1991* (Washington, DC: Government Printing Office, 1992), 714.

60. See Heidegger, "The Question Concerning Technology," 321, 324. See also Mark A. Wrathall, *Heidegger and Unconcealment: Truth, Language and History* (Cambridge: Cambridge University Press, 2011); and Aaron James Wendland, Christopher Merwin, and Christos Hadjioannou, eds., *Heidegger on Technology* (London: Routledge, 2019).

61. Anthony Giddens, *The Runaway World: How Globalization Is Reshaping Our Lives* (London: Profile Books, 1999). See also Sheryl N. Hamilton, "Traces of the Future: Biotechnology, Science Fiction, and the Media," *Science Fiction Studies* 30 (July 2003): 267–282.

62. Rose, *The Politics of Life Itself*, 3.

63. Rose, *The Politics of Life Itself*, 4–5. On somatic individualism, see Nikolas Rose, *Inventing Ourselves: Psychology, Power, and Personhood* (Cambridge: Cambridge University Press, 1996); and Nikolas Rose, "Governing the Will in a Neurochemical Age," in *On Willing Selves: Neoliberal Politics vis-à-vis the Neuroscientific Challenge*, ed. Sabine Massen and Barbara Sutter (London: Palgrave Macmillan, 2007), 81–99.

64. Rose, *The Politics of Life Itself*, 76.

65. Thomas Osborne and Nikolas Rose, "Against Posthumanism: Notes towards an Ethopolitics of Personhood," *Theory, Culture & Society* 40 (June 2023): 2–3. See also Thomas Osborne and Nikolas Rose, *Questioning Humanity: Being Human in a Posthuman Age* (Northampton, MA: Edward Elgar, 2024).

66. See Eric T. Juengst, "Can Enhancement Be Distinguished from Prevention in Genetic Medicine?," *Journal of Medicine and Philosophy* 22 (April 1997): 125–142.

67. Rose, *The Politics of Life Itself*, 252, 254.

68. Rose, *The Politics of Life Itself*, 26.

69. Melinda C. Hall, *The Bioethics of Enhancement: Transhumanism, Disability, and Biopolitics* (Lanham, MD: Lexington Books, 2017), x.

70. See Jon Turney, "Inhuman, Superhuman or Posthuman? Images of Genetic Futures," in *Crossing Over: Genomics in the Public Arena*, ed. Edna Einsiedel and Frank Timmermans (Calgary: University of Calgary Press, 2005), 225–235; and Turney's earlier book, *Frankenstein's Footsteps: Science, Genetics, and Popular Culture* (New Haven, CT: Yale University Press, 1998).

71. Richard Rorty, "Philosophy as Science, as Metaphor, and as Politics" (1986), in Rorty, *Essays on Heidegger and Others: Philosophical Papers*, vol. 2 (New York: Cambridge University Press, 1991), 23.

72. "Statement of Principles," Project for a New American Century, June 3, 1997, https://web.archive.org/web/20050205041635/http://www.newamericancentury.org/statementofprinciples.htm.

73. Gregory Stock, *Redesigning Humans: Choosing Our Children's Genes* (New York: Houghton Mifflin, 2002), 1.

74. Stock, *Redesigning Humans*, 3.

75. Ted Chiang, "The Evolution of Human Science" (2000), in Chiang, *Stories of Your Life and Others* (New York: Picador, 2014), 239.

76. Gregory Stock, *Metaman: The Merging of Humans and Machines into a Global Superorganism* (New York: Simon & Schuster, 1993), 31–32.

77. Stock, *Redesigning Humans*, 17.

78. Stock, *Redesigning Humans*, 70. On bone marrow donations, see Catherine Waldby and Robert Mitchell, *Tissue Economies: Blood, Organs, and Cell Lines in Late Capitalism* (Durham, NC: Duke University Press, 2006), 111–113.

79. Nicholas Zurbrugg, ed., *Jean Baudrillard: Art and Artefact* (London: Sage, 1997), 24.

80. "Biotechnology," episode of *Talk of the Nation*, aired April 15, 2002, on NPR, https://www.npr.org/templates/story/story.php?storyId=1141610. For Kass's views, see Leon R. Kass and James Q. Wilson, *The Ethics of Human Cloning* (Washington, DC: AEI Press, 1998); and Leon R. Kass, *Life, Liberty, and the Defense of Dignity: The Challenge for Bioethics* (San Francisco: Encounter, 2002). Stock responded to both Kass and Fukuyama in "Preface," in *Redesigning Humans* (Boston: Houghton Mifflin, 2003), xi–xiv.

81. Francis Fukuyama, *Our Posthuman Future: Consequences of the Biotechnology Revolution* (New York: Farrar, Straus and Giroux, 2002), 7.

82. George W. Bush, "Address to the Nation on Stem Cell Research," August 9, 2001, in *Public Papers of the Presidents of the United States: George W. Bush, 2001*, Book 2, *July 1 to December 31, 2001* (Washington, DC: Government Printing Office, 2003), 953–956; Leon R. Kass, "Preventing a Brave New World," *New Republic*, June 21, 2001; "The Sanctity of Life in a Brave New World: A Manifesto on Biotechnology and Human Dignity," Febru-

ary 5, 2003, https://www.kritischebioethik.de/us-manifest-english.pdf; *Issues Raised by Human Cloning Research: Hearing Before the Subcommittee on Oversight and Investigations, Committee on Energy and Commerce, House of Representatives, 107th Congress, 1st Session, 28 March 2001* (Washington, DC: Government Printing Office, 2001), https://www.govinfo.gov/content/pkg/CHRG-107hhrg71495/html/CHRG-107hhrg71495.htm.

83. Margaret Atwood, "Of the Madness of Mad Scientists" (2011), in Atwood, *In Other Worlds: SF and the Human Imagination* (London: Virago, 2011), 205, 211; Donna J. Haraway, *Staying with the Trouble: Making Kin in the Chthulucene* (Durham, NC: Duke University Press, 2016), 3.

84. On the precautionary principle and policy, see Adam D. Sheingate, "Promotion Versus Precaution: The Evolution of Biotechnology Policy in the United States," *British Journal of Political Science* 36 (March 2006): 243–268.

85. Lee M. Silver, *Remaking Eden: How Genetic Engineering and Cloning will Transform the American Family* (1998; repr., New York: Harper Perennial, 2007), 4–8.

86. Francis Fukuyama, *The End of History and the Last Man* (New York: Free Press, 1992).

87. Francis Fukuyama, *The Great Disruption: Human Nature and the Reconstitution of Social Order* (New York: The Free Press, 1999), 5.

88. Stock, *Redesigning Humans,* 151.

89. Fukuyama, *Our Posthuman Future,* 218; Fukuyama, *The Great Disruption,* 6.

90. Harold T. Shapiro to President Clinton, June 9, 1997, included as a preface to volume 1 of National Bioethics Advisory Commission, *Cloning Human Beings: Report and Recommendations of the National Bioethics Advisory Commission* (Rockville, MD: U.S. National Bioethics Advisory Commission, [1997]); Francis Fukuyama, "Biotechnology and the Threat of a Posthuman Future," in *Genetics: Science, Ethics, and Public Policy: A Reader,* ed. Thomas A. Shannon (Lanham, MD: Rowman & Littlefield, 2005), 9.

91. Stock, "Preface," xiii.

92. Max More, "The Philosophy of Transhumanism," in *The Transhumanist Reader: Classical and Contemporary Essays on the Science, Technology, and Philosophy of the Human Future,* ed. Max More and Natasha Vita-More (Chichester: John Wiley, 2013), 4. On the techno-progressive aspects of transhumanism, see Allen Porter, "Bioethics and Transhumanism," *Journal of Medicine and Philosophy* 3 (June 2017): 237–260.

93. For the proactionary principle, see the Extropy Institute website: https://www.extropy.org/proactionaryprinciple.htm, accessed April 14, 2024, and Max More, "The Proactionary Principle: Optimizing Technological Outcomes," in *The Transhumanist Reader: Classical and Contemporary Essays on the Science, Technology, and Philosophy of the Human Future,* ed. Max More and Natasha Vita-More (Chichester: John Wiley, 2013), 258–267.

94. Richard Powers, *Generosity* (New York: Farrar, Straus, and Giroux, 2009), 19. See Nick Bostrom, "Existential Risks: Analyzing Human Extinction Scenarios and Related Hazards," *Journal of Evolution and Technology,* 9 (March 2002), https://jetpress.org

/volume9/risks.pdf; and Nick Bostrom, *Deep Utopia: Life and Meaning in a Solved World* (Washington DC: IdeaPress, 2024).

95. Gregory Stock, "The Battle for the Future," in *The Transhumanist Reader: Classical and Contemporary Essays on the Science, Technology, and Philosophy of the Human Future*, ed. Max More and Natasha Vita-More (Chichester: John Wiley, 2013), 315.

96. Donna Haraway, *Primate Visions: Gender, Race and Nature in the World of Modern Science* (London: Verso, 1992), 54.

97. Donna Haraway, "Ecce Homo, Ain't (Ar'n't) I a Woman, and Inappropriate/d Others: The Human in a Posthumanist Landscape," in *The Haraway Reader* (New York: Routledge, 2004), 47–48.

98. Donna Haraway, *Modest_Witness@Second_Millennium.FemaleMan©_Meets_Onco-MouseTM: Feminism and Technoscience* (New York: Routledge, 1997), 51; Donna Haraway, *Primate Visions: Gender, Race and Nature in the World of Modern Science* (New York: Routledge, 1989), 5.

99. Haraway, "Ecco Homo," 48.

100. Haraway, "Ecco Homo," 47.

101. Haraway, *Primate Visions*, 287.

102. Julietta Singh, "Disposable Objects: Ethecology, Waste, and Maternal After-lives," *Studies in Gender and Sexuality* 19 (2018): 49.

103. Singh, "Disposable Objects," 49; Julietta Singh, *Unthinking Mastery: Dehumanism and Decolonial Entanglements* (Durham, NC: Duke University Press, 2018), 4.

104. For the perils of overpredicting or underpredicting biotechnological impact, see Eric Cohen, "The Real Meaning of Genetics," *New Atlantis* 9 (Summer 2005): 29–41.

105. Schwab, *The Fourth Industrial Revolution*, 99–100.

106. Paul J. H. Schoemaker and Joyce A. Schoemaker, *Chips, Clones, and Living Beyond 100: How Far Will the Biosciences Take Us?* (Upper Saddle River, NJ: Financial Times Press, 2009), 11.

107. See Bill McKibben, *The Age of Missing Information* (New York: Random House, 1992); and Richard Restak, *The New Brain: How the Modern Age Is Rewiring Your Mind* (Emmaus, PA: Rodale, 2003).

108. McKibben, *Age of Missing Information*, 198.

109. Paul Virilio, *The Administration of Fear* (New York: Semiotext(e), 2012), 27, 15.

110. David W. Hill, "Speed and Pessimism: Moral Experience in the Work of Paul Virilio," *Journal for Cultural Research* 23 (2019): 411; Anna Tsing, Nils Bubandt, Elaine Gan, and Heather Ann Swanson, *Arts of Living on a Damaged Planet: Ghosts and Monsters of the Anthropocene* (Minneapolis: University of Minnesota Press, 2017).

111. Richard Rorty, *Achieving Our Country: Leftist Thought in Twentieth-Century America* (Cambridge, MA: Harvard University Press, 1998).

112. On the pragmatic and positivist wings of scientific humanism, see Stephen P. Weldon, *The Scientific Spirt of American Humanism* (Baltimore, MD: Johns Hopkins University Press, 2020).

113. Thomas L. Friedman, *Thank You for Being Late: An Optimist's Guide to Thriving in the Age of Accelerations* (New York: Farrar, Straus and Giroux, 2016), 450.

114. Friedman, *Thank You for Being Late*, 450–451.

115. Robert N. Bellah, Richard Madsen, William M. Sullivan, Ann Swidler, and Steven M. Tipton, *The Good Society* (New York: Vintage, 1991).

116. Rorty, "Heidegger, Contingency, and Pragmatism," in *Essays on Heidegger and Others: Philosophical Papers*, vol. 2 (New York: Cambridge University Press, 1991), 49.

117. Robert N. Bellah, "A Symposium: What Is to Be Done?," *New Republic* 204 (May 1991): 28.

118. Bruce Booth, "The Biotech Paradox of 2020: A Year in Review," *Forbes*, January 4, 2021.

CHAPTER I — GENOMICS, DIVERSITY, AND THE
MILLENNIAL IMAGINATION

1. William J. Clinton, "Commencement Address at Morgan State University in Baltimore, Maryland," May 18, 1997, in *Public Papers of the Presidents of the United States, William J. Clinton, 1997, Book 1, January 1 to June 30, 1997* (Washington, DC: Government Printing Office, 1998), 613.

2. Clinton, "Commencement Address at Morgan State University," 614.

3. Office of Speechwriting and James (Terry) Edmonds, "Morgan State," May 1997, Clinton Digital Library, https://clinton.presidentiallibraries.us/items/show/36547.

4. Office of Science and Technology Policy, *Science and Technology Shaping the Twenty-First Century: A Report to the Congress* (Washington, DC: Government Printing Office, 1997).

5. On the One America in the 21st Century initiative, see Clinton, "Commencement Address at the University of California San Diego in La Jolla, California," June 14, 1997, in *Public Papers of the Presidents of the United States: William J. Clinton, 1997, Book 1, January 1 to June 30, 1997* (Washington, DC: Government Printing Office, 1998), 739–740.

6. Clinton, "Remarks in Portland, Maine," October 7, 1996, in *Public Papers of the Presidents of the United States: William J. Clinton, 1996, Book 2, July 1 to December 31, 1996* (Washington, DC: Government Printing Office, 1997), 1792.

7. Robert N. Bellah, Richard Madsen, William M. Sullivan, Ann Swidler, and Steven M. Tipton, *The Good Society* (New York: Vintage, 1991), 56. Clinton awarded Bellah the National Humanities Medal in December 2000 "for raising issues" about community "at the very heart of our national identity"; Office of Speechwriting and James (Terry) Edmonds, "Arts and Humanities," December 20, 2000, Clinton Digital Library, https://clinton.presidentiallibraries.us/items/show/34091.

8. Bellah et al., *The Good Society*, 271. For Clinton's engagement with Bellah's work, see Matteo Bortolini, *A Joyfully Serious Man: The Life of Robert Bellah* (Princeton, NJ: Princeton University Press, 2021), 295–296. For an echo of Bellah's position, see Bill Clinton, *Between Hope and History: Meeting America's Challenges for the 21st Century* (New York: Random House, 1996), 119, 141.

9. George Bush, "Remarks at the University of Michigan Commencement Ceremony in Ann Arbor," May 4, 1991, in *Public Papers of the Presidents of the United States, George H. W. Bush, 1991*, Book 1, *January 1 to June 30, 1991* (Washington, DC: Government Printing Office, 1992), 472.

10. Bill Clinton to Hiram Eastland, February 2, 1997, Office of Speechwriting and Michael Waldman, "Good Society," Clinton Digital Library, https://clinton .presidentiallibraries.us/items/show/45532; Robert N. Bellah, "A Symposium: What Is to Be Done?," *New Republic* 204 (May 1991): 28.

11. John Kenneth Galbraith, *The Good Society: The Humane Agenda* (Boston: Houghton Mifflin, 1996), 143. Clinton awarded Galbraith the Medal of Freedom on his ninetieth birthday for his service and for embodying "the dynamism and drive of the twentieth century"; Office of Speechwriting and Jeff Shesol, "Medal of Freedom, Galbraith [John Kenneth]," August 9, 2000, Clinton Digital Library, https://clinton.presidentiallibraries .us/items/show/12187.

12. "National Science & Technology Council [1]," Carol Rasco, and Subject Series, Domestic Policy Council, Clinton Digital Library, https://clinton.presidentiallibraries .us/items/show/22163; William J. Clinton and Albert Gore Jr., *Science in the National Interest* (Washington, DC: Office of Science and Technology Policy, 1994), 1, 27; Clinton, "Remarks at the California Institute of Technology in Pasadena, California," January 21, 2000, in *Public Papers of the Presidents of the United States: William J. Clinton, 2000–2001*, Book 1, *January 1 to June 26, 2000* (Washington, DC: Government Printing Office, 2001), 98–99.

13. Al Gore, "Planning a New Biotechnology Policy," *Harvard Journal of Law and Technology* 5 (Fall 1991): 19, 21. For industry opinion on what the Clinton administration meant for biotechnology, see Jeffrey L. Fox, "A Clinton–Gore Take on Biotech," *Biotechnology* 10 (December 1992): 1514–1516.

14. For Bellah's criticism of Clinton and his support of Al Gore's presidential campaign of 2000 and John Kerry's in 2004, see Bortolini, *A Joyfully Serious Man*, 310, 320.

15. Gore, "Planning a New Biotechnology Policy," 20.

16. Clinton, "Remarks at the California Institute of Technology," 100; Al Gore, *The Future: Six Drivers of Global Change* (New York: Random House, 2013), 208–211.

17. See "Genentech: Putting Science First," Participants' Working Papers— Rodriguez, Louise—Literature and Graphs from Biotech Industry, Box 478, OA/ID 1471, White House Health Care Interdepartmental Working Group: Participants Working Papers, William J. Clinton Presidential Library, Little Rock, Arkansas; U.S. Congress, Office of Technology Assessment, *Pharmaceutical R&D: Costs, Risks and Rewards*

(Washington, DC: Government Printing Office, 1993); Henry I. Miller, "When Politics Drives Science: Lysenko, Gore, and U.S. Biotechnology Policy," *Social Philosophy and Policy* 13, no. 2 (1996): 96–112.

18. Michael Dexter, director of the UK's Wellcome Trust, compared the Human Genome Project to moon exploration and the achievements of Copernicus and Darwin; Michael Dexter, Human Genome Project press conference, June 26, 2000, "Human Genome Project Press Conference Papers," June 2000, WT/B/7/6/1/2, Wellcome Collection, Wellcome Library, London (hereafter Wellcome Collection). For links between Cold War nuclear research and biomedicine, see Robert Cook-Deegan, *The Gene Wars: Science, Politics, and the Human Genome* (New York: Norton, 1995), 92–106; and Timothy Lenoir and Marguerite Hays, "The Manhattan Project for Biomedicine," in *Controlling Our Destinies: Historical, Philosophical, Ethical, and Theological Perspectives on the Human Genome Project*, ed. Philip R. Sloan (Notre Dame, IN: University of Notre Dame Press, 2000), 29–62.

19. "Dolly the Sheep Is Cloned," BBC, February 22, 1997; "Will There Ever Be Another You?," *Time*, March 10, 1997. The headline is from the *New York Times*, February 23, 1997. See also Jeanette Edwards, "Why Dolly Matters: Kinship, Culture, and Cloning," *Ethnos* 64, no. 3/4 (1999): 301–24; and Iina Hellsten, "Dolly: Scientific Breakthrough or Frankenstein's Monster? Journalistic and Scientific Metaphors of Cloning," *Metaphor and Symbol* 15 (December 2000): 213–21.

20. Tania M. Bubela and Timothy Caulfield, "Media Representations of Genetic Research," in *Crossing Over: Genomics in the Public Arena*, ed. Edna Einsiedel and Frank Timmermans (Calgary: University of Calgary Press, 2005), 117–130.

21. For a pro-cloning perspective, see "Declaration in Defense of Cloning and the Integrity of Scientific Research," *Free Inquiry* 17 (Summer 1997): 11–12.

22. "A New Creation: The Path to Cloning," *New York Times*, March 3, 1997, quoted in Gina Kolata, *Clone: The Road to Dolly and the Path Ahead* (London: Penguin, 1997), 22. For Wilmut's views of cloning and media sensationalism, see Ian Wilmut and Roger Highfield, *After Dolly: The Uses and Misuses of Human Cloning* (New York: Little, Brown, 2006); and Ian Wilmut, "The Limits of Cloning," *New Perspectives* 31, no. 1 (2014): 38–42.

23. Rudolf Jaenisch and Ian Wilmut, "Don't Clone Humans!," *Science* 291 (March 30, 2001): 5513.

24. See National Research Council, *Scientific and Medical Aspects of Human Reproductive Cloning* (Washington, DC: National Academies Press, 2002).

25. See Thomas Banchoff, *Embryo Politics: Ethics and Policy in Atlantic Democracies* (Ithaca, NY: Cornell University Press, 2011), 170–175. Toward the end of his administration, Jimmy Carter formed the President's Commission for the Study of Ethical Problems in Medicine and Biomedical and Behavioral Research. The commission released a number of reports in the early 1980s, including *Protecting Human Subjects* (1981) and *Splicing Life* (1982). On the 1988 Biomedical Ethical Advisory Committee, see John H. Evans, *Playing God? Human Genetic Engineering and the Rationalization of Public Bioethical Debate* (Chicago: University of Chicago Press, 2002), 83–134.

26. Leon R. Kass, "Brave New Biology: The Challenge for Human Dignity," Institute of United States Studies, University of London, March 19, 2002, included in "Cloning," Box 46, Jay Lefkowitz—Subject Files, Domestic Policy Council, George W. Bush Presidential Library, Dallas, Texas.

27. President's Council on Bioethics, *Human Cloning and Human Dignity: The Report of the President's Council on Bioethics* (New York: Public Affairs, 2002), xl–xli. For George W. Bush's limited and troubled engagement with science, see Chris Mooney, *The Republican War on Science*, rev. ed. (New York: Perseus Books, 2006), 2–13, 238–261; and Seth Shulman, *Undermining Science: Suppression and Distortion in the Bush Administration* (Berkeley: University of California Press, 2008), 130–137.

28. See, for example, Alondra Nelson and Thuy Nguyen Tu, eds., *TechniColor: Race, Technology, and Everyday Life* (New York: New York University Press, 2001).

29. Steve Jones, *The Language of Genes*, rev. ed. (London: Flamingo, 2000), xiii. See also Gregory E. Pence, *Who's Afraid of Human Cloning?* (Lanham, MD: Rowman & Littlefield, 1998), Pence, *Brave New Bioethics* (Lanham, MD: Rowman & Littlefield, 2003), and Pence, *Cloning after Dolly: Who's Still Afraid?* (Lanham, MD: Rowman & Littlefield, 2004).

30. British prime minister Tony Blair used this phrase in a 10 Downing Street Press Notice: Human Genome Project press pack, February 12, 2001, WT/B/7/6/1/3, Wellcome Collection.

31. Bush, "Letter to Congressional Leaders Transmitting the Annual Report on International Activities in Science and Technology," March 23, 1990, and "Remarks to the National Academy of Sciences," April 23, 1990, in *Public Papers of the Presidents of the United States: George H. W. Bush, 1990, Book 1, January 1 to June 30, 1991* (Washington, DC: Government Printing Office, 1991), 412, 545, respectively.

32. Memorandum from Allan Bromley to John H. Sununu, May 18, 1989, "Science and Technology (1989) [1]" and "Technology and the American Standard of Living," December 7, 1990, "Science and Technology (1990) [1]," Box 98, John Sununu Files, White House Office of Chief of Staff, George H. W. Bush Presidential Records, George H. W. Bush Presidential Library, College Station, TX. It is notable that NIH director Bernadine Healy, as vice chair, was the only woman in a group of twelve experts on the Presidential Council of Advisors on Science and Technology at its launch in 1990.

33. Bush, "Letter to Congressional Leaders Transmitting the Annual Report on International Activities in Science and Technology," 413. See also President's Council of Advisors on Science and Technology, *Megaprojects in the Sciences* (December 1992), 10–11.

34. President's Council on Competitiveness, *Report on National Biotechnology Policy* (February 1991), 4, 1; Bush, "Remarks to the National Academy of Sciences," 546. On the democratizing power of science and technology, see Bush, "Remarks to the American Association for the Advancement of Science," February 15, 1991, in *Public Papers of the Presidents of the United States, George H. W. Bush, 1991, Book 1, January 1 to June 30, 1991* (Washington, DC: Government Printing Office, 1992), 145–147.

35. "Facilitating Access to Science and Technology," Proclamation No. 12591, April 10, 1987, 52 Fed. Reg. 13414 (April 22, 1987).

36. This quotation is from Robert Sinsheimer's lecture "The End of the Beginning" of October 26, 1966, at California Institute of Technology, published in *Bulletin of the Atomic Scientists of Chicago* 23 (February 1967): 8–12.

37. "Human Genome Symposium: Panel Discussion," University of California at Santa Cruz, August 25, 2001, YouTube video, accessed April 12, 2024, https://www.youtube.com/watch?v=oE35hjLiZqY&feature=youtu.be.

38. "Gene Therapy Poised for Takeoff," *Insight*, November 7, 1988, 54. On early media coverage see, for example, "The Genome Project," *New York Times Magazine*, December 13, 1987; "The Gene Hunt," *Time*, March 20, 1989; and Jerry E. Bishop and Michael Waldholz, *Genome: The Story of the Astonishing Attempt to Map All the Genes in the Human Body* (New York: Simon and Schuster, 1991). On federal investment in biotechnology, see William P. Browne, "Biotechnology, State Economic Development, and Interest Politics: A Troublesome Trinity," *Politics and the Life Sciences* 9 (February 1991): 245–250.

39. Cook-Deegan, *Gene Wars*, 149.

40. U.S. Congress, Office of Technology Assessment, *Mapping Our Genes: The Genome Projects: How Big? How Fast?* (Washington, DC: Government Printing Office, 1988).

41. Cook-Deegan, *Gene Wars*, 11.

42. See Robert Cook-Deegan and James Watson, "The Human Genome Project and International Health," *JAMA* 263 (June 1990): 3222–3224. On Cook-Deegan's views, see Jenny Reardon, *Race to the Finish: Identity and Governance in an Age of Genomics* (Princeton, NJ: Princeton University Press, 2005), 47–52.

43. On the coordinating role of the Human Genome Organization, see John Sulston, *The Common Thread: Science, Politics, Ethics and the Human Genome* (London: Corgi, 2003), 171–195.

44. Tom Wilkie, *Perilous Knowledge: The Human Genome Project and Its Implications* (London: Faber and Faber, 1993), 1. See also M. Buchwald, L. C. Tsui, and J. R. Riordan, "The Search for the Cystic Fibrosis Gene," *New Scientist*, October 21, 1989, 54–58; and Daniel Pollen, *Hannah's Heirs: The Quest for the Genetic Origins of Alzheimer's Disease* (New York: Oxford University Press, 1993).

45. Daniel Koshland, "Sequences and Consequences of the Human Genome," *Science* 246 (October 13, 1989): 189.

46. See, for example, José Santiago, "The Fate of Mental Health Services in Health Care Reform: I. A System in Crisis," *Hospital and Community Psychiatry* 43 (November 1992): 1091–1094.

47. J. Craig Venter, *A Life Decoded: My Genome, My Life* (New York: Penguin, 2008), 171, 3. See also Venter, *Life at the Speed of Light: From the Double Helix to the Dawn of Digital Life* (New York: Viking, 2013), 47–62.

48. "The Race Is Over," *Time*, July 3, 2000. The cover headline was "Cracking the Code!"

49. See Collins's comments in U.S. Committee on Science, *The Human Genome Project, How Private Sector Developments Affect the Government Program: Hearing Before the Subcommittee on Energy and Environment of the Committee on Science, U.S. House of Representatives,*

One Hundred Fifth Congress, Second Session, June 17, 1998 (Washington, DC: Government Printing Office, 1998), 57, 80. See also Brigitte Nerlich, Robert Dingwall, and David D. Clarke, "The Book of Life: How the Completion of the Human Genome Project was Revealed to the Public," *Health: An Interdisciplinary Journal of the Social Study of Health, Illness and Medicine* 6 (October 2002): 445–469. On intellectual property protection, see President's Council of Advisors on Science and Technology, *Achieving the Promise of the Bioscience Revolution: The Role of the Federal Government* ([Washington, DC]: President's Council of Advisors on Science and Technology, 1992), 6.

50. Rodney Loeppky, *Encoding Capital: The Political Economy of the Human Genome Project* (New York: Routledge, 2005), 2.

51. Loeppky, *Encoding Capital*, 3.

52. See Bernard D. Davis, "The Human Genome and Other Initiatives," *Science* 249 (July 27, 1990): 342–343. On the NIH's biomedical agenda, see Daniel Callahan, *The Roots of Bioethics: Health, Progress, Technology, Death* (Oxford: Oxford University Press, 2012).

53. Charles Cantor, "The Challenges to Technology and Informatics," in *The Code of Codes: Scientific and Social Issues in the Human Genome Project*, ed. Daniel J. Kevles and Leroy Hood (Cambridge, MA: Harvard University Press, 1992), 99.

54. Catherine Waldby, *The Visible Human Project: Informatic Bodies and Posthuman Medicine* (London: Routledge, 2000), 37.

55. Waldby, *The Visible Human Project*, 27–33.

56. Clinton, "Annual Message to a Joint Session of Congress," January 27, 2000, in *Public Papers of the Presidents of the United States, William J. Clinton, 2000–2001*, Book 1, *January 1 to June 26, 2000* (Washington, DC: Government Printing Office, 2001), 138. See also Bill Clinton, *My Life* (New York: Random House, 2004), 1429, 1463; and Rick Weiss, "Genome Project Completed," *Washington Post*, April 14, 2003.

57. For the quotation, see Watson's comments in United States Congress, Senate, Committee on Energy and Natural Resources, Subcommittee on Energy Research and Development, *The Human Genome Project: Hearing before the Subcommittee on Energy Research and Development of the Committee on Energy and Natural Resources, United States Senate, One Hundred First Congress, Second Session on the Human Genome Project, July 11, 1990* (Washington, DC: Government Printing Office, 1990), 23–24.

58. Thomas H. Murray, Mark A. Rothstein, and Robert F. Murray Jr., *The Human Genome Project and the Future of Health Care* (Bloomington: Indiana University Press, 1996), vii–viii.

59. Necia Grant Cooper, ed., *The Human Genome Project: Deciphering the Blueprint of Heredity* (Mill Valley, CA: University Science Books, 1994), 167.

60. Santiago Grisolía, "Introduction," in Fundación BBV, *Human Genome Project: Ethics* (Bilbao: Fundación BBV, 1992), 16.

61. Workshop on International Cooperation for the Human Genome Project, "Valencia Declaration," in Fundación BBV, *Human Genome Project: Ethics* (Bilbao: Fundación BBV, 1992), 19; Cook-Deegan, *Gene Wars*, 205–206.

62. Workshop on International Cooperation for the Human Genome Project, "Valencia Declaration," 21. See also John Harris, "Cloning and Human Dignity," *Cambridge Quarterly of Healthcare* 7 (Spring 1988), 163–167.

63. See Diane B. Paul, "Genetic Engineering and Eugenics: The Uses of History," in *Is Human Nature Obsolete? Genetics, Bioengineering, and the Future of the Human Condition*, ed. Harold W. Baillie and Timothy K. Casey (Cambridge, MA: MIT Press, 2005), 123–151.

64. Clinton, "Remarks at the California Institute of Technology," 101.

65. Catrina Dennis, Richard Gallagher, and Philip Campbell, "Everyone's Genome," *Nature* 409 (February 15, 2001): 813.

66. Alan Swedlund, quoted in Roger Lewin, "Genes from a Disappearing World," *New Scientist*, May 29, 1993, 25–29. See also Reardon, *Race to the Finish*, 92–4. On diversity and genomics, see David S. Goodsell, *The Machinery of Life*, 2nd ed. (New York: Copernicus, 2009); Raymond A. Zilinskas and Peter J. Balint, *The Human Genome Project and Minority Communities: Ethical, Social, and Political Dilemmas* (Westport, CT: Praeger, 2001); and Kim TallBear, *Native American DNA: Tribal Belonging and the False Promise of Genetic Science* (Minneapolis: University of Minnesota Press, 2013).

67. Reardon, *Race to the Finish*, 3.

68. Reardon, *Race to the Finish*, 9.

69. Reardon, *Race to the Finish*, 16. The quotation is from global health expert Charles Rotini of the U.S. National Human Genome Research Institute and one of the leaders of H3Africa. He is quoted in "10 Years After the Genome, Africa Finally to Reap Reward of the Genetics," *Times* (London), June 23, 2010.

70. Alondra Nelson, *The Social Life of DNA: Race, Reparations, and Reconciliation after the Genome* (Boston: Beacon, 2016), 4–8.

71. Brian D. Smedley, Adrienne Y. Sith, and Alan R. Nelson, eds., *Unequal Treatment: Confronting Racial and Ethnic Disparities in Health Care* (Washington, DC: National Academy Press, 2002); Louis W. Sullivan, *Breaking Ground: My Life in Medicine* (Athens: University of Georgia Press, 2014), 212.

72. See Dorothy Roberts, *Fatal Invention: How Science, Politics, and Big Business Re-Create Race in the Twenty-First Century* (New York: New Press, 2012).

73. Debra Harry and Jonathan Marks, "Human Population Genetics versus the HGDP," *Politics and the Life Sciences* 18 (September 1999): 305.

74. Cantor, "The Challenges to Technology and Informatics," 105.

75. See Leslie Roberts, "A Genetic Survey of Vanishing Peoples," *Science* 252 (June 21, 1991): 1614–1617.

76. On the rhetoric of scientific revolutions, see Thomas Lee, *Gene Future: The Promise and Peril of the New Biology* (New York: Plenum 1993); and John Parrington, *Redesigning Life: How Genome Editing Will Transform the World* (Oxford: Oxford University Press, 2016).

77. Wilkie, *Perilous Knowledge*, 95.

78. Watson quoted in Wilkie, *Perilous Knowledge*, 96.

79. James D. Watson, "The Human Genome Project: Past, Present, and Future," *Science* 248 (April 6, 1990): 44.

80. Steven Pinker, *The Blank Slate: The Modern Denial of Human Nature* (New York: Allen Lane, 2002), 76–78.

81. Wilmut and Highfield, *After Dolly*, 45.

82. Wilmut and Highfield, *After Dolly*, 44–47, 95.

83. Wilmut and Highfield, *After Dolly*, 120–122.

84. Cynthia Fox, *Cell of Cells: The Global Race to Capture and Control the Stem Cell* (New York: Norton, 2007), 155–207; David Brin, *Kiln People* (New York: Tor Books, 2002); Neil Astley, *The Sheep Who Changed the World* (Hexham: Flambard Press, 2015).

85. Adam Phillips, "Sameness Is All," in *Clones and Clones: Facts and Fantasies about Human Cloning*, ed. Martha C. Nussbaum and Cass R. Sunstein (New York: Norton, 1998), 88. See also Dorothy Nelkin and M. Susan Lindee, "Cloning in the Popular Imagination," *Cambridge Quarterly of Healthcare* 7 (Spring 1988): 145–149.

86. Phillips, "Sameness Is All," 94. See Stephen E. Levick, *Clone Being: Exploring the Psychological and Social Dimensions* (Lanham, MD: Rowman & Littlefield, 2004), 126, 231, 255.

87. James D. Watson, "Moving Toward the Clonal Man: Is This What We Want?," *The Atlantic*, May 1971, 51–53.

88. On biofacturing, see Andrew Kimbrell, *The Human Body Shop: The Engineering and Marketing of Life* (San Francisco, CA: HarperCollins, 1994), 214.

89. Harold T. Shapiro to President Clinton, June 9, 1997, in National Bioethics Advisory Commission, *Cloning Human Beings: Report and Recommendations of the National Bioethics Advisory Commission* (Rockville, MD: The Commission, 1997), n.p.

90. See World Health Organization, "Ethical, Scientific and Social Implications of Cloning in Human Health," Agenda item 20, WHA51.10, Fifty-First World Health Assembly, May 16, 1998.

91. National Bioethics Advisory Commission, *Cloning Human Beings*, iii. Clinton echoed these views in his public speeches in 1997–1998. Examples include "Remarks Announcing the Prohibition on Federal Funding for Cloning Human Beings and an Exchange with Reporters," March 4, 1997, in *Public Papers of the Presidents of the United States: William J. Clinton, 1997*, Book 1, *January 1 to June 30, 1997* (Washington, DC: Government Printing Office, 1998), 230–231. For the argument that the National Bioethics Advisory Commission report was too cautious, see Ronald M. Green, "Much Ado about Mutton: An Ethical Review of the Cloning Controversy," in *Cloning and the Future of Human Embryo Research*, ed. Paul Lauritzen (Oxford: Oxford University Press, 2001), 127–131.

92. Leon R. Kass and James Q. Wilson, *The Ethics of Human Cloning* (Washington, DC: American Enterprise Institute, 1998).

93. Letter from James H. Scully Jr. to Leon R. Kass, May 12, 2003, "Mental Health: American Psychiatric Association," Box 20, Jay Lefkowitz—Subject Files, Domestic Policy Council, George W. Bush Presidential Library.

94. Leon R. Kass, "The Wisdom of Repugnance," *New Republic*, June 2, 1997, 17–26, reprinted in Leon R. Kass and James Q. Wilson, *The Ethics of Human Cloning* (Washington, DC: American Enterprise Institute, 1998), 3–60.

95. George W. Bush, "Remarks on Human Cloning Prohibition Legislation," April 10, 2002, in *Public Papers of the Presidents of the United States: George W. Bush, 2002*, Book 1, *January 1 to June 30, 2002* (Washington, DC: Government Printing Office, 2004), 597–599.

96. Memo from Leon R. Kass to George W. Bush, March 9, 2005, quoted in Rick Weiss, "Conservatives Draft a 'Bioethics Agenda' for President," *Washington Post*, March 8, 2005. On Kass's memo, see Kathryn Hinsch, "Bioethics: The New Conservative Crusade," in *Progress in Bioethics: Science, Policy and Politics*, ed. Jonathan D. Moreno and Sam Berger (Cambridge, MA: MIT Press, 2009), 70–71. On the American Competitiveness Initiative, see "Office of Science and Technology Policy: A Timeline (2001–2008)," Box 3, While House Office of the Staff Secretary, Thomas (Tommy) von der Heydt—Bush Record Policy Memos, George W. Bush Presidential Library and Museum.

97. Memo from Yuval Levin to April 7th bioethics strategy meeting participants, April 6, 2005, "Bioethics," 5992, Claude Allen—Subject Files, Domestic Policy Council, George W. Bush Presidential Library.

98. Kass, "Brave New Biology."

99. United Nations Declaration on Human Cloning: Resolution Adopted by the General Assembly, A/Res/59/280, March 23, 2005, accessed February 1, 2003, https://digitallibrary.un.org/record/543570?ln=en; Kass, "The Wisdom of Repugnance," 19; Leon R. Kass, "Family Needs Its Natural Roots," in Leon R. Kass and James Q. Wilson, *The Ethics of Human Cloning* (Washington, DC: American Enterprise Institute, 1998), 87.

100. See Catherine Mills, "In Defence of Repugnance," in *The Future of Bioethics: International Dialogues*, ed. Akira Akabayashi (Oxford: Oxford University Press, 2014), 366–70.

101. Martha Nussbaum, "Nussbaum on Disgust as Cause of Action," University of Chicago Law School, October 1, 2004, accessed February 1, 2023, https://www.law.uchicago.edu/news/nussbaum-disgust-cause-action.

102. Adam Briggle, *A Rich Bioethics: Public Policy, Biotechnology, and the Kass Council* (Notre Dame, IN: University of Notre Dame Press, 2010), 3.

103. Briggle, *A Rich Bioethics*, 36.

104. Briggle, *A Rich Bioethics*, 37.

105. President's Council on Bioethics, *Human Cloning and Human Dignity*, xvii.

106. President's Council on Bioethics, *Human Cloning and Human Dignity*, xxii.

107. Evelyn Fox Keller, *The Century of the Gene* (Cambridge, MA: Harvard University Press, 2000), 148; Evelyn Fox Keller, "Nature, Nurture, and the Human Genome

Project," in *The Code of Codes: Scientific and Social Issues in the Human Genome Project*, ed. Daniel J. Kevles and Leroy Hood (Cambridge, MA: Harvard University Press, 1992), 281–99.

108. "The Cemetery Dance Interview: Michael Marshall Smith," Cemetery Dance Online, August 2, 2019, accessed November 1, 2022, https://www.cemeterydance.com/extras/interview-michael-marshall-smith.

109. Michael Marshall Smith, *Spares* (New York: HarperCollins, 1996), 4–5, 10.

110. See Renée C. Fox and Judith P. Swazey, *Spare Parts: Organ Replacement in American Society* (New York: Oxford University Press, 1992), 7–13.

111. Smith, *Spares*, 42.

112. Kaushik Sunder Rajan, "Two Tales of Genomics: Capital, Epistemology, and Global Constitutions of the Biomedical Subject," in *Reframing Rights: Bioconstitutionalism in the Genetic Age*, ed. Sheila Jasanoff (Cambridge, MA: MIT Press, 2011), 202.

113. Smith, *Spares*, 44–45.

114. See Benjamin Capps, "Redefining Property in Human Body Parts: An Ethical Enquiry," in *The Future of Bioethics: International Dialogues*, ed. Akira Akabayashi (Oxford: Oxford University Press, 2014), 235–263; Alys Eve Weinbaum, "The Slave Episteme in Biocapitalism," *Catalyst: Feminism, Theory, Technoscience* 8, no. 1 (2022): 1–25.

115. Smith, *Spares*, 45.

116. Kazuo Ishiguro, *Never Let Me Go* (London: Faber & Faber, 2005), 248, 239. See also John Marks, "Clone Stories: 'Shallow Are the Souls that Have Forgotten How to Shudder'," *Paragraph* 33, no. 3 (2010): 331–353; Josie Gill, *Biofictions: Race, Genetics and the Contemporary Novel* (London: Bloomsbury, 2020).

117. Smith, *Spares*, 53–54.

118. Nelson Harris, *Roanoke Valley in the 1940s* (Charleston, SC: The History Press, 2020), 23.

119. Smith, "The Cemetery Dance Interview."

120. See Nessa Carey, *Hacking the Code of Life: How Gene Editing Will Rewrite Our Futures* (London: Icon, 2019).

121. Margaret Atwood, *Oryx and Crake: A Novel* (New York: Anchor, 2003), 296.

122. Margaret Atwood, "*The Handmaid's Tale* and *Oryx and Crake* in Context," *PMLA*, 119 (May 2004): 515. Atwood coined the term "Ustopia" based on a belief that utopia and dystopia "each contains a latent version of the other"; Margaret Atwood, "Dire Cartographies: The Roads to Ustopia," *In Other Worlds: SF and the Human Imagination* (London: Virago, 2011), 66.

123. Atwood, *Oryx and Crake*, 376. On the novel's satirical elements, see J. Brooks Bouson, "'It's Game Over Forever': Atwood's Satiric Vision of a Bioengineered Posthuman Future in *Oryx and Crake*," *Journal of Commonwealth Literature* 39 (September 2004): 139–156.

124. Margaret Atwood, "An End to Audience?" (1980), in *Second Words: Selected Critical Prose 1960–1982* (Toronto: Anansi, 1982), 346. See also Amelia DeFalco, "MaddAddam, Biocapitalism, and Affective Things," *Contemporary Women's Writing* 11 (November 2017): 432–451.

125. Atwood, *Oryx and Crake*, 305. See Hanan Muzaffer, "Margaret Atwood's Crakers and the Posthuman Future of Humanity," in *Bodies in Flux: Embodiments at the End of Anthropocentrism*, ed. Hanan Muzaffar and Barbara Braid (Leiden: Brill/Rodopi, 2019), 149–164.

126. Margaret Atwood, "Letter to America," *The Nation*, April 14, 2003, 22–23, reprinted in Atwood, *Moving Targets: Writing with Intent, 1982–2004* (Toronto: Anansi, 2004), 324–327.

127. Atwood, *Oryx and Crake*, 305.

128. Donna Haraway, *Modest_Witness@Second_Millennium.FemaleMan©Meets_OncomouseTM* (New York: Routledge, 1997), 43.

129. Atwood, *In Other Worlds*, 140.

130. See Sarah Parry, "Interspecies Entities and the Politics of Nature," in *Nature after the Genome*, ed. Sarah Parry and John Dupré (London: Wiley-Blackwell, 2010), 113–129.

131. Atwood, *Oryx and Crake*, 5.

132. Atwood, *Oryx and Crake*, 3.

133. Atwood, *Oryx and Crake*, 25. See also Jay Sanderson, "Pigoons, Rakunks and Crakers: Margaret Atwood's *Oryx and Crake* and Genetically Engineered Animals in a (Latourian) Hybrid World," *Law and Humanities* 7, no. 2 (2013): 218–240.

134. Atwood, *Oryx and Crake*, 166.

135. Atwood, *Oryx and Crake*, 303–305.

136. Robert Bohrer, "Future Fall-Out from the Genetic Revolution," *Futures* 24 (September 1992): 681–688.

137. Atwood, *In Other Worlds*, 67. See *Art's Work in the Age of Biotechnology: Shaping Our Genetic Future* (Chapel Hill: University of North Carolina Press, 2019), based on the exhibition of the same title at North Carolina State University Libraries, October 2019–March 2020.

138. "Part-Human, Part-Pig Embryos Created by Scientists to Grow Human Organs in Pigs," *USA Today*, June 6, 2016; "Embryo Experiments Take 'Baby Steps' toward Growing Human Organs in Livestock," *Science*, June 26, 2019. For the quotation, see Isoo Hyun, "What's Wrong with Human/Nonhuman Chimera Research?," *PLoS Biology* 14 (August 2016), https://www.ncbi.nlm.nih.gov/pmc/articles/PMC5004893. For chimeric research across Asia, see Steven P. McGiffen, *Biotechnology: Corporate Power versus the Public Interest* (London: Pluto, 2005), 119–129; and Darrell M. West, *Biotechnology Policy across National Boundaries: The Science-Industrial Complex* (New York: Palgrave Macmillan, 2007), 109–112.

139. Francis Collins, talk given at the Science Museum, London, June 24, 2010, quoted in Steven Connor, "Ten Years Ago Today, It Was Revealed that the Human Genome Had Been Decoded," *The Independent* (London), June 26, 2010.

140. Denise Grady, "Crispr Takes Its First Steps in Editing Genes to Fight Cancer," *New York Times*, November 6, 2019. See also Britt Wray, *Rise of the Necrofauna: The Science, Ethics, and Risks of De-Extinction* (Vancouver: Greystone, 2019), 49–53.

141. Alice Park, "A Powerful New Tool for 'Editing' the Human Genome," *Time*, February 4, 2016.

142. Editorial Board, "Should Scientists Toy with the Secret to Life?," *New York Times*, January 28, 2019; Mark Buchanan, "Gene Editing Might Alter Our DNA and Destroy Our Humanity," *Japan Times*, November 26, 2019.

143. Robin Cook, *Pandemic: A Novel* (New York: Random House, 2018), 2.

144. David Cyranoski, "First Crispr Babies: Six Questions that Remain," *Nature*, November 30, 2018, https://www.nature.com/articles/d41586-018-07607-3. See also Torill Kornfeldt, *The Unnatural Selection of Our Species: At the Frontier of Gene Editing*, trans. Fiona Graham (London: Hero, 2021).

145. On Lulu's and Nana's births, see Bill McKibben, *Falter: Has the Human Game Begun to Play Itself Out?* (London: Headline, 2019), 144–145; Emily Baumgaertner, "As D.I.Y. Gene Editing Gains Popularity, 'Someone Is Going to Get Hurt,'" *New York Times*, May 14, 2018; Jon Cohen, "Moratorium for Germline Editing Splits Biologists," *Science* 363 (May 15, 2019); David Cyranoski, "What CRISPR-Baby Prison Sentences Mean for Research," *Nature* 577 (January 9, 2020).

146. Sam Brownback to Tommy Thompson, May 13, 2002, "Human Cloning," Box 47, Jay Lefkowitz—Subject Files, Domestic Policy Council, George W. Bush Presidential Library. The slippery slope metaphor was used in Charles Krauthammer, "Mounting the Slippery Slope," *Time*, July 23, 2001; and Wesley J. Smith, "Closing in on Cloning," *Weekly Standard*, January 14, 2002.

147. Leon Kass delivered "A More Perfect Human: The Promise and Peril of Modern Science" at the Holocaust Memorial Museum on March 17, 2005, YouTube video: https://www.youtube.com/watch?v=bqhbWxflNzs. On chimera research and bioethics, see Stuart J. Youngner, "Why Would It Be Morally Wrong to Create a Human-Animal Chimera?," in *The Future of Bioethics: International Dialogues*, ed. Akira Akabayashi (Oxford: Oxford University Press, 2014), 358–365; Ronald Bailey, *Liberation Biology: The Scientific and Moral Case for the Biotech Revolution* (New York: Prometheus Books, 2005), 109–118.

148. See Jochen Taupitz and Marion Weschka, eds., *CHIMBRIDS: Chimeras and Hybrids in Comparative European and International Research: Scientific, Ethical, Philosophical and Legal Aspects* (Heidelberg: Springer, 2009).

149. Sarah Parry and John Dupré, eds., *Nature after the Genome* (London: Wiley-Blackwell, 2010), 5–6.

150. Jenny Reardon, "Human Population Genomics and the Dilemma of Difference," in *Reframing Rights: Bioconstitutionalism in the Genetic Age*, ed. Sheila Jasanoff (Cambridge, MA: MIT Press, 2011), 233.

CHAPTER 2 — EMBRYONIC ENTANGLEMENTS

1. William J. Clinton, "Remarks on Signing Memorandums on Medical Research and Reproductive Health and an Exchange with Reporters," January 22, 1993, in *Public Papers of the Presidents of the United States: William J. Clinton, 1993*, Book 1, *January 1 to June 30, 1993* (Washington, DC: Government Printing Office, 1994), 7.

2. Clinton used the phrase "safe, legal, and rare" four times in policy speeches in 1995 and periodically over the next five years. On Clinton's shifting abortion stance, see Felicity Barringer, "Campaign Issues: Clinton and Gore Shifted on Abortion," *New York Times*, July 20, 1992. For its longer arc, see Alexandra DeSanctis, "How Democrats Purged 'Safe, Legal, Rare' from the Party," *Washington Post*, November 15, 2019.

3. Clinton, "Remarks on Signing Memorandums, 7. On the 1994 proposal on fetal experimentation of the National Institutes of Health, see Eliot Marshall, "Rules on Embryo Research Due Out," *Science* 265 (August 19, 1994): 1024–1026. See also Advisory Committee to the Director, National Institutes of Health, *Report of the Human Embryo Research Panel* (Bethesda, MD: National Institute of Health, 1994); and William J. Clinton, "Statement on Federal Funding of Research on Human Embryos," December 2, 1994, in *Public Papers of the Presidents of the United States: William J. Clinton, 1994*, Book 2, *August 1 to December 31, 1994* (Washington, DC: Government Printing Office, 1995), 2142.

4. William J. Clinton, "Joint Statement by President Clinton and Prime Minister Tony Blair of the United Kingdom on Availability of Human Genome Data," March 14, 2000, in *Public Papers of the Presidents of the United States: William J. Clinton, 2000–2001*, Book 1, *January 1 to June 26, 2000* (Washington, DC: Government Printing Office, 2001), 462.

5. See, for example, Nisha Verma and Daniel Grossman, "Self-Managed Abortion in the United States," *Current Obstetrics and Gynecology Reports* 12 (2023): 70–75.

6. On the Equal Rights Amendment (and its failure to be ratified in 1982) within the pro-life/pro-choice culture wars, see N. E. H. Hull and Peter Charles Hoffer, *Roe v. Wade: The Abortion Rights Controversy in American History* (Lawrence: University Press of Kansas, 2001).

7. Leon Kass, "Reflections on Public Bioethics: A View from the Trenches," *Kennedy Institute of Ethics Journal* 15 (September 2005): 223. On the politicization of abortion, see Eva R. Rubin, *Abortion, Politics, and the Courts: Roe v. Wade and Its Aftermath*, rev. ed. (New York: Greenwood, 1987), 89–113; Laurence H. Tribe, *Abortion: The Clash of Absolutes* (New York: Norton, 1990), 77–112; Gilbert Steiner, ed., *The Abortion Dispute and the American System* (Washington, DC: Brookings Institution, 2010); and Judith Orr, *Abortion Wars: The Fight for Reproductive Rights* (London: Policy Press, 2017), 83–106.

8. Clinton, "Remarks on Signing Memorandums," 7–8; George W. Bush, "Statement to Participants in the March for Life," January 22, 2001, in *Public Papers of the Presidents of the United States: George W. Bush, 2001*, Book 1, *January 20 to June 30, 2001* (Washington, DC: Government Printing Office, 2003), 9; Caryle Murphy, "Abortion Foes Gather for 27th Annual Rally," *Washington Post*, January 22, 2001; Kurt Kleiner, "US to Sanction Embryo Research," *New Scientist* 144 (October 8, 1994). On the NBC *Today* interview of

January 18, 2001, see Laura Welch Bush, *Spoken from the Heart* (New York: Simon & Schuster, 2010), 302–303. See also Seth Shulman, *Undermining Science: Suppression and Distortion in the Bush Administration* (Berkeley: University of California Press, 2008).

9. For a definition of compassionate conservatism see Stephen Goldsmith, "What Compassionate Conservatism Is—and What It Is Not," The Hoover Institution, October 30, 2002, https://www.hoover.org/research/what-compassionate-conservatism-and-not.

10. Steve Chabot, "Introduction of the 'Partial-Birth Abortion Ban Act of 2002,'" House of Representatives, June 19, 2022, Congressional Record, E1096, https://www.govinfo.gov/content/pkg/CREC-2002-06-19/pdf/CREC-2002-06-19-pt1-PgE1096-5.pdf. Chabot's speech and coverage is collated in "Abortion: Partial Birth Abortion Ban Act 2002," Box 1, Diana Schacht—Subject Files, Domestic Policy Council, George W. Bush Presidential Library, Dallas, Texas.

11. Ann Devroy, "Late-Term Abortion Ban Vetoed," *Washington Post*, April 11, 1996. Director Jonathan Flora made a supernatural courtroom film titled *A Distant Thunder* about partial-birth abortion in 2005 after meeting with Chabot and his congressional coauthor, Rick Santorum.

12. Leon R. Kass, *Toward a More Natural Science: Biology and Human Affairs* (New York: Free Press, 1986), 124. On pro-life opposition to science, see "Cellular Divide" and "Battle for Bush's Soul," *Newsweek*, July 9, 2001.

13. George W. Bush, "Telephone Remarks to Participants in the March for Life," January 22, 2002, in *Public Papers of the Presidents of the United States, George W. Bush, 2002*, Book 1, *January 1 to June 30, 2002* (Washington, DC: Government Printing Office, 2004), 96.

14. See "Pro-Life Legacy: A Timeline (2001–2008)," Box 3, While House Office of the Staff Secretary, Thomas (Tommy) von der Heydt—Bush Record Policy Memos, George W. Bush Presidential Library.

15. Roe v. Wade, 410 U.S. 113 (1973), 91.

16. Harold T. Shapiro to President Clinton, June 9, 1997, in *Cloning Human Beings: Report and Recommendations of the National Bioethics Advisory Commission* (Rockland, MD: Government Printing Office, 1997), n.p. For presidential concerns about human cloning, see "Memorandum on the Prohibition on Federal Funding for Cloning of Human Beings," March 4, 1997, in *Public Papers of the Presidents of the United States: William J. Clinton, 1997*, Book 1, *January 1 to June 30, 1997* (Washington, DC: Government Printing Office, 1998), 233; "Statement on House of Representatives Action on Legislation to Prohibit Human Cloning," February 27, 2003, in *Public Papers of the Presidents of the United States: George W. Bush, 2003*, Book 1, *January 1 to June 30, 2003* (Washington, DC: Government Printing Office, 2004), 224–225.

17. Advisory Committee to the Director, National Institutes of Health, *Report of the Human Embryo Research Panel*, vol. 1 (Bethesda, MD: National Institutes of Health, 1994).

18. The White House, "President Bush Signs Partial-Birth Abortion Ban Act of 2003," November 5, 2003, https://georgewbush-whitehouse.archives.gov/news/releases/2003/11/20031105-1.html. Christopher Smith used the phrase "culture of death" at the Janu-

ary 2002 March for Life, a year after he had read President Bush's prepared remarks to the pro-life rally; "March for Life" Rally, C-SPAN, January 22, 2002, accessed November 11, 2022, https://www.c-span.org/video/?168314-1/march-life-rally. On antiabortion activism, see Johanna Schoen, *Abortion after Roe* (Chapel Hill: University of North Carolina Press, 2015), 155–198.

19. Bioethics agenda memo from Yuval Levin to George W. Bush (through Claude Allen), May 12, 2005, "Bioethics Policy," 6007, Anna Lisa Holand—Chron Files, Domestic Policy Council, George W. Bush Presidential Library.

20. On Laura Bush's interview in the September 18, 2001 episode of the *Oprah Winfrey Show*, see Laura Bush, *Spoken from the Heart*, 211, 231.

21. George W. Bush, "Telephone Remarks to the March for Life," January 22, 2007, in *Public Papers of the Presidents of the United States, George W. Bush, 2007*, Book 1, *January 1 to June 30, 2007* (Washington, DC: Government Printing Office, 2007), 41; and "Remarks to March for Life Participants," January 22, 2008, in *Public Papers of the Presidents of the United States, George W. Bush, 2008*, Book 1, *January 1 to June 30, 2008* (Washington, DC: Government Printing Office, 2012), 101. On the response of the Family Research Council, see the letter from its president, Kenneth L. Connor, to George W. Bush, July 9, 2002, "Stem Cells [3]," Box 52, Jay Lefkowitz—Subject Files, Domestic Policy Council, George W. Bush Presidential Library.

22. Gretchen Vogel, "Bush Squeezes between the Lines on Stem Cells," *Science* 293 (August 17, 2001): 1242–1245. For James Dobson's collected correspondence with the White House, see the George W. Bush Presidential Library, 2015-0037 F.

23. See Chris Mooney, "Research and Destroy," *Washington Monthly*, October 2004.

24. Bush "Remarks to March for Life Participants," 101. See also Lynn Morgan, *Icons of Life: A Cultural History of Human Embryos* (Berkeley: University of California Press, 2009), 236–242; Thomas Banchoff, *Embryo Politics: Ethics and Policy in Atlantic Democracies* (Ithaca, NY: Cornell University Press, 2011), 175–181. On fetal rights and personhood, see Robert M. Baird and Stuart E. Rosenbaum, *The Ethics of Abortion: Pro-Life vs. Pro-Choice* (Buffalo, NY: Prometheus, 1993), 249–267; and Carol Sanger, *About Abortion: Terminating Pregnancy in Twenty-First-Century America* (Cambridge, MA: Harvard University Press, 2017), 71–76.

25. Stefanie R. Fishel, *The Microbial State: Global Thriving and the Body Politic* (Minneapolis: University of Minnesota Press, 2017), 3–6; Andrew Kimbrell, *The Human Body Shop: The Engineering and Marketing of Life* (San Francisco: Harper, 1993), 66, 73.

26. "2 Charge 'Jealous' Doctor Killed 'Test-Tube Baby,'" *New York Times*, July 18, 1978; "The First Test Tube Baby," *Time*, July 31, 1978; "Life in the Test Tube," *New York Times*, August 6, 1978. See also Margaret Marsh and Wanda Ronner, *The Pursuit of Parenthood: Reproductive Technology from Test-Tube Babies to Uterus Transplants* (Baltimore, MD: Johns Hopkins University Press, 2019).

27. See Rosalind Pollack Petchesky, "Fetal Images: The Power of Visual Culture in the Politics of Reproduction," *Feminist Studies* 13 (Summer 1987): 263–292.

28. Kimbrell, *The Human Body Shop*, 54–56. See also Susan Tawia, "When Is the Capacity for Sentience Acquired during Human Fetal Development?," *Journal of Maternal-Fetal Medicine* 1 (July 1992): 153–165.

29. Morgan, *Icons of Life*, 217–221. See also Rosalind Pollack Petchesky, "Fetal Images and the Power of Visual Culture in the Politics of Reproduction," *Feminist Studies* 13 (Summer 1987): 263–92; and Alexander Tsiaris and Barry Wirth, *From Conception to Birth* (New York: Doubleday, 2002). Bush dedicates a whole chapter to stem cells in his post-presidential memoir: George W. Bush, *Decision Points* (New York: Crown), 105–125.

30. On mothers as "central moral subjects of the abortion question," see Catriona Mackenzie, "Abortion and Embodiment," in *Troubled Bodies: Critical Perspectives on Post-modernism, Medical Ethics, and the Body*, ed. Paul A. Komesaroff (Durham, NC: Duke University Press, 1995), 38–61.

31. See Dion Farquhar, *The Other Machine: Discourse and Reproductive Technologies* (New York: Routledge, 1996); and Rickie Solinger, *Reproductive Politics: What Everyone Needs to Know* (New York: Oxford University Press, 2013).

32. Gay Becker, *The Elusive Embryo: How Women and Men Approach New Reproductive Technologies* (Berkeley: University of California Press, 2000), 12, 16. On health data, see George Annas, "Protecting Privacy in the Genetics Age," in *Justice and the Human Genome Project*, ed. Timothy F. Murphy and Marc A. Lappé (Berkeley: University of California Press, 1994), 75–89.

33. Robin Marantz Henig, *Pandora's Baby: How the First Test Tube Babies Sparked the Reproductive Revolution* (Boston: Houghton Mifflin, 2004), 9.

34. Kass, "Reflections on Public Bioethics," 223.

35. Kass, "Family Needs Its Natural Roots," in Leon R. Kass and James Q. Wilson, *The Ethics of Human Cloning* (Washington, DC: American Enterprise Institute, 1998), 87.

36. Kimbrell, *The Human Body Shop*, 73–74; Samuel B. Condic and Maureen L. Condic, *Human Embryos, Human Beings: A Scientific and Philosophical Approach* (Washington, DC: Catholic University of American Press, 2018), 260. See also Gay Becker, *The Elusive Embryo: How Women and Men Approach New Reproductive Technologies* (Berkeley: University of California Press, 2001); and Lauren Jade Martin, *Reproductive Tourism in the United States: Creating Family in the Mother Country* (New York: Routledge, 2015).

37. Carlos Novas and Nikolas Rose, "Genetic Risk and the Birth of the Somatic Individual," *Economy and Society* 29 (November 2000): 485–513.

38. Denise Grady, "Son Conceived to Provide Blood Cells for Daughter," *New York Times*, October 4, 2000; Pam Belluck, "Gene Editing for 'Designer Babies'? Highly Unlikely, Scientists Say," *New York Times*, August 4, 2017.

39. See Bonnie Steinbock, "Respect for Human Embryos," in *Cloning and the Future of Human Embryo Research*, ed. Paul Lauritzen (Oxford: Oxford University Press, 2001); and Brigitte Nerlich, Susan Johnson, and David D. Clarke, "The First 'Designer Baby': The Role of Narratives, Clichés and Metaphors in the Year 2000 Media Debate," *Science as Culture* 12 (December 2003): 471–498.

40. Laura Briggs, *How All Politics Became Reproductive Politics: From Welfare Reform to Foreclosure to Trump* (Berkeley: University of California Press, 2017), 4.

41. Roe v. Wade, 410 U.S., 91.

42. See Jonathan S. Swartz, "The Human Cloning Prohibition Act of 2001: Vagueness and Federalism," *Jurimetrics* 43 (Fall 2002): 79–90; and Margaret R. McLean, "Stem Cells: Shaping the Future in Public Policy," in *The Human Embryonic Stem Cell Debate: Science, Ethics, and Public Policy,* ed. Suzanne Holland, Karen Lebacqz, and Laurie Zoloth (Cambridge, MA: MIT Press, 2001), 2007), 197–207.

43. James D. Watson, "Potential Consequences of Experimentation with Human Eggs," address to the 12th meeting of the Panel on Science and Astronautics, U.S. House of Representatives, 92nd Congress, 1st Session, January 28, 1971, JDW/2/4/1/13, James D. Watson Collection, Wellcome Collection, Wellcome Library, London.

44. James D. Watson, "Moving Toward the Clonal Man: Is This What We Want?," *Atlantic,* May 1971, 51–53.

45. National Commission on Health Science and Society, *Hearings before the Subcommittee on Government Research of the Committee on Government Operations, United States Senate, Ninetieth Congress, Second Session, on S.J. Res. 145* (Washington, DC: Government Printing Office, 1968), 47; E. J. Mishan, "On Making the Future Safe for Mankind," *Public Interest,* Summer 1971, 33–61; Irving Kristol, "Is Technology a Threat to Liberal Society?," *Public Interest,* Spring 2001, 45–52. Kristol originally gave this as a lecture in March 1975.

46. "The Promise and Peril of the New Genetics," *Time,* April 19, 1971.

47. Paul Ramsey, *Fabricated Man: The Ethics of Genetic Control* (New Haven, CT: Yale University Press, 1970), 60–103; Leon R. Kass, "Making Babies—The New Biology and the 'Old' Morality," *Public Interest* 26 (Winter 1972): 18–56; Joseph Fletcher: *The Ethics of Genetic Control: Ending Reproductive Roulette* (New York: Anchor, 1974). See also Eric Cohen and William Kristol, *The Future Is Now: America Confronts the New Genetics* (Lanhan, MD: Rowman & Littlefield, 2002); Kass, *Toward a More Natural Science,* 48–55; and Banchoff, *Embryo Politics,* 28–34.

48. Shulamith Firestone, *The Dialectic of Sex: The Case for Feminist Revolution* (1970; repr., London: Verso, 2015), 174–209; Joan Rothschild, *The Dream of the Perfect Child* (Bloomington: Indiana University Press, 2005), 226; Ramsey, *Fabricated Man,* 151–160.

49. Willard Gaylin, "The Frankenstein Myth Becomes a Reality—We Have the Awful Knowledge to Make Exact Copies of Human Beings," *New York Times Magazine,* March 5, 1973. For a cultural study of this period, see Sophie A. Jones, *The Reproductive Politics of American Literature and Film, 1959–73* (Edinburgh: Edinburgh University Press, 2025).

50. See Jael Silliman, Marlene Gerber Fried, Loretta Ross, and Elena R. Gutiérrez, *Undivided Rights: Women of Color Organize for Reproductive Justice* (2004; repr., Chicago: Haymarket, 2016). See also Dorothy Roberts, *Killing the Black Body: Race, Reproduction, and the Meaning of Liberty* (New York: Vintage, 1999).

51. See Jon W. Gordon, *The Science and Ethics of Engineering the Human Germ Line: Mendel's Maze* (Hoboken, NJ: Wiley, 2003), 116–118.

52. Dion Farquhar, *The Other Machine: Discourse and Reproductive Technologies* (New York: Routledge, 1996), 133.

53. Sarah Franklin, *Biological Relatives: IVF, Stem Cells, and the Future of Kinship* (Durham, NC: Duke University Press, 2013), 4.

54. U.S. Congress, Committee on Small Business, *Consumer Protection Issues involving In Vitro Fertilization Clinics* (Washington, DC: Government Printing Office, 1988). See also Andrea Bonnicksen, *In Vitro Fertilization: Building Policy from Laboratories to Legislatures* (New York: Columbia University Press, 1991); Lisa Harris, "Challenging Conception: A Clinical and Cultural History of In Vitro Fertilization in the United States" (PhD diss., University of Michigan, 2006); and Future Baby Productions, *Unbornox9*, publication associated with art installation of the same name, Science Gallery London, accessed July 20, 2023, https://unbornox9.labomedia.org/wp-content /uploads/2021/08/UNBORNox9_BOOKLET_2020.pdf.

55. Franklin, *Biological Relatives*, 31–32.

56. On feminist concerns about prenatal diagnosis, see Adrienne Asch and Gail Geller, "Feminism, Bioethics, and Genetics," in *Feminism and Bioethics: Beyond Reproduction*, ed. Susan M. Wolf (Oxford: Oxford University Press, 1996), 335–340.

57. See Andrew Pollack, "Sequenom Fires Chief and Others over Handling of Data," *New York Times*, September 28, 2009; George Estreich, *Fables and Futures: Biotechnology, Disability, and the Stories We Tell Ourselves* (Cambridge, MA: MIT Press, 2019), 52–53, 71. See also Ruth Schwartz Cowan, "Genetic Technology and Reproductive Choice: An Ethics of Autonomy," in *The Code of Codes: Scientific and Social Issues in the Human Genome Project*, ed. Daniel J. Kevles and Leroy Hood (Cambridge, MA: Harvard University Press, 1992), 244–263; and Lynn M. Morgan and Meredith W. Michaels, *Fetal Subjects, Feminist Positions* (Philadelphia: University of Pennsylvania Press, 1999), 291–294. For postmillennial discussions of Down syndrome in the public sphere, see Bonnie Rochman, "Early Decision," *Time*, February 27, 2012; and Sarah Zhang, "The Last Children of Down Syndrome," *Atlantic*, December 2020.

58. See Finn Bowring, *Science, Seeds and Cyborgs: Biotechnology and the Appropriation of Life* (London: Verso, 2003), 193–196.

59. Thomas H. Murray, Mark A. Rothstein, and Robert F. Murray Jr., *The Human Genome Project and the Future of Health Care* (Bloomington: Indiana University Press, 1996), 84. On parental fears, see George Estreich, *The Shape of an Eye: A Memoir* (New York: Penguin, 2013); and Scott Gilbert and Clare Pinto-Correia, *Fear, Wonder, and Science in the New Age of Reproductive Biotechnology* (New York: Columbia University Press, 2017).

60. Union of Concerned Scientists, "2004 Scientist Statement on Restoring Scientific Integrity to Federal Policy Making," updated July 13, 2008, https://www.ucsusa.org /resources/2004-scientist-statement-scientific-integrity.

61. See Mooney, *The Republican War on Science*, 238–239.

62. Joel W. Adelson and Joanna K. Weinberg, "The California Stem Cell Initiative: Persuasion, Politics, and Public Service," *American Journal of Public Health* 100 (March 2010): 444–451.

63. See the President's Commission for the Study of Ethical Problems in Medicine and Biomedical and Behavioral Research, *Splicing Life: The Social and Ethical Issues of Genetic Engineering with Human Beings* (Washington, DC: Government Printing Office, 1982), Appendix B, 95.

64. Bush, "Telephone Remarks to Participants in the March for Life," 96. See also Leslie J. Reagan, *Dangerous Pregnancies: Mothers, Disabilities, and Abortion in Modern America* (Berkeley: University of California Press, 2010).

65. James A. Thomson, J. Itskovitz-Eldor, S. S. Shapiro, M. A. Waknitz, J. J. Swiergiel, V. S. Marshall, and J. M. Jones, "Embryonic Stem Cell Lines Derived from Human Blastocysts," *Science* 282 (November 6, 1998): 1145–1147; Chris Mooney, *The Republican War on Science*, rev. ed. (New York: Perseus Books, 2006), 196–197. See also Barack Obama, "Remarks on Signing an Executive Order Removing Barriers to Responsible Scientific Research Involving Human Stem Cells and a Memorandum on Scientific Integrity," March 9, 2009, in *Public Papers of the Presidents of the United States: Barack Obama, 2009*, Book 1, *January 20 to June 30, 2009* (Washington, DC: Government Printing Office, 2010), 199–200. See also Jon Parrington, *Redesigning Life: How Genome Editing Will Transform the World* (Oxford: Oxford University Press, 2016), 183.

66. Nicholas Wade, "Obama Plans to Replace Bush's Bioethics Panel," *New York Times*, June 17, 2009.

67. See Shaila Dewan, "After Change in Federal Policy, Some States Take Steps to Limit Stem Cell Research," *New York Times*, March 13, 2009.

68. "Symposium, Biotechnology: A House Divided," *Public Interest* 150 (Winter 2003): 38–63; Vogel, "Bush Squeezes between the Lines on Stem Cells," 1242–1245.

69. See Jonathan R. Cohen, "In God's Garden: Creation and Cloning in Jewish Thought," in *The Human Cloning Debate*, ed. Gleen McGee (Berkeley, CA: Berkeley Hills Books, 2002), 261, 264; and Brent Waters and Ronald Cole-Turner, eds., *God and the Embryo: Religious Voices on Stem Cells and Cloning* (Washington, DC: Georgetown University Press, 2003), 11–12.

70. Silver, *Remaking Eden*, 275. For these faith-based resolutions, see Waters and Cole-Turner, *God and the Embryo*, 163–203.

71. For Nellie Gray's speech that opened the January 22, 2001, March for Life, see "'March for Life' Rally," C-SPAN, January 22, 2001, accessed December 10, 2021, https://www.c-span.org/video/?162083-1/march-life-rally.

72. Jakobus Vorster, "A Christian Ethical Perspective on the Moral Status of the Human Embryo," *Acta Theologica* 31 (2011): 189–204. For a more nuanced reading of embryonic design, see Spencer S. Stober and Donna Yarri, *God, Science, and Designer Genes: An Exploration of Emerging Genetic Technologies* (Santa Barbara, CA: ABC Clio, 2009), 71–103.

73. Warren E. Leary, "Koop Says Abortion Report Couldn't Survive Challenge," *New York Times*, March 17, 1989; Nada L. Stotland, "The Myth of the Abortion Trauma Syndrome," *Journal of the American Medical Association* 268 (October 1992): 2078–2079; Nada L. Stotland, "The Myth of Abortion Trauma Syndrome: Update, 2007," *Psychiatric*

News, July 20, 2007; Emily Bazelon, "Is There a Post-Abortion Syndrome?," *New York Times*, January 21, 2007; Karissa Haugeberg, *Women Against Abortion: Inside the Largest Moral Reform Movement of the Twentieth Century* (Urbana: University of Illinois Press, 2017), 35–55; David C. Reardon, "The Abortion and Mental Health Controversy," *SAGE Open Medicine* 6 (2018): 1–38. In 2021, the pro-life Colorado representative Lauren Boebert misquoted the headline figure of a decade-long study that suggests that women undergoing an abortion have an 81 percent increased risk of mental health challenges (she did not mention that only 10 percent of these cases were attributable to abortion). See Priscilla K. Coleman, "Abortion and Mental Health: Quantitative Synthesis and Analysis of Research Published 1995–2009," *British Journal of Psychiatry* 199 (September 2011): 180–186; "User Clip: Lauren Boebert on Abortion," U.S. House of Representatives Session, C-SPAN, September 21, 2021, accessed November 1, 2022, https://www.c -span.org/video/?c5003450/user-clip-lauren-boebert-abortion.

74. Silver, *Remaking Eden*, 276.

75. On race and abortion, see Linda Beckman and S. Marie Harvey, *The New Civil War: The Psychology, Culture, and Politics of Abortion* (Washington, DC: American Psychological Association, 1998). For the argument that pro-lifers should engage with biotechnology, see Paige Comstock Cunningham, "Learning from Our Mistakes: The Pro-Life Cause and the New Bioethics," in *Human Dignity in the Biotech Century: A Christian Vision for Public Policy*, ed. Charles W. Colson and Nigel M. de S. Cameron (Downers Grove, IL: InterVarsity Press, 2004), 136–159.

76. Kass, "Reflections on Public Bioethics," 223–224.

77. Nicholas Wade, "Leon Kass; Moralist of Science Ponders Its Power," *New York Times*, March 19, 2002. For a critique of Kass, see Gaymon Bennett, *Technicians of Human Dignity: Bodies, Souls, and the Making of Intrinsic Worth* (New York: Fordham University Press, 2016), 201–274.

78. Elizabeth Blackburn, "Bioethics and the Political Distortion of Biomedical Science," *New England Journal of Medicine* 350 (April 1, 2004): 1379–1380. For complaints about Bush officials interfering in nominations, see Leigh Turner, "Science, Politics and the President's Council on Bioethics," *Nature Biotechnology* 22 (May 2004): 509–510; Emma Marris, "Bush Accused of Trying to Foist Favourites on Health Agency," *Nature* 430 (July 2004); Mooney, *The Republican War on Science*, 208–214; Shulman, *Undermining Science*, 35–36, 128–130. Georgetown University medical ethicist Edmund Pellegrino succeeded Kass as chair in September 2004.

79. President's Council on Bioethics, *Human Cloning and Human Dignity: An Ethical Inquiry* (Washington, DC: President's Council on Bioethics, 2002), 80.

80. President's Council on Bioethics, *Human Cloning and Human Dignity*, 91.

81. President's Council on Bioethics, *Human Cloning and Human Dignity*, 108–109.

82. See Thomas H. Murray, Mark A. Rothstein, and Robert F. Murray Jr., eds., *The Human Genome Project and the Future of Health Care* (Bloomington: Indiana University Press, 1996), 68–70, 158–172, 231–232; and McGee, *Perfect Baby*, 95–97.

83. For the quotation, see "S. 1416—Genetic Privacy and Nondiscrimination Act of 1995," 104th Congress, 1995–1996, https://www.congress.gov/bill/104th-congress/senate-bill/1416.

84. President's Information Technology Advisory Committee, "Transforming Health Care through Information Technology," February 2001, in "Health Care [1]," Box 12, Jay Lefkowitz—Subject Files, Domestic Policy Council, George W. Bush Presidential Library. The 2003 report of the President's New Freedom Commission, *Achieving the Promise: Transforming Mental Health Care in America*, emphasized the transformative potential of technology on access to health care and health care recordkeeping.

85. Sara Dubow, *Ourselves Unborn*, 184.

86. On design fictions, see Julian Bleecker, "Design Fiction: A Short Essay on Design, Science, Fact and Fiction," Near Future Laboratory, March 2009, https://nearfuture laboratory.myshopify.com/products/design-fiction-a-short-essay-on-design-science-fact-and-fiction.

87. Lee M. Silver, *Remaking Eden: How Genetic Engineering and Cloning Will Transform the American Family* (New York: Harper, 1997); President's Council on Bioethics, *Human Cloning and Human Dignity*, 85.

88. Michael Bérubé, "Disability, Democracy, and the New Genetics," in *The Disability Studies Reader*, ed. Lennard J. Davis, 4th ed. (London: Routledge, 2013), 102–103.

89. Martine Rothblatt, *Unzipped Genes: Taking Charge of Baby Making in the New Millennium* (Philadelphia, PA: Temple University Press, 1997).

90. For an effort to correct the scientific biases of *Gattaca* and *Beggars in Spain*, see Ronald M. Green, *Babies by Design: The Ethics of Genetic Choice* (New Haven, CT: Yale University Press, 2007), 5–7, 112–113, 146–147.

91. Andrew Solomon, *Far from the Tree: Parents, Children, and the Search for Identity* (New York: Scribner's, 2012), 4.

92. On genetic discrimination (or genoism) see Jon Frauley, *Criminology, Deviance and the Silver Screen: The Fictional Reality and the Criminological Imagination* (New York: Palgrave Macmillan, 2010), 195–216.

93. Everett Hamner, *Editing the Soul: Science and Fiction in the Genome Age* (Philadelphia: Pennsylvania State University Press, 2017), 31.

94. Hamner, *Editing the Soul*, 32–33.

95. David A. Kirby, "The New Eugenics in Cinema: Genetic Determinism and Gene Therapy in *Gattaca*," *Science Fiction Studies* 27 (July 2000): 193–215. See also Colin Gavaghan, "'No Gene for Fate': Luck, Harm, and Justice in *Gattaca*," in *Bioethics in the Movies*, ed. Sandra Shapshay (Baltimore, MD: Johns Hopkins University Press, 2009), 75–86.

96. For this 2021 statistic from the European Society of Human Reproduction and Embryology, see Mary Ann Mason and Tom Ekman, *Babies of Technology: Assisted Reproduction and the Rights of the Child* (New Haven, CT: Yale University Press, 2017), 3.

97. For research informing *Change Agent*, see Daniel Suarez, "Talks at Google," Los Angeles, April 21, 2017, YouTube video, https://m.youtube.com/watch?v=TvM9DWjk-bSI. See also Suarez's list for further reading at the back of *Change Agent*.

98. See Suarez's tweet @itsDanielSuarez of December 20, 2018, in response to Michael Le Page, "We've Been Using Crispr for Years—Now We Know How It Really Works," *New Scientist*, December 13, 2018. See also Fankang Meng and Tom Ellis, "The Second Decade of Synthetic Biology: 2010–2020," *Nature Communications* 11 (October 14, 2020): article 5174, retweeted by @itsDanielSuarez on October 17, 2020.

99. See *Unnatural Selection*, dir. Joe Egender and Leeor Kaufman (2019).

100. See Kalindi Vora, *Life Support: Biocapital and the New History of Outsourced Labor* (Minneapolis: University of Minnesota Press, 2015); Lisa Chiyemi Ikemoto, 'Reproductive Tourism: Equality Concerns in the Global Market for Fertility Services," in *Beyond Bioethics: Toward a New Biopolitics*, ed. Osagie B. Obasogie and Marcy Darnovsky (Berkeley: University of California Press, 2018), 339–349. Despite setting *Change Agent* in Singapore, Suarez arguably overlooked the work of the Singapore government's Bioethics Advisory Committee, established in 2000: see John M. Elliott, W. Calvin Ho, and Sylvia S. N. Lim, eds, *Bioethics in Singapore: The Ethical Microcosm* (New Jersey: World Scientific, 2010); and Aiwha Ong and Nancy N. Chen, eds, *Asian Biotech: Ethics and Communities of Fate* (Durham, NC: Duke University Press, 2010).

101. Daniel Suarez, *Change Agent* (New York: Dutton, 2018), 279–280.

102. Suarez, *Change Agent*, 2; Estreich, *Fables and Futures*, 42.

103. Suarez, *Change Agent*, 3–4.

104. Suarez, *Change Agent*, 9.

105. Suarez, *Change Agent*, 4, 8.

106. See Catherine Waldby, "Oocyte Markets: Women's Reproductive Work in Embryonic Stem Cell Research," *New Genetics and Society* 27 (May 2008): 26. See also Lori Andrews and Dorothy Nelkin, *Body Bazaar: The Market for Human Tissue in the Biotechnology Age* (New York: Crown, 2001); and Catherine Waldby and Robert Mitchell, *Tissue Economies: Blood, Organs, and Cell Lines in Late Capitalism* (Durham, NC: Duke University Press, 2006).

107. Suarez, *Change Agent*, 25.

108. George Church and Ed Regis, *Regenesis: How Synthetic Biology Will Reinvent Nature and Ourselves* (New York: Basic Books, 2012), 243.

109. Suarez, *Change Agent*, 279.

110. Suarez, *Change Agent*, 22, 6.

111. Suarez, *Change Agent*, 23.

112. Suarez, *Change Agent*, 30.

113. Suarez, *Change Agent*, 209, 319.

114. Suarez, *Change Agent*, 218.

115. Suarez, *Change Agent*, 219.

116. Suarez, *Change Agent*, 219–220, 225.

117. Suarez, *Change Agent*, 222.

118. Suarez, *Change Agent*, 339, 394.

119. Suarez, *Change Agent*, 223.

120. Interview with Daniel Suarez, *Phantastisch Magazine* 62 (May 2015), accessed November 11, 2022, http://daniel-suarez.com/PhantastischinterviewinEnglish.html.

121. Michael A. Goldman, "Calamity Gene: When Biotechnology Spins out of Control," *Nature* 445 (February 2007): 819. See also Jorge L. Contreras, "*Next* and Michael's Crichton's Five-Step Program for Biotechnology Law Reform," *Jurimetrics* 48 (Spring 2008): 337–348.

122. See Ross D. Parke, Christine Ward Galley, Scott Coltrane, and M. Robin DiMatteo, "The Pursuit of Perfection," in *Clones, Fakes and Posthumans: Cultures of Replication*, ed. Philomena Essed and Garbiele Schwab (Amsterdam: Rodopi, 2012), 111–126.

123. See Sigmund Freud, "The Family Romances" (1909), in *On Sexuality: Three Essays on the Theory of Sexuality and Other Works, The Penguin Freud Library*, vol. 7, trans. James Strachey, ed. Angela Richards (London: Penguin, 1977), 217–225. Whereas Freud was primarily interested in infantile sexuality, *Perfect People* focuses on a genetic struggle within the family.

124. James Q. Wilson, "Paradox of Cloning," in Leon R. Kass and James Q. Wilson, *Ethics of Human Cloning* (Washington, DC: American Enterprise Institute, 1998), 66.

125. Peter James, *Perfect People* (London: Macmillan, 2011), 10.

126. James, *Perfect People*, 59, 279.

127. Mike Pence viewed the March of Life as a "solemn protest": Mike Pence, *So Help Me God* (New York: Simon and Schuster, 2022), 88, 208–209. On hate crime against abortionists, see Joe Stumpe and Monica Davey, "Abortion Doctor Shot to Death in Kansas Church," *Washington Post*, May 31, 2009.

128. James, *Perfect People*, 1–2, 5.

129. James, *Perfect People*, 89–90, 16.

130. Elias A. Zerhouni to Diana DeGette and Michael Castle, May 14, 2004, "Stem Cell [1]," Box 25, Claude Allen—Subject Files, Domestic Policy Council, George W. Bush Presidential Library.

131. James, *Perfect People*, 16.

132. James, *Perfect People*, 17.

133. James, *Perfect People*, 12–13, 36–37.

134. James, *Perfect People*, 29.

135. Ken Macleod, *Intrusion* (London: Orbit, 2012); Rothschild, *Dream of the Perfect Child*, 214.

136. Stephen E. Levick, *Clone Being: Exploring the Psychological and Social Dimensions* (Lanham, MD: Rowman & Littlefield, 2004), 11.

137. James, *Perfect People*, 240.

138. Ralph Adolphs and Daivd J. Anderson, *The Neuroscience of Emotion: A New Synthesis* (Princeton, NJ: Princeton University Press, 2018), 6.

139. James, *Perfect People*, 312.

140. James, *Perfect People*, 350, 357.

141. James, *Perfect People*, 504, 512.

142. James, *Perfect People*, 551.

143. On progeria, see Robert N. Butler, *The Longevity Revolution: The Benefits and Challenges of Living a Long Life* (New York: Public Affairs, 2008), 156–158.

144. Richard F. Storrow, "Therapeutic Reproduction and Human Dignity," *Law and Literature* 21 (Summer 2009): 257.

145. Novas and Rose, "Genetic Risk and the Birth of the Somatic Individual," 507; President's Council on Bioethics, *Human Cloning and Human Dignity*, xvii.

146. See Alondra Nelson, *The Social Life of DNA: Race, Reparations, and Reconciliation after the Genome* (Boston: Beacon, 2017); Ruha Benjamin, *Race after Technology: Abolitionist Tools for the New Jim Code* (Cambridge: Polity, 2019).

147. Rothschild, *Dream of the Perfect Child*, 227.

CHAPTER 3 — HEALTH IN THE NEURONAL WORKSPACE

1. Frances H. Rauscher, Gordon L. Shaw, and Katherine N. Ky, "Music and Spatial Task Performance," *Nature* 365 (October 14, 1993): 611.

2. Kevin Sack, "Georgia's Governor Seeks Musical Start for Babies," *New York Times*, January 15, 1998; Nikhil Swaminathan, "Fact or Fiction? Babies Exposed to Classical Music End Up Smarter," *Scientific American*, September 13, 2007; Don Campbell, *The Mozart Effect: Tapping the Power of Music to Heal the Body, Strengthen the Mind, and Unlock the Creative Spirit* (New York: Avon, 1997).

3. Julie Passanante Elman, *Chronic Youth: Disability, Sexuality, and U.S. Media Cultures of Rehabilitation* (New York: New York University Press, 2014), 132; Jonathan Franzen, *The Corrections* (New York: Picador, 2001), 156.

4. William J. Clinton, "Interview with Matt Lauer of NBC's 'Today' Show in New York City," June 16, 2000, in *Public Papers of the Presidents of the United States: William J. Clinton, 2000, Book 1, January 1 to June 26, 2001* (Washington, DC: Government Printing Office, 2001), 1153–7. See also Jacqueline Trescott, "'Arts Education' Colors Debate," *Washington Post*, August 5, 1997; Ellen Winner and Lois Hetland, "Mozart and the S.A.T.'s," *New York Times*, March 4, 1999; and Roberta Hershenson, "Debating the Mozart Theory," *New York Times*, August 6, 2000.

5. See Peter G. Hepper, "An Examination of Fetal Learning before and after Birth," *Irish Journal of Psychology* 12, no. 2 (1991): 95–107. See also Aniruddh D. Patel, *Music, Language, and the Brain* (Oxford: Oxford University Press, 2007), 382–387.

6. Christopher F. Chabris, "Prelude or Requiem for the 'Mozart Effect'?," *Nature* 400 (August 1999): 826–827; James S. Catterall and Frances H. Rauscher, "Unpacking the

Impact of Music on Intelligence," in *Neurosciences in Music Pedagogy*, ed. Wilfried Gruhn and Frances Rauscher (New York: Oxford University Press, 2008), 171.

7. Oliver Sacks, *Musicophilia: Tales of Music and the Brain* (London: Picador, 2007), 95.

8. Philip Ball, *The Music Instinct* (London: Bodley Head, 2010), 251. Both Sacks and Ball cite Glenn Schellenberg's work. See, for example, E. Glenn Schellenberg's essays "Music Lessons Enhance IQ," *Psychological Science* 15 (August 2004): 511–514; "Music and Cognitive Abilities," *Current Directions in Psychological Science* 14 (December 2005): 317–320; and "Long-Term Positive Associations between Music Lessons and IQ," *Journal of Educational Psychology* 98 (May 2006): 457–468.

9. On media accounts see Adrian Bangerter and Chip Heath, "The Mozart Effect: Tracking the Evolution of a Scientific Legend," *British Journal of Social Psychology*, 43(4) (December 2004), 605–23.

10. See Mark Tramo, "Music of the Hemispheres," *Science* 291 (January 2001): 54–56; Eckart Altenmüller, M. Wiesendanger, and J. Kesselring, *Music, Motor Control and the Brain* (Oxford: Oxford University Press, 2006); and Eckart Altenmüller and Gottfried Schlaug, "Music, Brain, and Health: Exploring Biological Foundations of Music's Health Effects," in *Music, Health, and Well-Being*, ed. Raymond MacDonald, Gunter Kreutz, and Laura Mitchell (Oxford: Oxford University Press, 2012), 12–24.

11. See Nikolas Rose and Joelle M. Abi-Rached, *Neuro: The New Brain Sciences and the Management of the Mind* (Princeton, NJ: Princeton University Press, 2013), 25–52.

12. Rose and Abi-Rached, *Neuro*, 17.

13. Kewal K. Jain, *Applications of Biotechnology in Neurology* (New York: Humana Press, 2013), 575.

14. Jain, *Applications of Biotechnology in Neurology*, v, 4; memorandum from Louis W. Sullivan to President George H. W. Bush, March 3, 1990, "Briefings 4/90–3/91: Decade of the Brain," OA/IS 018144, Molly Osborne Files, White House Office of Public Liaison, George H. W. Bush Presidential Records, George Bush Presidential Library, College Station, Texas.

15. Jain, *Applications of Biotechnology*, 50.

16. Jain, *Applications of Biotechnology*, 50.

17. For profile-raising pieces, see Sharon Begley, "Mapping the Brain" and Newsweek Staff, "Is the Mind an Illusion?," both in *Newsweek*, April 20, 1992; and "The Decade of the Brain: Where to Find More Information," *Scientific American* 267 (September 1992): BR13–14.

18. H. J. Res. 174, "To Designate the Decade beginning January 1, 1990, as the 'Decade of the Brain,'" July 25, 1989, 101st Congress, https://www.congress.gov/bill/101st-congress/house-joint-resolution/174?q=%7B%22search%22%3A%22actionCode%3A%288000+OR+17000%29%22%7D&s=1&r=34.

19. Subcommittee on Brain and Behavioral Sciences, *Decade of the Brain 1990–2000: Maximizing Human Potential* ([Washington, DC]: Subcommittee on Brain and Behavioral Sciences, 1991), https://files.eric.ed.gov/fulltext/ED410480.pdf.

20. Susan Koester, "Renewal of the Silvio O. Conte Centers for Basic Neuroscience or Translational Mental Health Research," National Institute of Mental Health, May 30, 2019: https://www.nimh.nih.gov/funding/grant-writing-and-application-process/concept -clearances/2019/renewal-of-the-silvio-o-conte-centers-for-basic-neuroscience-or -translational-mental-health-research. See also Johanna Schneider, "Neuroscience at NIH," *Science* 258 (December 4, 1992); National Institute of Mental Health, "Silvio O. Conte Centers for the Neuroscience of Mental Disorders," press release, April 17, 1998, https://grants.nih.gov/grants/guide/pa-files/PAR-98-058.html. The first volume in the Decade of the Brain series was dedicated to Conte; see Richard D. Broadwell, ed., *Neuro-science, Memory, and Language* (Washington, DC: Library of Congress, 1995).

21. James H. Billington and Frederick K. Goodwin, "Preface," in *Neuroscience, Mem-ory, and Language*, ed. Richard D. Broadwell (Washington, DC: Library of Congress, 1995), xviii.

22. "Mental Illness Awareness Week," Proclamation No. 6196, 55 Fed. Reg. 197 (Octo-ber 11, 1990), 41329; "Research Supports Call for Earlier Attention to Disorders," *Los Angeles Times*, October 9, 1990.

23. George H. W. Bush, "Remarks at the Dedication Ceremony for the Michael Bilira-kis Alzheimer's Center in Palm Harbor, Florida," April 27, 1989, in *Public Papers of the Presidents of the United States: George H. W. Bush, 1989, Book 1, January 20 to June 30, 1989* (Washington, DC: Government Printing Office, 1990), 490. The Alliance for the Men-tally Ill wrote to President Bush to criticize his language and sentiment toward mental ill health in the ABC *Prime Time* interview of September 21, 1989; see John Holodak to George Bush, October 2, 1989, ID# 081646, HE001–05, OA/ID 17991, White House Office of Records Management, George H. W. Bush Presidential Library, College Station, TX.

24. George H. W. Bush, "Statement on Signing the ADAMHA Reorganization Act," July 13, 1992, in *Public Papers of the Presidents of the United States: George H. W. Bush, 1992, Book 1, January 1 to July 31, 1992* (Washington, DC: Government Printing Office, 1993), 1109.

25. Robert M. Cook-Deegan and United States Congress Office of Technology Assess-ment, *Confronting Alzheimer's Disease and Other Dementias* (Philadelphia, PA: Lippincott, 1988), 4.

26. World Health Organization and Alzheimer's Disease International, *Dementia—A Public Health Priority* (Geneva: World Health Organization, 2012), 90.

27. Henry T. Greely, "The Neuroscience Revolution, Ethics and the Law," Markkula Center for Applied Ethics, Santa Clara University, April 20, 2004, https://www.scu.edu /ethics/focus-areas/bioethics/resources/the-neuroscience-revolution-ethics-and-the-law.

28. See Dennett, *Brainchildren: Essays on Designing Minds* (Cambridge, MA: MIT Press, 1998).

29. Richard Dawkins, *Unweaving the Rainbow: Science, Delusion, and the Appetite for Wonder* (Boston: Houghton Mifflin, 1998). For Dennett's anti-religious arguments, see Daniel C. Dennett, *Breaking the Spell: Religion as a Natural Phenomenon* (London: Penguin, 2009).

30. Dennett C. Dennett, *Consciousness Explained* (London: Penguin, 1991), 65–67, 228. See also Daniel C. Dennett, *Darwin's Dangerous Idea: Evolution and the Meanings of Life* (London: Penguin, 1995), 393.

31. Francis Crick, *The Astonishing Hypothesis: The Scientific Search for the Soul* (London: Touchstone, 1994), 282.

32. Richard Rorty, "Blunder around for a While," *London Review of Books*, November 21, 1991.

33. Dennett, *Consciousness Explained*, 39.

34. Dennett, *Consciousness Explained*, 111.

35. Dennett, *Consciousness Explained*, 432.

36. See Andy Clark, "That Special Something: The Making of Minds and Selves," in *Daniel Dennett*, ed. Andrew Brook and Don Ross (Cambridge: Cambridge University Press, 2002), 187–205.

37. Dennett, *Consciousness Explained*, 425.

38. Crick, *Astonishing Hypothesis*, 283.

39. John R. Searle, *The Rediscovery of Mind* (Cambridge, MA: MIT Press, 1992), 2, 34.

40. Searle, *The Rediscovery of Mind*, 17. See also John R. Searle, "Some Relations between Mind and Brain," in *Neuroscience, Memory, and Language*, ed. Richard D. Broadwell (Washington, DC: Library of Congress, 1995), 25–34.

41. Gerald M. Edelman, *Bright Air, Brilliant Fire* (New York: Penguin, 1992), 9.

42. See Gerald M. Edelman, "Bright Air, Brilliant Fire: Neurobiology and the Mind," in *Neuroscience, Memory, and Language*, ed. Richard D. Broadwell (Washington, DC: Library of Congress, 1995), 3–9; Gerald M. Edelman and Giulio Tononi, *A Universe of Consciousness* (New York: Basic Books, 2000).

43. John R. Searle, *Freedom and Neurobiology: Reflections on Free Will, Language, and Political Power* (New York: Columbia University Press, 2008), 15.

44. John R. Searle, "The Mystery of Consciousness," Part 1, *New York Review of Books*, November 16, 1995; and Searle, "The Mystery of Consciousness," Part 2, *New York Review of Books*, December 21, 1995; Daniel C. Dennett's reply to Searle, "'The Mystery of Consciousness': An Exchange," *New York Review of Books*, December 21, 1995.

45. Daniel C. Dennett, "Are We Explaining Consciousness Yet?," *Cognition* 79 (April 2001): 231. For his attack on ontology, see Daniel C. Dennett, "Real Patterns," *Journal of Philosophy* 88 (January 1991): 27–51.

46. Searle, *Rediscovery of Mind*, 247.

47. Thomas Nagel, *The View from Nowhere* (New York: Oxford University Press, 1986), 214–215. Searle aligns with Nagel's view of the irreducibility of consciousness in *Rediscovery of the Mind*, 116–118.

48. Nagel, *View from Nowhere*, 216.

49. Thomas Nagel, "Is Consciousness an Illusion?," *New York Review of Books*, March 9, 2017. See also Nagel, *Mind and Cosmos: Why the Materialist Neo-Darwinian Conception of Nature Is Almost Certainly False* (New York: Oxford University Press, 2012), 13.

50. John Searle, *Minds, Brains and Science* (1984; repr., London: Penguin, 1991), 86.

51. Nagel, *View from Nowhere*, 222–223.

52. Larry Churchill, "The Human Experience of Dying: The Moral Primacy of Stories over Stages," *Soundings* 62 (Spring 1979): 24–37.

53. See David Flood and Rhonda L. Soricelli, "Development of the Physician's Narrative Voice in the Medical Case History," *Literature and Medicine* 11 (1992): 67, 71.

54. See Anil K. Seth, "Consciousness: The Last 50 Years (and the Next)," *Brain and Neuroscience Advances* 2 (November 2018): 1–6; Anil K. Seth and Tim Bayne, "Theories of Consciousness," *Nature Reviews Neuroscience*, May 2022, https://www.nature.com/articles/s41583-022-00587-4; and Anil K. Seth, *Being You: A New Science of Consciousness* (London: Faber & Faber, 2022).

55. Oliver Sacks, *The Man Who Mistook His Wife for a Hat* (London: Picador, 1986), 163–167.

56. Oliver Sacks, "Clinical Tales," *Literature and Medicine* 5 (1986): 17.

57. See Angela Woods, "Beyond the Wounded Storyteller: Rethinking Narrativity, Illness and Embodied Self-Experience," in *Health, Illness and Disease: Philosophical Essays*, ed. Havi Carel and Rachel Cooper (Newcastle: Acumen, 2012), 113–128.

58. See Oliver Sacks, *The River of Consciousness* (New York: Picador, 2018), 169, 176, 183. The title essay of this posthumous collection first appeared in the *New York Review of Books* on January 15, 2004.

59. Dennett, *Consciousness Explained*, 197–198.

60. Dennett, *Consciousness Explained*, 300. Dennett and Sacks featured in a philosophical roundtable discussion for the 1993 series *A Glorious Accident*, filmed for Dutch television and aired on PBS on June 12, 1994. See "A Glorious Accident (7 of 7) Coming Together: We Wonder, Ever Wonder Why We Found Us Here," YouTube video, accessed March 1, 2023, https://www.youtube.com/watch?v=RVrnn7QW6Jg&list=PLzLGaX_JvmJoIGJFR_1Mo88pMz68qUtnc&index=7.

61. Jerome Bruner, *Actual Minds, Possible Worlds* (Cambridge, MA: Harvard University Press, 1986), 21.

62. Jerome Bruner, *Acts of Meaning* (Cambridge, MA: Harvard University Press, 1990), 53. See also Bruner, "Frames for Thinking: Ways of Making Meaning," in *Modes of Thought: Explorations in Culture and Cognition*, ed. David R. Olson and Nancy Torrance (Cambridge: Cambridge University Press, 1996), 93–105.

63. See Antonio R. Damasio, *The Feeling of What Happens: Body, Emotion and the Making of Consciousness* (New York: Vintage, 1999), 17–18.

64. Antonio R. Damasio and Hanna Damasio, "Emotion and Decision in the Adaptable Brain," in *The Adaptable Brain*, ed. Sherry Levy-Reiner (Washington, DC: Library of

Congress, 1999), 3–9; Antonio R. Damasio, *Self Comes to Mind: Constructing the Conscious Brain* (London: Vintage, 2012), 22–23. On consciousness and sociability, see Damasio, *The Strange Order of Things: Life, Feeling, and the Making of Cultures* (New York: Random House, 2018) and Damasio, *Feeling, Being and Knowing: Making Minds Conscious* (New York: Ballantine Books, 2021).

65. See Benard J. Baars, *In the Theater of Consciousness: The Workspace of the Mind* (New York: Oxford University Press, 1997).

66. Dennett, "Are We Explaining Consciousness Yet?," 222. See also Stanislas Dehaene and Lionel Naccache, "Towards a Cognitive Neuroscience of Consciousness: Basic Evidence and a Workspace Framework," *Cognition* 79 (April 2001): 1–37.

67. Damasio, *The Feeling of What Happens*, 188. See Gerald M. Edelman, *Second Nature: Brain Science and Human Knowledge* (New Haven, CT: Yale University Press, 2006).

68. Robin Gandy, "Human versus Mechanical Intelligence," in *The Legacy of Alan Turing*, vol. 1, *Machines and Thought*, ed. Peter Millican and Andy Clark (Oxford: Oxford University Press, 1996), 125.

69. Daniel C. Dennett, "The Self as a Responding—and Responsible—Artifact," *Annals of the New York Academy of Sciences* 1001 (October 2003): 39–50.

70. Dennett, "The Self as a Responding—and Responsible—Artifact," 48. See also Dennett, *Freedom Evolves* (New York: Viking, 2003).

71. Gerald M. Edelman, Joseph A. Gally, and Bernard J. Baars, "Biology of Consciousness," *Frontiers in Psychology* 2 (January 25, 2011): 1–7.

72. For a critique of Edelman's model of consciousness, see Martine Rothblatt, *Virtually Human: The Promise—and the Peril—of Digital Immortality* (New York: St. Martin's Press, 2014), 21–25. See also Luiz Pessoa, *The Entangled Brain: How Perception, Cognition, and Emotion Are Woven Together* (Cambridge, MA: MIT Press, 2022).

73. James H. Billington and Steven E. Hyman, "Discovering Ourselves: The Science of Emotions," Executive Summary, The Decade of the Brain, 1990–2000, May 1998, https://www.loc.gov/loc/brain/emotion/Intro.html.

74. Lewis L. Judd to George W. Owings III (Maryland House of Delegates), February 9, 1989, ID# 005564, FA005 Public Health, White House Office of Records Management, George H. W. Bush Presidential Library.

75. Tipper Gore, "Toward Understanding Our Total Health," The Decade of the Brain, 1990–2000, May 6, 1998, https://www.loc.gov/loc/brain/emotion/MrsGore.html.

76. See Debra Rosenberg, "Tipper Steps Out," *Newsweek*, May 24, 1999; and JoAnn Bren Guernsey, *Tipper Gore: Voice for the Voiceless* (Minneapolis, MN: Lerner, 1994), 26, 40, 43.

77. Gore, "Toward Understanding Our Total Health." On the search for organic biomarkers of mental ill health, see Amy Ellis Nutt, "The Mind's Biology," *Washington Post*, February 19, 2016.

78. Stanley I. Greenspan, "Emotional Origins of Intelligence," The Decade of the Brain, 1990–2000, May 6, 1998, https://www.loc.gov/loc/brain/emotion/Greenspa.html.

79. Stanley I. Greenspan, "Emotional Intelligence," in *Learning and Education: Psychoanalytic Perspectives*, ed. Kay Field, Bertram Cohler, and Glorye Wool (Madison, CT: International Universities Press, 1989), 209–243.

80. Stanley I. Greenspan with Beryl Lieff Benderly, *The Growth of the Mind and the Endangered Origins of Intelligence* (Cambridge, MA: Perseus, 1997), 8. See also Stanley I. Greenspan, *The Growth of the Mind and the Endangered Origins of Intelligence* (Boston: Da Capo, 1998).

81. Richard J. Hernstein and Charles Murray, "Race, Genes, and IQ—An Apologia," *New Republic*, October 31, 1994.

82. See Richard J. Hernstein and Charles Murray, *The Bell Curve: Intelligence and Class Structure in American Life* (New York: Free Press, 1994); and Charles Murray, "IQ and Economic Success," *The Public Interest* 128 (Summer 1997): 21–45.

83. Hernstein and Murray, *The Bell Curve*, 21.

84. Henry Louise Gates Jr., "Why Now?" in *The Bell Curve Wars: Race, Intelligence and the Future of America*, ed. Steven Fraser (New York: Basic Books, 1995), 95. See also Malcolm W. Browne, "What Is Intelligence, and Who Has It?," *New York Times*, October 16, 1994; and David Reich, "How Genetics Is Changing Our Understanding of 'Race,'" *New York Times*, March 23, 2018.

85. Cole Cohen, *Head Case: My Brain and Other Wonders* (New York: Henry Holt, 2015), 26.

86. Stephen Jay Gould, *The Mismeasure of Man*, rev. and expanded ed. (New York: Norton, 1996), 368. The piece was first published as "Curveball," *New Yorker*, November 28, 1994, 139–149.

87. Gould, *The Mismeasure of Man*, 34.

88. Gould, *The Mismeasure of Man*, 376.

89. See Alan Glynn, *The Dark Fields* (New York: Little, Brown, 2001). MDT-48 is renamed NZT-48 in the 2011 film. See also Robert Kolker, "The Real *Limitless* Drug Isn't Just for Lifehackers Anymore," *New York*, March 29, 2013; Hub Zwart, "*Limitless* as a Neuro-Pharmaceutical Experiment and as a *Daseinanalyse*: On the Use of Fiction in Preparatory Debates on Cognitive Enhancement," *Medical Health Care and Philosophy* 17 (2014): 29–38; and Arran Frood, "Use of 'Smart Drugs' on the Rise,'" *Nature*, July 5, 2018.

90. See Nick Bostrom, *Superintelligence: Paths, Dangers, Strategies* (Oxford: Oxford University Press, 2014), 48–54. For a parody in which class remains consequential despite cognitive enhancements, see Ted Chiang, "It's 2059, and the Rich Kids Are Still Winning," *New York Times*, May 27, 2019.

91. See James D. Watson, *Avoid Boring People: Lessons from a Life in Science* (Oxford: Oxford University Press, 2007).

92. Gould, *The Mismeasure of Man*, 33.

93. John Horgan, "Oliver Sacks and the Binding Power of Rhythm," *Scientific American*, May 18, 2015. On music therapy for aphasic and Parkinson's patients, see Sacks, *Musicophilia*, 214–223, 248–258.

94. Oliver Sacks, *An Anthropologist on Mars* (London: Penguin, 1995), 62. 'The Last Hippie' was first published in the *New York Review of Books*, March 26, 1992.

95. Edelman, *Second Nature*, 39.

96. See Jessica Hamzelou, "The Checkup: What Minimally Conscious Brains Can Do," *MIT Technology Review*, September 16, 2022.

97. Damasio, *The Feeling of What Happens*, 109.

98. See Sacks, "Speed: Aberrations of Time and Movement," *New Yorker*, August 23, 2004.

99. Sacks, *Man Who Mistook His Wife for a Hat*, 184.

100. See Bruce H. Dobkin, "The Medical Assault on Stroke," *New York Times*, April 29, 1990; Kil-Byung Lim, Yong-Kyun Kim, Hong-Jae Lee, Jeehyun Yoo, Ji Youn Hwang, Jeong-Ah Kim, and Sung-Kyun Kim, "The Therapeutic Effect of Neurologic Music Therapy and Speech Language Therapy in Post-Stroke Aphasic Patients," *Annals of Rehabilitation Medicine* 37 (August 2013): 556–562; and Dawn L. Merrett, Anna Zumbansen, and Isabelle Peretz, "A Theoretical and Clinical Account of Music and Aphasia," *Aphasiology* 33 (February 2019): 379–381.

101. Sacks, "The Creative Self," in Sacks, *The River of Consciousness* (New York: Picador, 2018), 147.

102. Oliver Sacks, *Everything in Its Place: First Loves and Last Tales* (London: Picador, 2019), 228.

103. On the entwining of the neurosciences and humanities, see Jon Leefman and Elisabeth Hildt, *The Human Sciences and the Decade of the Brain* (London: Academic Press, 2017).

104. Greenspan, *The Growth of the Mind*, 8.

105. Barbara Arrowsmith-Young, *The Woman Who Changed Her Brain: How We Can Shape Our Minds and Other Tales of Cognitive Transformation* (New York: Vintage, 2013), 8, 152.

106. Rose and Abi-Rached, *Neuro*, 15.

107. Arrowsmith-Young, *The Woman Who Changed Her Brain*, 32–33.

108. Arrowsmith-Young, *The Woman Who Changed Her Brain*, 29. On Barry Kaufman's Son-Rise program, see Martin Halliwell, *Voices of Mental Health: Medicine, Politics, and American Culture, 1970–2000* (New Brunswick, NJ: Rutgers University Press, 2017), 133–138. See also Norman Doidge, *The Brain that Changes Itself: Stories of Personal Triumph from the Frontiers of Brain Science* (New York: Penguin, 2008). As a champion of the Arrowsmith program, Doidge wrote the foreword to *The Woman Who Changed Her Brain*.

109. Elman, *Chronic Youth*, 132.

110. Bill Clinton, "Remarks and a Question-and-Answer Session at a Democratic National Committee Luncheon in Palm Beach, Florida," October 31, 1997, in *Public Papers of the Presidents of the United States: William J. Clinton, 1997*, Book 2, *July 1 to December 31, 1997* (Washington, DC: Government Printing Office, 1999), 1468–1469; George W. Bush, "Remarks and a Question-and-Answer Session at Griegos Elementary School in

Albuquerque," August 15, 2001, in *Public Papers of the Presidents of the United States: George H. W. Bush, 2001*, Book 2, *July 1 to December 31, 2001* (Washington, DC: Government Printing Office, 2003), 976–978.

111. Arrowsmith-Young, *The Woman Who Changed Her Brain*, 43. See also "Barbara Arrowsmith-Young: Transforming Learning Disabilities through the Power of the Brain," Just Education Podcast, May 11, 2020, https://www.buzzsprout.com/251698/3711578.

112. For Soundsory, see "The Soundsory Program," https://soundsory.com/learn -more/program/, accessed March 18, 2024.

113. See Jill Scott's 2014 Aural Roots project: https://isea-archives.siggraph.org/wp -content/uploads/2019/06/2016_Scott_AURALROOTS.pdf.

114. See, for example, Diane A. Toigo, "Autism: Integrating a Personal Perspective with Music Therapy Practice," *Music Therapy Perspectives* 10 (May 1992): 13–20; Gordon Graham, "Music and Autism," *Journal of Aesthetic Education* 35 (Summer 2001): 39–47; Michael Bakan, *Speaking for Ourselves: Conversations on Life, Music, and Autism* (Oxford: Oxford University Press, 2018).

115. Mindvalley: www.mindvalley.com; Neuralink: https://neuralink.com (both accessed December 1, 2022). See also the Mindvalley cofounder Vishen Lakhiani's *The Code of the Extraordinary Mind* (New York: Rodale, 2016).

116. Lisa Genova, *Still Alice* (New York: Simon & Schuster, 2007), 1.

117. Genova, *Still Alice*, 316.

118. A. O. Scott, "Losing Her Bearings in Familiar Places," *New York Times*, December 4, 2014.

119. See Lucy Burke, "The Locus of our Dis-ease: Narratives of Family Life in the Age of Alzheimer's," in *Popularizing Dementia: Public Expressions and Representations of Forgetfulness*, ed. Mark Schweda and Aagje Swinnen (Berlin: Verlag, 2015), 23–42.

120. Advisory Panel on Alzheimer's Disease, *Fourth Report of the Advisory Panel on Alzheimer's Disease*, NIH 93–3520 (Washington, DC: Government Printing Office, 1992), 31–50.

121. On biomarkers, see Margaret Lock, *The Alzheimer Conundrum: Entanglements of Dementia and Aging* (Princeton, NJ: Princeton University Press, 2013), 132–155. See also Sarah Falcus and Katsura Sako, *Contemporary Narratives of Dementia: Ethics, Ageing, Politics* (New York: Routledge, 2019); Cristina Garrigós, ed., *Alzheimer's Disease in Contemporary U.S. Fiction* (New York: Routledge, 2021); and Irmela Marei Krüger-Fürhoff, Nina Schmidt, and Sue Vice, eds., *The Politics of Dementia: Forgetting and Remembering the Violent Past in Literature, Film and Graphic Narratives* (Berlin: De Gruyter, 2021).

122. Genova, *Still Alice*, 229.

123. Genova, *Still Alice*, 281.

124. Genova, *Still Alice*, 335.

125. Michael Ignatieff, *Scar Tissue* (London: Vintage, 1993), 47. On life worlds and dementia, see Jaber F. Grubium, "Narrative Practice and the Inner Worlds of the Alzheimer Disease Experience," in *Concepts of Alzheimer Disease: Biological, Clinical and*

Cultural Perspectives, ed. Peter J. Whitehouse, Konrad Maurer, and Jesse F. Ballinger (Baltimore, MD: Johns Hopkins University Press, 2000), 181–203; Annette Leibing, "Divided Gazes: Alzheimer's Disease, the Person within and Death in Life," in *Thinking about Dementia: Culture, Loss, and the Anthropology of Senility*, ed. Annette Leibing and Lawrence Cohen (New Brunswick, NJ: Rutgers University Press, 2006), 240–268.

126. David Auburn's play *Proof* (2000), about mathematics and mental illness, takes the place of Chekhov in Genova's novel.

127. Janelle S. Taylor, "Should Old Acquaintance Be Forgot? Friendship in the Face of Dementia," in *Successful Aging as a Contemporary Obsession: Global Perspectives*, ed. Sarah Lamb (New Brunswick, NJ: Rutgers University Press, 2017), 130.

128. See Vittorio Gallese, "Mirror Neurons, Embodied Simulation, and the Neural Basis of Social Identification," *Psychoanalytic Dialogues* 19 (October 2009): 528.

129. This scene forms the novel's epilogue, but the playtext Lydia reads to Alice is not revealed; Genova, *Still Alice*, 327.

130. See, for example, H. B. Svansdottir and J. Snaedal, "Music Therapy in Moderate and Severe Dementia of Alzheimer's Type: A Case Control Study," *International Psycho-geriatrics* 18 (December 2006): 613–621. See also Genova's 2018 novel of a pianist's experience of neurodegenerative disease, *Every Note Played* (New York: Allen & Unwin, 2018).

131. Genova, *Still Alice*, 79. See also "Early Onset Familial AD," interview with Lisa Genova, Alzforum: Working for a Cure, accessed July 1, 2022, https://www.alzforum .org/early-onset-familial-ad/profiles/interview-lisa-genova.

132. Genova, *Still Alice*, 131.

133. Genova, "Early Onset Famililal AD." On tensions between medical paternalism and self-medication, see Jessica Flanigan, *Pharmaceutical Freedom: Why Patients Have a Right to Self-Medicate* (New York: Oxford University Press, 2017).

134. Genova, *Still Alice*, 155, 321. In her postscript, Genova explains why she included a fictional drug but does not note that a new company with almost the same name, Amy-lyx (est. 2013), had started to investigate a drug that might slow the neurodegenerative process (329).

135. Genova, *Still Alice*, 77.

136. Genova, *Still Alice*, 269, 271. See Helen Sweeting and Mary Gilhooly, "Dementia and the Phenomenon of Social Death," *Sociology of Health and Illness* 19 (January 1997): 93–117; Dragana Lukić, "Multiple Ontologies of Alzheimer's Disease in *Still Alice* and *A Song for Martin*: A Feminist Visual Studies of Technoscience Perspective," *European Journal of Women's Studies* 26 (November 2019): 375–389.

137. David Foster Wallace, "Consider the Lobster," *Gourmet*, August 2004, 50–64; Genova, *Still Alice*, 82.

138. Elizabeth Bishop, "One Art," *New Yorker*, April 26, 1976. See also "U.S. Government Sets Out Alzheimer's Plan," *Scientific American*, May 23, 2012, quoted in Lock, *The Alzheimer Conundrum*, 4. Caregiving is a topic of *The Alzheimer's Project: Caregivers* (HBO, 2009) and *Alzheimer's: The Caregiver's Perspective* (PBS, 2016).

139. Tim Armstrong, "'A Transfinite Syntax': Modernism and Mathematics," *Affirmations: of the modern* 6 (Spring 2019): 1–29.

140. See Lisa Genova, *Remember: The Science of Memory and the Art of Forgetting* (New York: Harmony, 2021). On happiness pills, see David Herzberg, *Happy Pills in America: From Miltown to Prozac* (Baltimore. MD: Johns Hopkins University Press, 2010). On zombification, see Susan M. Behuniak, "The Living Dead? The Construction of People with Alzheimer's Disease as Zombies," *Ageing and Society* 31 (January 2011): 70–92.

141. Scott Selberg, *Mediating Alzheimer's: Cognition and Personhood* (Minneapolis: University of Minnesota Press, 2022), 214.

142. "Alzheimer's Drug Slows Mental Decline in Trial—But Is It a Breakthrough?," *Nature* 609 (September 29, 2022); Pam Belluck, "New Federal Decisions Make Alzheimer's Drug Leqembi Widely Accessible," *New York Times*, July 6, 2023.

CHAPTER 4 — AUGMENTED LIVES

1. William J. Clinton and Albert Gore Jr., *Science in the National Interest* (Washington, DC: Office of Science and Technology Policy, 1994), 1.

2. Clinton and Gore, *Science in the National Interest*, 5.

3. Clinton and Gore, *Science in the National Interest*, 3–4. The frontier theme of the 2016 Pittsburgh conference was highlighted in a "White House Frontiers" briefing of October 7. See Cristin Dorgelo and Kristen Lee, "White House Frontiers: Robots, Space Exploration, and the Future of American Innovation," The White House: President Barack Obama, October 7, 2016, https://obamawhitehouse.archives.gov/blog/2016/10/07/white-house-frontiers-conference-robots-space-exploration-and-future-american.

4. Barack Obama, "Remarks during a Panel Discussion at the White House Frontiers Conference at Carnegie Mellon University in Pittsburgh, Pennsylvania," October 13, 2016, in *Public Papers of the Presidents of the United States: Barack Obama, 2016*, Book 2, *July 1, 2016 to January 20, 2017* (Washington, DC: Government Printing Office, 2016), 1320.

5. Barack Obama, "Inaugural Address," January 20, 2009, in *Public Papers of the Presidents of the United States: Barack Obama, 2009*, Book 1, *January 20 to June 30, 2009* (Washington, DC: Government Printing Office, 2010), 2.

6. Obama, "Remarks during a Panel at the White House Frontiers Conference," 1321; Chris Mooney, *The Republican War on Science* (New York: Perseus, 2006). See also Rush Holt, "Reversing the Congressional Science Lobotomy," *Wired*, April 29, 2009.

7. "Scientists Bring the Sense of Touch to a Robotic Arm," NPR, May 20, 2021, https://www.npr.org/sections/health-shots/2021/05/20/998725924/a-sense-of-touch-boosts-speed-accuracy-of-mind-controlled-robotic-arm. See also "The Pentagon's Bionic Arm," CBS News, April 10, 2009, https://www.cbsnews.com/news/the-pentagons-bionic-arm/; Sharlene N. Flesher, John E. Downey, Jeffrey M. Weiss, Christopher L. Hughes, Angelica J. Herrera, Elizabeth C. Tyler-Kabara, Michael L. Boninger, et al., "A Brain-Computer Interface that Evokes Tactile Sensations Improves Robotic Arm Control," *Science* 372 (May 21, 2021): 831–836.

8. Michael Weisskopf, *Blood Brothers: Among the Soldiers of Ward 57* (New York: Holt, 2007), 125. See also Michael Belifore, *The Department of Mad Scientists* (New York: HarperCollins, 2009), 3, 11.

9. U.S. Congress, *The Dawn of Artificial Intelligence: Hearing before the Subcommittee on Space, Science, and Competitiveness of the Committee on Commerce, Science, and Transportation, 114th Congress, 2nd Session, November 30, 2016* (Washington, DC: Government Printing Office, 2017); U.S. House of Representatives, *The Disrupter Series: Advanced Robotics: Hearing before the Subcommittee on Commerce, Manufacturing Trade of the Committee on Energy and Commerce, 114th Congress, 2nd Session, September 14, 2016* (Washington, DC: Government Printing Office, 2016).

10. U.S. Congress, *The Dawn of Artificial Intelligence*, 3.

11. Barack Obama, "Address Before a Joint Session of the Congress on the State of the Union, February 12, 2013," and "Remarks on Science and Technology," April 2, 2013, both in *Public Papers of the Presidents of the United States: Barack Obama, 2013*, Book 1, *January 1 to June 30, 2013* (Washington, DC: Government Printing Office, 2018), 99, 258–261, respectively. See also John Markoff, "Obama Seeking to Boost Study of Human Brain," *New York Times*, February 17, 2003.

12. Obama, "Remarks at the National Conference on Mental Health," June 3, 2013, in *Public Papers of the Presidents of the United States: Barack Obama, 2013*, Book 1, *January 1 to June 30, 2013* (Washington, DC: Government Printing Office, 2018), 516–519.

13. Malcolm Gay, *The Brain Electric: The Dramatic High-Tech Race to Merge Minds and Machines* (New York: Farrar, Straus and Giroux, 2015), 51.

14. Rachel Mabe, "What Is It Like to Regain a Sense of Touch, Only to Lose It Again?," *Atlantic*, April 10, 2017, https://www.theatlantic.com/science/archive/2017/04/mind-controlled-robot-arm/522315/.

15. U.S. Congress, *The Dawn of Artificial Intelligence*, 7, 10.

16. U.S. Congress, *The Dawn of Artificial Intelligence*, 38. For the Musk quotation, see Matt MacFarland, "Elon Musk: 'With Artificial Intelligence We Are Summoning the Demon,'" *Washington Post*, October 24, 2014. It is important to recognize that Musk does not speak for the variety of opinion in Silicon Valley on the promises and perils of AI: see Nitasha Tiku, "Doomsday to Utopia: Meet AI's Rival Factions," *Washington Post*, April 10, 2023.

17. U.S. Congress, *The Dawn of Artificial Intelligence*, 38. Speakers at the hearing argued that user error and network failure of weak AI applications were more pressing issues than the ontological dangers of strong, ultra-intelligent AI. See also Luciana Floridi, "The Ethics of Artificial Intelligence," in *Megatech: Technology in 2050*, ed. Daniel Franklin (New York: Public Affairs, 2017), 155–161.

18. Murray Shanahan, *The Technological Singularity* (Cambridge, MA: MIT Press, 2013), 1; Martin Ford, *The Rise of the Robots: Technology and the Threat of Mass Unemployment* (London: One World, 2016), 230.

19. Robert H. Carlson, "Biotechnology's Possibilities," in *Megatech: Technology in 2050*, ed. Daniel Franklin (New York: Public Affairs, 2017), 43. See also Robert H. Carlson,

Biology Is Technology: The Promise, Peril, and New Business of Engineering Life (Cambridge, MA: Harvard University Press, 2010). For the prediction, see Raymond Kurzweil, *The Singularity Is Near: When Humans Transcend Biology* (New York: Penguin, 2005).

20. U.S. House of Representatives, *Beyond I, Robot: Ethics, Artificial Intelligence, and the Digital Age: Hearing before the Task Force on Artificial Intelligence of the Committee on Financial Services, 117th Congress, 1st Session, October 13, 2021* (Washington, DC: Government Printing Office, 2021). The Task Force on Artificial Intelligence was launched on June 10, 2021; "The Biden Administration Launches the National Artificial Intelligence Research Resource Task Force," The White House, June 10, 2021, https://www.whitehouse.gov /ostp/news-updates/2021/06/10/the-biden-administration-launches-the-national -artificial-intelligence-research-resource-task-force.

21. Neda Atanasoski and Kalindi Vora, *Surrogate Humanity: Race, Robots, and the Politics of Technological Futures* (Durham, NC: Duke University Press, 2019), 3.

22. Robert M. Geraci, *Apocalyptic AI: Visions of Heaven in Robotics, Artificial Intelligence, and Virtual Reality* (Oxford: Oxford University Press, 2010), 1–3.

23. Atanasoski and Vora, *Surrogate Humanity*, 3.

24. On digital eugenics, see Martine Rothblatt, *Virtually Human: The Promise—and the Peril—of Digital Immortality* (New York: St Martin's Press, 2014), 91–119.

25. John Markoff, "The Coming Superbrain," *New York Times*, May 23, 2009.

26. Asimov's laws were first stated in his 1942 short story "Runaround" and were reprinted in Isaac Asimov, *I, Robot* (New York: Gnome Press, 1950).

27. See Dylan Evans and Walter de Beck, "Evolutionary Robotics," in *Applied Evolutionary Psychology*, ed. S. Craig Roberts (Oxford: Oxford University Press, 2012), 414–425.

28. U.S. Congress, *The Dawn of Artificial Intelligence*, 54.

29. U.S. Congress, *The Dawn of Artificial Intelligence*, 53.

30. Ford, *The Rise of the Robots*, 151–168.

31. Robert Kirk, *Robots, Zombies and Us: Understanding Consciousness* (London: Bloomsbury, 2017), 28.

32. Kirk, *Robots, Zombies and Us*, 29–30.

33. David Ewing Duncan, *Talking to Robots: A Brief Guide to Our Human-Robot Futures* (London: Robinson, 2019), 3.

34. See Geraci, *Apocalyptic AI*, 50–53.

35. Tether quoted in Michael Belfiore, *Department of Mad Scientists: How DARPA is Remaking Our World, from the Internet to Artificial Limbs* (New York: Harper, 2010), 180. See also Barack Obama, "Remarks at Carnegie Mellon University in Pittsburgh, Pennsylvania," June 24, 2011, in *Public Papers of the Presidents of the United States: Barack Obama, 2011, Book 1, January 1 to June 30, 2011* (Washington, DC: Government Printing Office, 2014), 707.

36. On Japanese robotics, see "Better than People: Japan's Humanoid Robots," *The Economist*, December 24, 2005; and Amelia DeFalco, "Beyond Prosthetic Memory: Post-

humanism, Embodiment, and Caregiving Robots," *Age, Culture, Humanities: An Interdisciplinary Journal* 3 (January 2018): 1–31.

37. Daniel C. Dennett, "Where Am I?," in *The Mind's I: Fantasies and Reflections on Self and Soul*, ed. Douglas R. Hofstadter and Daniel C. Dennett (London: Penguin, 1981), 224–225.

38. See Jonathan Glover, *I: The Philosophy and Psychology of Personal Identity* (New York: Viking, 1988).

39. Daniel C. Dennett, "2015: What Do You Think about Machines that Think?," *Edge*, [2015], https://www.edge.org/response-detail/26035.

40. Tim Requarth, "Bringing a Virtual Brain to Life," *New York Times*, March 18, 2013.

41. John R. Seale, "Minds, Brains, and Programs," in *The Mind's I: Fantasies and Reflections on Self and Soul*, ed. Douglas R. Hofstadter and Daniel C. Dennett (London: Penguin, 1981), 352. Searle's "Minds, Brains, and Programs" was first published in *Behavioral and Brain Sciences* 3 (September 1980): 417–424.

42. Marvin Minsky, "Steps toward Artificial Intelligence," *Proceedings of the IRE* 49 (January 1961): 27.

43. On boundary issues of synthetic lives, see Deborah Knight and George McKnight, "What Is It to Be Human? *Blade Runner* and *Dark City*," in *The Philosophy of Science Fiction Film*, ed. Steven M. Sanders (Lexington: University Press of Kentucky, 2008), 21–37; and Despina Kakoudaki, *Anatomy of a Robot: Literature, Cinema, and the Cultural Work of Artificial People* (New Brunswick, NJ: Rutgers University Press 2014), 183–185.

44. Philip K. Dick, "The Android and the Human" (1972), in *The Shifting Realities of Philip K. Dick: Selected Literary and Philosophical Writings*, ed. Lawrence Sutin (New York: Pantheon, 1995), 183–210.

45. See Timothy Shanahan, *Philosophy and Blade Runner* (London: Palgrave Macmillan, 2014).

46. N. Katherine Hayles, *How We Became Posthuman: Virtual Bodies in Cybernetics, Literature and Informatics* (Chicago: University of Chicago Press, 1999), xii,

47. See, for example, Arielle A. J. Scoglio, Erin D. Reilly, Jay A. Gorman, and Charles E. Drebing, "Use of Social Robots in Mental Health and Well-Being Research: Systematic Review," *Journal of Medical Internet Research* 21 (July 2019), https://www.jmir.org/2019/7/e13322.

48. Laurel D. Riek, "Robotics Technology in Mental Healthcare," in *Artificial Intelligence in Behavioral Health and Mental Health Care*, ed. David D. Luxton (Amsterdam: Elsevier, 2015), 187–188; "Computer AI Passes Turing Test in 'World First,'" BBC, June 9, 2014, https://www.bbc.com/news/technology-27762088; Gary Marcus, "What Comes After the Turing Test?," *New Yorker*, June 9, 2014.

49. See Lambèr Royakkers and Rinie van Est, *Just Ordinary Robots: Automation from Love to War* (Boca Raton, FL: CRC Press, 2016), 10–14.

50. Andrew O'Hehir, "Dark Secrets of the Sex Robot," *Salon*, April 22, 2015. See also Julie Wosk, *My Fair Ladies: Female Robots, Androids, and Other Artificial Eves* (New

Brunswick, NJ: Rutgers University Press, 2015); and Jude Browne, Stephen Cave, Eleanor Drage, and Kerry McInerney, eds., *Feminist AI* (Oxford: Oxford University Press, 2023).

51. Murray Shnahan, *"Ex Machina* and the Question of Consciousness," in *Cybermedia: Explorations in Science, Sound, and Vision,* ed. Carol Vernallis, Holly Rogers, Selmin Kara, and Jonathan Leal (New York: Bloomsbury, 2022), 145.

52. See Despina Kakoudaki, "Unmaking People: The Politics of Negation in Franken-stein and Ex Machina," *Science Fiction Studies* 45 (July 2018): 289–307; and Jean Alvares and Patricia Salzman-Mitchell, "The Succession Myth and the Rebellious AI Creation: Classical Narratives in the 2015 Film *Ex Machina," Arethusa* 52 (Spring 2019): 181–202.

53. Franny Choi, "Queerness, Cyborgs, and Cephalopods: An Interview with Franny Choi," *Paris Review,* May 21, 2019, https://www.theparisreview.org/blog/2019/05/21/queerness-cyborgs-and-cephalopods-an-interview-with-franny-choi.

54. For an exploration of broken androids, see Franny Choi, "Chi," in Choi, *Soft Science: Poems* (Farmington, ME: Alice James Books, 2019), 39–44. See also Choi's "A Brief History of Cyborgs" and "Kyoko's Language Files Are Recovered Following Extensive Damage to her CPU," both also in *Soft Science,* 14–15, 86–89, respectively.

55. See Jan Harlan and Jane M. Struthers, eds., *AI: Artificial Intelligence from Stanley Kubrick to Steven Spielberg: The Vision behind the Film* (London: Thames & Hudson, 2009), 10, 12.

56. Riek, "Robotics Technology in Mental Healthcare," 188. Hans Moravec's 1988 *Mind Children* was one of the key sources of *A.I. Artificial Intelligence.*

57. Daniel H. Wilson, *Amped* (New York: Simon & Schuster, 2018), 8.

58. Kim Stanley Robinson, *2312* (New York: Orbit, 2012), 468.

59. Wilson, *Amped,* 18, 26.

60. Wilson, *Amped,* 83, 20.

61. Adam Piore, *The Body Builders: Inside the Science of the Engineered Human* (New York: HarperCollins, 2017), 5. See also Michel Marriott, "Robo-Legs," *New York Times,* June 20, 2005.

62. Piore, *Body Builders,* 5.

63. Piore, *Body Builders,* 21. On robotization, see Leopoldina Fortunati, "More than the Modeling of Emotions," in *Toward Robotic Socially Believable Behaving Systems,* vol. 1, *Modeling Emotions,* ed. Anna Esposito and Lakhmi C. Jain (Geneva: Springer, 2016), 1–8.

64. Adam Piore, "Triumph of the Bionic Limbs," *Discover,* January 31, 2013, https://www.discovermagazine.com/technology/94-triumph-of-the-bionic-limbs.

65. On the ethics of athletic enhancement, see Ronald M. Green, *Babies by Design: The Ethics of Genetic Choice* (New Haven, CT: Yale University Press, 2007), 17–32.

66. Piore, *Body Builders,* 52.

67. Piore, *Body Builders,* 342.

68. Piore, *Body Builders,* 344.

69. Barack Obama, "Statement on the 10th Anniversary of the Iraq War," March 19, 2013, in *Public Papers of the Presidents of the United States: Barack Obama, 2013*, Book 1, *January 1 to June 30, 2013* (Washington, DC: Government Printing Office, 2018), 201.

70. Barack Obama, "Remarks on the National Conference on Mental Health," June 3, 2013, in *Public Papers of the Presidents of the United States: Barack Obama, 2013*, Book 1, *January 1 to June 30, 2013* (Washington, DC: Government Printing Office, 2018), 518.

71. See U.S. House of Representatives, *Post Traumatic Stress Disorder and Personality Disorders: Challenges for the U.S. Department of Veterans Affairs: Hearing before the Committee of Veterans Affairs, 110th Congress, 1st Session, July 25, 2007* (Washington, DC: Government Printing Office, 2008), https://www.govinfo.gov/content/pkg/CHRG-110hhrg37475/pdf/CHRG-110hhrg37475.pdf.

72. Tony Tether, "DARPATech 2002 Welcoming Speech," Anaheim, California, July 30, 2002, accessed March 1, 2023, https://www.linkedin.com/pulse/darpatech-2002-welcoming-speech-tony-tether. On Tether's speech, see also Woody Evans, "Swarms Are Hell: Warfare as an Anti-Transhuman Choice," *Journal of Evolution and Technology* 23 (December 2013): 56–60.

73. Statement by Tony Tether to the U.S. Senate Subcommittee on Emerging Threats and Capabilities, Armed Services Committee, April 10, 2002, https://www.darpa.mil/attachments/TestimonyArchived(April%2010%202002).pdf. On unmanned warfare, see P. W. Singer, *Wired for War: The Robotics Revolution and Conflict in the 21st Century* (New York: Penguin, 2010).

74. Belfiore, *Department of Mad Scientists*, 176; Jai Galliott and Mianna Lotz, *Super Soldiers* (London: Routledge, 2016), 2. See also Jai Galliott, *Military Robots: Mapping the Moral Landscape* (Ashgate: Farnham, 2015).

75. The federal emphasis on AI was underlined by President Trump's executive order 13859, "Maintaining American Leadership in Artificial Intelligence," 83 Fed. Reg. 31 (February 11, 2019), 3967–3972.

76. Galliott and Lotz, *Super Soldiers*, 1. See also Gregory T. Huang, "Mind-Machine Merger," *Technology Review* 106 (May 2003): 38–46. For the argument that the Department of Defense is wary about adopting innovative technologies, see Eric Lipton, "Start-Ups Bring Silicon Valley Ethos to a Lumbering Military-Industrial Complex," *New York Times*, May 21, 2023.

77. See DARPA Biological Technologies Office Programs, accessed March 1, 2023, https://www.darpa.mil/about-us/offices/bto#OfficeProgramsList.

78. Arun Kundnani, "Wired for War: Military Technology and the Politics of Fear," *Race & Class* 46 (July 2004): 117. See also Richard O'Meara, *Governing Military Technologies in the 21st Century: Ethics and Operations* (London: Palgrave, 2016).

79. Piore, *Body Builders*, 182, 186.

80. Piore, *Body Builders*, 190.

81. Piore, *Body Builders*, 198–199.

82. Jonathan Moreno, *Mind Wars: Brain Science and the Military in the 21st Century* (New York: Bellevue Literary Press, 2012), 29, 33.

83. On AI and narrative continuity, see Cody Turner and Susan Schneider, "Could You Merge with AI? Reflections on the Singularity and Radical Brain Enhancement," in *The Oxford Handbook of Ethics of AI*, ed. Markus D. Dubber (Oxford: Oxford University Press, 2020), 307–324.

84. Tether quoted in Moreno, *Mind Wars*, 25; Michael Callahan quoted in Patrick Lin, Max Mehlman, Keith Abney, and Jai Galliott, "Super Soldiers (Part 1): What Is Military Human Enhancement?," in *Global Issues and Ethical Considerations in Human Enhancement Technologies*, ed. Steven John Thompson (Hershey, PA: Medical Information Science Reference, 2014), 123–124. See also "Engineering Humans for War," *Atlantic*, September 23, 2015.

85. R. H. Stretch, D. H. Marlowe, K. M. Wright, P. D. Bliese, K. H. Knudson, and C. H. Hoover, "Post-Traumatic Stress Disorder Symptoms among Gulf War Veterans," *Military Medicine* 161 (July 1996): 407–410.

86. U.S. Congress, *The Traumatic Brain Injury Act of 1992: Committee on Labor and Human Resources, 102nd Congress, 2nd Session, September 23, 1992* (Washington, DC: Government Printing Office, 1992).

87. See Institute of Medicine, *Gulf War and Health*, vol. 4, *Health Effects of Serving in the Gulf War* (Washington, DC: National Academies, 2006).

88. George W. Bush, "Remarks of a Groundbreaking Ceremony for the Walter Reed National Military Medical Center in Bethesda, Maryland," July 3, 2008, in *Public Papers of the Presidents of the United States: George W. Bush, 2008, Book 2, July 1 to December 31, 2008* (Washington, DC: Government Printing Office, 2012), 975.

89. U.S. House of Representatives, *Access to Mental Health Care and Traumatic Brain Injury Services: Addressing the Challenges and Barriers for Veterans: Subcommittee on Oversight and Investigation of the Committee on Veterans Affairs, 113th Congress, 2nd Session* (Washington, DC: Government Printing Office, 2014), 4–5.

90. Jean-François Caron, *A Theory of the Super Soldier: The Morality of Capacity-Increasing Technologies in the Military* (Manchester: Manchester University Press, 2018), 20, 77.

91. See J. Douglas Bremner, "Traumatic Stress: Effects on the Brain," *Dialogues in Clinical Neuroscience* 8 (December 2006): 445–461.

92. Bessel van der Kolk, *The Body Keeps the Score: Brain, Mind, and Body in the Healing of Trauma* (New York: Penguin, 2014), 246–247.

93. Van der Kolk, *The Body Keeps the Score*, 247.

94. Van der Kolk, *The Body Keeps the Score*, 249.

95. Van der Kolk, *The Body Keeps the Score*, 224–228. The 2010 report is Karen H. Seal, Shira Maguen, Beth Cohen, Kristian S Gima, Thomas J Metzler, Li Ren, Daniel Bertenthal, and Charles R Marmar, "VA Mental Health Services Utilization in Iraq and Afghanistan Veterans in the First Year of Receiving New Mental Health Diagnoses," *Journal of Traumatic Stress* 23 (February 2010): 5–16.

96. Paul Gaita, "Scene Dissection: Screenwriter Mark Boal Breaks Down One of 'The Hurt Locker's' Most Pivotal Moments," *Los Angeles Times*, February 20, 2010.

97. Mark Boal, "The Man in the Bomb Suit," *Playboy*, September 2005. See also Boal, "The Real Cost of War," *Playboy*, March 2007.

98. For Bigelow on the film's aesthetics and politics, see Peter Keough, ed., *Kathryn Bigelow: Interviews* (Jackson: University of Mississippi Press, 2013), 201.

99. Sara A. Alzahrani, "Dialectics of Humanism: Thematic Readings of the Literature of the Vietnam and Iraq Wars" (PhD thesis, University of Leicester, 2020), 73. See also Robert Sparrow, "Killer Robots," *Journal of Applied Philosophy* 24 (March 2007): 62–77; and Janet S. Robinson, "The Gendered Geometry of War in Kathryn Bigelow's *The Hurt Locker* (2008)," in *Heroism and Gender in War Films*, ed. Karen A. Ritzenhoff and Jakub Kazecki (London: Palgrave Macmillan, 2014), 153–171.

100. See Florentina C. Andreescu, "War, Trauma and the Militarized Body," *Subjectivity* 9 (July 2016): 205–233.

101. Cameron quoted in Frank Rose, *The Art of Immersion: How the Digital Generation Is Remaking Hollywood, Madison Avenue, and the Way We Tell Stories* (New York: Norton, 2011), 49. See also *James Cameron: Interviews*, ed. Brent Dunham (Jackson: University Press of Mississippi, 2012), 189–199.

102. James Clarke, *The Cinema of James Cameron: Bodies in Heroic Motion* (London: Wallflower Press, 2014), 129.

103. Steven Spielberg "Foreword," in *A.I.: Artificial Intelligence from Stanley Kubrick to Steven Spielberg*, ed. Jan Harlan, Jane M. Struthers, and Chris Baker (London: Thames & Hudson, 2009), 7. See also Julian Rice, *Kubrick's Story, Spielberg's Film: A.I. Artificial Intelligence* (Lanham, MD: Rowman & Littlefield, 2017).

104. Orin Starn, "Here Come the Anthros (Again): The Strange Marriage of Anthropology and Native Americans," *Cultural Anthropology* 26 (April 2011): 197; Todd McGowan, "Maternity Divided: *Avatar* and Enjoyment of Nature," *Jump Cut*, Summer 2010, https://www.ejumpcut.org/archive/jc52.2010/mcGowanAvatar/index.html; Mark T. Decker, *Industrial Society and the Science Fiction Blockbuster: Social Critique in Films of Lucas, Scott and Cameron* (Jefferson, NC: McFarland, 2016), 154–168.

105. "Talking the Amazon Rainforest with *Avatar*'s James Cameron," *Mongabay*, May 11, 2010, https://news.mongabay.com/2010/05/talking-the-amazon-rainforest-with -avatars-james-cameron.

106. See the discussion of Asimov's *Foundation's Edge* (1982) in Dustin A. Abnet, *The American Robot: A Cultural History* (Chicago: University of Chicago Press, 2020), 292–293.

107. Lennard J. Davis, *The End of Normal: Identity in a Biocultural Era* (Ann Arbor: University of Michigan Press, 2013), 43; Sami Schalk, "Wounded Warriors of the Future: Disability Hierarchy in *Avatar* and *Source Code*," *Journal of Literary and Cultural Disability Studies* 14 (November 2020): 403–419.

108. James Cameron, *Avatar*, filmscript, accessed March 1, 2023, http://roteirodecinema .com.br/scripts/reader/files/AVATAR_JamesCameron.pdf.

109. Cameron, "Project 880," Avatar Wiki, accessed March 1, 2023, https://james-camerons-avatar.fandom.com/wiki/Project_880.

110. Barack Obama, "Remarks on Military Operations in Iraq at Camp Lejeune, North Carolina," February 27, 2009, in *Public Papers of the Presidents of the United States: Barack Obama, 2009,* Book 1, *January 20 to June 30, 2009* (Washington, DC: Government Printing Office, 2011), 162. The development of "warrior transition units" during Obama's first term was a response to inadequate care facilities for Afghanistan- and Iraq-era veterans. See Dana Priest and Ann Hull, "Soldiers Face Neglect, Frustration at Army's Top Medical Facility," *Washington Post,* February 18, 2007; and John M. Kinder, *Paying with Their Bodies: American War and the Problem of the Disabled Veteran* (Chicago: University of Chicago Press, 2015), 293–295.

111. Michael Bess, *Our Grandchildren Redesigned: Life in the Bioengineered Society of the Near Future* (Boston: Beacon Press, 2015), 87.

112. Barack Obama, "Remarks at the Wounded Warrior Project Soldier Ride Opening Ceremony," April 30, 2009, in *Public Papers of the Presidents of the United States: Barack Obama, 2009,* Book 1, *January 20 to June 30, 2009* (Washington, DC: Government Printing Office, 2011), 599.

113. Ellen Grabiner, *I See You: The Shifting Paradigms of James Cameron's* Avatar (Jefferson, NC: McFarland & Co., 2012), 197.

114. See Hamish Dalley, "The Deaths of Settler Colonialism: Extinction as a Metaphor of Decolonization in Contemporary Settler Literature," *Settler Colonial Studies* 8 (October 2016): 30–46.

115. Dana Fore, "The Tracks of Sully's Tears: Disability in James Cameron's *Avatar,*" *Jump Cut,* Summer 2011, https://www.ejumpcut.org/archive/jc53.2011/foreAvatar/index.html.

116. Piore, *Body Builders,* 134.

117. Eugene Thacker, "Bio-X: Removing Bodily Contingency in Regenerative Medicine," *Journal of Medical Humanities* 23 (Winter 2002): 241.

118. Obama, "Remarks at the Wounded Warrior Project Soldier Ride Opening Ceremony," 599; Schalk, "Wounded Warriors of the Future," 406–407.

119. Grabiner, *I See You,* 138.

120. See Matthew Belloni and Borys Kit, "James Cameron Sounds the Alarm on Artificial Intelligence and Unveils a 'Terminator' for the 21st Century," *Hollywood Reporter,* September 27, 2017. See also David B. Resnick, *Environmental Health Ethics* (Cambridge: Cambridge University Press, 2012), 51–53.

121. Jeffrey Ressner, "In Search of the Miraculous," *Directors Guild of America Quarterly,* Summer 2008, https://www.dga.org/Craft/DGAQ/All-Articles/0802-Summer-2008/DGA-Interview-James-Cameron.aspx.

122. On Pandora, see Maria Wilhelm and Dirk Mathison, *James Cameron's Avatar: A Confidential Report on the Biological and Social History of Pandora* (New York: It Books, 2009); Aylish Wood, "Where Codes Collide: The Emergent Ecology of *Avatar,*" *Animation: An Interdisciplinary Journal* 7 (November 2012): 309–322; Timothy Morton, "Pando-

ra's Box: *Avatar*, Ecology, Thought," in *Green Planets: Ecology and Science Fiction*, ed. Gerry Canavan and Kim Stanley Robinson (Middletown, CT: Wesleyan University Press, 2014), 206–225; and Steen Ledet Christiansen, *Drone Age Cinema: Action Film and Sensory Assault* (London: I. B. Tauris, 2017), 130–138.

123. Andrew M. Butler, *Cyberpunk* (Hertfordshire: Pocket Essentials, 2001), 14.

124. Dick, "Android and the Human," 191.

125. David J. Morris, *The Evil Hours: A Biography of Post-Traumatic Stress Disorder* (Boston: Houghton Mifflin, 2015), 57.

126. On Jake Sully as a disguised colonialist, see John James and Tom Ue, "'I See You': Colonial Narratives and the Act of Seeing in *Avatar*," in *The Films of James Cameron*, ed. Matthew Wilhelm Kapell and Stephen McVeigh (Jefferson, NC: McFarland & Co., 2011), 190–191.

127. Grabiner, *I See You*, 7.

128. Sean Redmond, ed., *Liquid Metal: The Science Fiction Film Reader* (London: Wallflower, 2004), 156–157.

129. Slavoj Žižek, "Avatar: Return of the Natives," *New Statesman*, March 4, 2010, https://zizek.uk/avatar-return-of-the-natives.

130. Kyla Schuller, "Avatar and the Movements of Neocolonial Sentimental Cinema," *Discourse* 35 (Spring 2013): 178; Clarke, *Cinema of James Cameron*, 129.

131. Rob White, "Only Connect," *Film Quarterly* 63 (Spring 2010): 4–5.

132. Decker, *Industrial Society and the Science Fiction Blockbuster*, 156, 160.

133. Jesscia Pierce, "Can Bioethics Survive in a Dying World?," *Journal of Medical Humanities* 23 (Spring 2002): 3–6.

CHAPTER 5 — KEEPING ON

1. Robert N. Butler, *Why Survive? Being Old in America* (New York: Harper and Row, 1975). George Bush, "Remarks at the Dedication Ceremony for the Michael Bilirakis Alzheimer's Center in Palm Harbor, Florida," April 27, 1989, in *Public Papers of the Presidents of the United States: George H. W. Bush, 1989*, Book 1, *January 20 to June 30, 1989* (Washington, DC: Government Printing Office, 1990), 490.

2. Arthur S. Flemming, "Foreword," in Robert N. Butler and Myrna I. Lewis, *Aging and Mental Health: Positive Psychosocial Approaches* (St. Louis, MO: C. V. Mosby, 1973), vii.

3. Robert N. Butler, *The Longevity Revolution: The Benefits and Challenges of Living a Long Life* (New York: Public Affairs, 2008), 15, 89–91.

4. Robert N. Butler, Myrna I. Lewis, and Trey Sunderland, *Aging and Mental Health: Positive Psychosocial and Biomedical Approaches*, 4th ed. (New York: Merrill, 1991), 129–132; W. Andrew Achenbaum, *Robert Butler, MD: Visioning of Healthy Aging* (New York: Columbia University Press, 2013), 192–193. On suicide rates, see Robert E. McKeown, Steven P. Cuffe, and Richard M. Schulz, "US Suicide Rates by Age Group, 1970–2002: An Examination of Recent Trends," *American Journal of Public Health* 96 (October 2006): 1744–1751.

5. American Public Health Association Task Force on Aging, "Health Policy Statement on Aging," October 21, 1977, American Public Health Association Memos, Chairman Kurt W. Deuschle, MD records, 1948–2000, Arthur H. Aufses, Jr., MD Archives, Icahn School of Medicine at Mount Sinai, New York City. In 1982, the Department of Health and Human Services published *A National Plan for Research on Aging*, which called for multidisciplinary research on emergent trends in the aging process.

6. Rosalynn Carter, "Foreword," in Robert N. Butler, Myrna I. Lewis, and Trey Sunderland, *Aging and Mental Health: Positive Psychosocial and Biomedical Approaches*, 4th ed. (New York: Merrill, 1991), ix. Rosalynn Carter was an honorary board member of the International Longevity Center USA. Jimmy Carter contributed his own reflections in *The Virtues of Aging* (New York: Random House, 1998).

7. Tipper Gore, keynote speech, in United States, Congress, Senate, Special Committee on Aging, *Mental Health and the Aging: Forum before the Special Committee on Aging, U.S. Senate, 103rd Congress, 1st Session, Washington, D.C., July 15, 1993* (Washington, DC: Government Printing Office, 1993), 3–5.

8. Butler, *Longevity Revolution*, 107–109; "Interview with Robert N. Butler, M.D.," *Rejuvenation Research* 11 (2008): 977–981.

9. Robert N. Bellah, Richard Madsen, William M. Sullivan, Ann Swidler, and Steven M. Tipton, *The Good Society* (New York: Knopf, 1991), 5–6; William J. Clinton, "The President's Radio Address," September 18, 1993, in *Public Papers of the Presidents of the United States: William J. Clinton, 1993, Book 2, August 31 to December 31, 1993* (Washington, DC: Government Printing Office, 1995), 1533.

10. William J. Clinton, "Remarks to the White House Conference on Aging," May 3, 1995, in *Public Papers of the Presidents of the United States: William J. Clinton, 1995, Book 1, January 1 to June 30, 1995* (Washington, DC: Government Printing Office, 1997), 629.

11. Senator David Pryor speaking at the White House Conference on Aging, May 3, 1995, at 13:02, www.c-span.org/video/?64889-1/white-house-conference-aging.

12. "Final Agenda for the 1995 White House Conference on Aging," 60 Fed. Reg. 22 (February 2, 1995), 6598.

13. See Donna Shalala's open letter to President Clinton of February 1996, reprinted as the frontispiece to *The Road to an Aging Policy for the 21st Century: Final Report, 1995 White House Conference on Aging* (Washington, DC: Government Printing Office, 1996).

14. Butler, *Longevity Revolution*, 315; *The Road to an Aging Policy for the 21st Century*, 353. A more optimistic account is Bob Blancato, "25 Years after the 1995 White House Aging Conference, Where We Are Now," Next Avenue, May 5, 2020, www.nextavenue.org/1995-white-house-aging-conference. Blancato was the executive director of the 1995 conference.

15. *The National Institute on Aging: Strategic Directions for Research, 2020–2025*, 11, accessed December 7, 2022, https://www.nia.nih.gov/sites/default/files/2020-05/nia-strategic-directions-2020-2025.pdf.

16. Robert N. Butler, "Combatting Ageism: A Matter of Human and Civil Rights," in International Longevity Center Anti-Ageism Taskforce, *Ageism in America* (New York: International Longevity Center–USA, 2006), 1.

17. On the stratification of aging, see Corey M. Abramson, *The End Game: How Inequity Shapes Our Final Years* (Cambridge, MA: Harvard University Press, 2015).

18. See Robert N. Butler's comments at the 1995 White House Conference on Aging, May 3, 1995, at 1:13:19, www.c-span.org/video/?64889-1/white-house-conference-aging.

19. Butler, *Why Survive?*, 1. The second funding priority of the NIA in the 1990s was the Claude D. Pepper Older Americans Independence Centers program (initiated in 1988), which aimed to establish a national network of centers focusing on geriatric research.

20. Robert N. Butler, "A Generation at Risk: When the Baby Boomers Reach Golden Pond," *Across the Board*, July/August 1983, 1–16. In 1997, the *Washington Post* explored the paradox of aging by contrasting the former president George H. W. Bush parachuting over Arizona with the baby boomer current president Bill Clinton on crutches after an operation to repair a knee tendon: Abigail Trafford, "President's Precedents Redefine Aging," *Washington Post*, April 1, 1997. Bush repeated the parachute jump every five years of his retirement, up to age ninety, despite having used a scooter since 2012 due to vascular Parkinson's.

21. Sarah Kliff, "The Small End of Ted Kennedy's Big CLASS Act Dream," *Washington Post*, September 18, 2013.

22. Jocelyn Kaiser, "The Alzheimer's Gamble," *Science*, August 30, 2018.

23. *The National Institute on Aging: Strategic Directions for Research, 2020–2025*, 1.

24. Robert N. Butler, "Age-ism: Another Form of Bigotry," *The Gerontologist* 9 (Winter 1969): 243. See also Louise Aronson, *Elderhood: Redefining Aging, Transforming Medicine, Reimagining Life* (New York: Bloomsbury, 2019), 69–74.

25. Butler, "Age-ism," 243–244.

26. *The National Institute on Aging: Strategic Directions for Research, 2020–2025*; Butler, *Longevity Revolution*, 89–91.

27. National Advisory Council on Aging, Report of the Panel on Biomedical Research, *Our Future Selves: A Research Plan toward Understanding Aging* (Washington, DC: Government Printing Office, 1980).

28. See Robert N. Butler's comments at the 1995 White House Conference on Aging at 1:21:10, www.c-span.org/video/?64889-1/white-house-conference-aging.

29. For a critique of the "successful aging" concept, see Sarah Lamb, ed., *Successful Aging as a Contemporary Obsession* (New Brunswick, NJ: Rutgers University Press, 2017), 1–40.

30. Butler, *Longevity Revolution*, 383.

31. Robert N. Butler, "Prologue or Introduction to Life Review" (2010), in Andrew Achenbaum, *Robert N. Butler, MD: Visioning of Healthy Aging* (New York: Columbia

University Press, 2013), 216; Robert N. Butler, "Declaration of the Rights of Older Persons," *The Gerontologist* 42 (April 2002): 152–153.

32. Butler, *Longevity Revolution*, 192; Lamb, *Successful Aging as a Contemporary Obsession*, 6–7. See also John W. Rowe and Robert L. Kahn, *Successful Aging* (New York: Pantheon, 1998); and Martha B. Holstein and Meredith Minkler, "Critical Gerontology: Reflections for the 21st Century," in *Critical Perspectives on Ageing Societies*, ed. Miriam Bernard and Thomas Sharf (Bristol: Policy Press, 2007), 15. For a critique of these concepts, see Nikolas Rose, *The Politics of Life Itself: Biomedicine, Power, and Subjectivity in the Twenty-First Century* (Princeton, NJ: Princeton University Press, 2007), 35.

33. Achenbaum, *Robert N. Butler*, 209; George Bush, "Remarks at the Dedication Ceremony for the Michael Bilirakis Alzheimer's Center," 490.

34. 2005 White House Conference on Aging, *Report to the President and the Congress*, 119, https://nicoa.org/wp-content/uploads/2014/05/2005-WHCOA-Final-Report.pdf; *2015 White House Conference on Aging: Final Report*, 27–28, https://whitehouseconferenceonaging.gov/2015-WHCOA-Final-Report.pdf. Butler was critical of Bush for not attending the 2005 White House conference. See Butler, *Longevity Revolution*, 315; and Achenbaum, *Robert N. Butler*, 149, 167.

35. Federal Coordinating Council for Science, Engineering and Technology, *Decade of the Brain 1990–2000: Maximizing Human Potential* (Washington, DC: Government Printing Office, 1991), 13–21, 35–37; Robert N. Butler, "Introduction," in Robert Fogel and Stanley Prusiner, *Health, Science, and Wealth* (New York: International Longevity Center–USA, 2007), 1.

36. Butler, Lewis, and Sunderland, *Aging and Mental Health*, 461–465; Butler, *Longevity Revolution*, 203.

37. Barbara Vobejda, "Elderly Find Alternatives to Institutions," *Washington Post*, June 28, 1993. On the benefits of technology for seniors, see Rodney Brooks, "Technology's Elder Boom," *Technology Review* 107 (April 1, 2004), https://www.technologyreview.com/2004/04/01/233084/technologys-elder-boom.

38. Butler, "Prologue or Introduction," 209.

39. Robert N. Butler, "The Longevity Revolutions," in *Proceedings of the First Brookdale Conference on Aging in America: Social and Health Care Needs of the Elderly: Public and Private Responsibility* ([New York]: [Brookdale Foundation], 1984), 13.

40. See Alzheimer's Association Special Report, *More than Normal Aging: Understanding Mild Cognitive Impairment* (2022), https://www.alz.org/media/Documents/alzheimers-facts-and-figures-special-report-2022.pdf.

41. Butler, *Longevity Revolution*, 139–144.

42. Butler, *Longevity Revolution*, 139, 130.

43. Butler, *Longevity Revolution*, 231, 313–314.

44. Achenbaum, *Robert N. Butler*, 161.

45. Michael Norman, "The Man Who Saw Old Anew," *New York Times*, March 9, 1997.

46. On the Salzburg seminar, see Robert N. Butler, "Health, Productivity, and Aging: An Overview," in *Enhancing Vitality in Later Life*, ed. Robert N. Butler and Herbert P. Gleason (New York: Springer, 1985), 1–14. See also Betty Friedan, "Postscript," in *Productive Aging: Enhancing Vitality in Later Life*, ed. Robert N. Butler and Herbert P. Gleason (New York: Springer, 1985), 121–122.

47. Betty Friedan, *The Fountain of Age* (New York: Simon & Schuster, 1993), 17. See also Freidan's essays "The Mystique of Age" and "Changing Sex Roles: Vital Aging" in *Productive Aging: Enhancing Vitality in Later Life*, ed. Robert N. Butler and Herbert P. Gleason (New York: Springer, 1985), 37–46, 93–104, respectively.

48. Friedan, *The Fountain of Age*, 538, 548.

49. Friedan, *The Fountain of Age*, 30.

50. U.S. Department of Health and Human Services, *Report to Congress: Aging Services Technology Study* (Washington, DC: Office of the Assistant Secretary for Planning and Evaluation, U.S. Department of Health and Human Services, 2012), https://aspe.hhs .gov/sites/default/files/migrated_legacy_files//175261/ASTSRptCong.pdf; *Tackling Diseases of Aging: Why Research Collaboration Matters: Roundtable before the Special Committee on Aging, October 29, 2013, U.S. Senate, 113th Congress, 1st Session* (Washington, DC: Government Printing Office, 2013).

51. President's Council of Advisors on Science and Technology, *Report to the President: Independence, Technology, and Connection in Older Age*, March 2016, https://www.broadinstitute .org/files/sections/about/PCAST/2016%20pcast-independence-tech-ging.pdf; *Aging and Disability in the 21st Century: How Technology Can Help Maintain Health and Quality of Life, May 22, 2019, U.S. Senate Hearing before the Special Committee on Aging, 116th Congress, 1st Session* (Washington, DC: Government Printing Office, 2022). The Senate also considered accessible technologies that might assist older and disabled Americans on July 28, 2022, at a hearing titled Accessible Federal Technology for People with Disabilities, Older Americans, and Veterans, https://www.aging.senate.gov/hearings/click -here-accessible-federal-technology-for-people-with-disabilities-older-americans-and -veterans.

52. Nick Mourtoupalas and Derek Hawkins, "The Average Age of Congress Is Rising. That's Unlikely to Change Soon," *Washington Post*, July 27, 2023.

53. See Edward Alan Miller, Pamela Nadash, and Michael K. Gusmano, eds., *Aging Policy and Politics in the Trump Era: Implications for Older Americans* (New York: Routledge, 2019).

54. See Sarah Campbell, "Will Biotechnology Stop Aging?: The Quest to Slow, Stop, or Turn Back the Body's Clock," *IEEE Pulse*, March/April 2019, 3–7.

55. Robin Marantz Henig, "Is Misplacing Your Glasses Alzheimer's," *New York Times*, April 24, 1994.

56. Stanley I. Rapoport and Larry D. Wright, "Alzheimer's: The Disease of the Century," Occasional Paper, International Longevity Center–USA, 2006, https://search .issuelab-dev.org/resource/alzheimers-the-disease-of-the-century; Patrick Fox, "From

Senility to Alzheimer's Disease: The Rise of the Alzheimer Disease Movement," *Milbank Quarterly* 67 (March 1989): 95, 59. See also Scott Selberg, *Mediating Alzheimer's: Cognition and Personhood* (Minneapolis: University of Minnesota Press, 2022).

57. Jessica N. Cooke-Bailey, Margaret A. Pericak-Vance, and Jonathan L. Haines, "The Impact of the Human Genome Project on Complex Disease," *Genes* 5 (September 2014): 522; Fox, "From Senility to Alzheimer Disease," 59.

58. Fox, "From Senility to Alzheimer Disease," 97.

59. For this bilateral ILC collaboration, see International Longevity Center Japan, *A Comparative Study of Values and Value Transmission between Japan and the U.S.* (March 1995), Robert N. Butler Columbia Aging Center Archives, Mailman School of Public Health, Columbia University.

60. S. Jay Olashansky, Daniel Perry, Richard A. Miller, and Robert N. Butler, "Pursuing the Longevity Dividend: Scientific Goals for an Aging World," *Annals of the New York Academy of Sciences* 1114 (2006): 11–13.

61. Richard C. Adelman, "The Alzheimerization of Aging," *The Gerontologist* 35 (August 1995): 526; Butler, *Longevity Revolution*, 132. See also Sid Gilman and Norman L. Foster, "'The Alzheimerization of Aging': A Response," *The Gerontologist* 36 (February 1996): 9–10.

62. Claudia Chaufan, Brook Hollister, Jennifer Nazareno, and Patrick Fox, "Medical Ideology as a Double-Edge Sword: The Politics of Cure and Care in the Making of Alzheimer's Disease," *Social Science and Medicine* 74 (2012): 788–795. For commentary on Fox, see Margaret Lock, *The Alzheimer Conundrum: Entanglements of Dementia and Aging* (Princeton, NJ: Princeton University Press, 2013), 40–41.

63. Michael G. Zey, *Ageless Nation: The Quest for Superlongevity and Physical Perfection* (Far Hills, NJ: New Horizon Press, 2007), 5, 130; Cooke-Bailey, Pericak-Vance, and Haines, "Impact of the Human Genome Project on Complex Disease," 522. See also Sheila M. Rothman and David J. Rothman, *The Pursuit of Perfection: The Promise and Perils of Medical Enhancement* (New York: Pantheon, 2003), 213–215.

64. David Schlessinger quoted in "What Is Aging?," *Washington Times*, June 14, 2005.

65. National Institute on Aging, "Alzheimer's Disease Genetics Fact Sheet," https://www.nia.nih.gov/health/alzheimers-disease-genetics-fact-sheet.

66. Alison M. Goate, Marie-Christine Chartier-Harlin, Mike Mullan, Jeremy Brown, Fiona Crawford, Liana Fidani, et al., "Segregation of a Missense Mutation in the Amyloid Precursor Protein Gene with Familial Alzheimer's Disease," *Nature* 349 (February 21, 1991): 704–706. See also "Third Gene Tied to Early Onset Alzheimer's: Researchers Move a Step Close to an Alzheimer's Drug," *New York Times*, August 18, 1995.

67. Huntington Potter, "Alzheimer Disease and Down Syndrome—Chromosome 21 Nondisjunction May Underlie Both Disorders," *American Journal of Human Genetics* 48 (1991): 1192–2000; Lisa Marshall, "Down Syndrome and Alzheimer's Disease Have a Lot in Common," *Scientific American*, July 1, 2014.

68. Bradley T. Hyman, "Alzheimer's Disease or Alzheimer's Diseases? Clues from Molecular Epidemiology," *Annals of Neurology* 40 (1996): 136. On memory retrieval, see Lisa Genova, *Remember: The Science of Memory and the Art of Forgetting* (New York: Harmony, 2021), 16.

69. See Lock, *The Alzheimer Conundrum.*

70. Andrew Steele, *Ageless: The New Science of Getting Older without Getting Old* (New York: Doubleday, 2020), 136.

71. "Dementia vs. Alzheimer's: Which Is It?," American Association of Retired Persons, June 15, 2020, https://www.aarp.org/health/dementia/info-2018/difference-between-dementia-alzheimers.html.

72. Alzheimer's Association, *Special Report: Race, Ethnicity, and Alzheimer's* (Chicago: Alzheimer's Association, 2021), www.ideas-study.org/-/media/Ideas/Files/Educational-Resources/Race-Ethnicity-and-Alzheimers-in-America.pdf. See also Butler, *Longevity Revolution*, 16.

73. See Rosa Seijo, Henry Gomez, and Judith Freidenberg, "Language as a Communication Barrier in Medical Care for Hispanic Patients," *Hispanic Journal of Behavioral Sciences*, 13 (November 1991): 363–376; Judith Freidenberg, *Growing Old in El Barrio* (New York: New York University Press, 2000).

74. "Health Disparities Framework," National Institute on Aging, February 2021, https://www.nia.nih.gov/research/osp/framework. On telomere research, see President's Council on Bioethics, *Beyond Therapy: Biotechnology and the Pursuit of Happiness* (Washington, DC: President's Council on Bioethics, 2003); 179–181; Diego A. Forero, "Meta-Analysis of Telomere Length in Alzheimer's Disease," *Journals of Gerontology Series A: Biological Sciences and Medical Sciences* 71 (August 2016): 1069–1073; Steele, *Ageless*, 86–89, 187–195.

75. President's Council on Bioethics, *Taking Care: Ethical Caregiving in our Aging Society* (Washington, DC: President's Council on Bioethics, 2005), 36.

76. Jonathan Franzen, "My Father's Brain" (2001), in Franzen, *How to Be Alone: Essays* (New York: Farrar, Straus and Giroux, 2002), 19.

77. Franzen, "My Father's Brain," 19.

78. Franzen, "My Father's Brain," 22.

79. Franzen singles out David Shenk's *The Forgetting: Alzheimer's Portrait of an Epidemic* (New York: Doubleday, 2001). On Roth's *Patrimony*, see Martin Halliwell, *Voices of Mental Health: Medicine, Politics, and Mental Health, 1970–2000* (New Brunswick, NJ: Rutgers University Press, 2017), 114–119.

80. Franzen, "My Father's Brain," 24, 12.

81. Franzen, "My Father's Brain," 24.

82. Franzen, "My Father's Brain," 31. See Bethany Coston and Michael Kimmel, "Aging Men, Masculinity and Alzheimer's: Caretaking and Caregiving in the New

Millennium," in *Aging Men, Masculinities and Modern Medicine*, ed. Antje Kampf, Barbara A. Marshall, and Alan Peterson (London: Routledge, 2013), 191–200.

83. Franzen, "My Father's Brain," 38.

84. Joseph Carroll, "Correcting for *The Corrections*: A Darwinian Critique of a Foucauldian Novel," *Style* 47 (Spring 2003): 87.

85. Franzen writes about his own depression in "Why Bother?" (1996), in *How to Be Alone*, 72–73, 87, 92–93.

86. Robert N. Butler and Myrna I. Lewis, *The New Love and Sex after 60*, rev. ed. (1976; repr., New York: Ballantine, 2002), 280.

87. Franzen, "Why Bother?," 95; Jonathan Franzen, "Pain Won't Kill You" (2011), in *Farther Away* (New York: Farrar, Straus, and Giroux, 2012), 7.

88. Jonathan Franzen, *The Corrections* (New York: Picador, 2001), 464.

89. Jesús Blanco Hidalga, *Jonathan Franzen and the Romance of Community: Narratives of Salvation* (New York: Bloomsbury, 2017), 150.

90. Franzen, "Scavenging," in *Tolstoy's Dictaphone: Technology and the Muse*, ed. Sven Birkets (Saint Paul, MN: Graywolf Press, 1996), 10. See also Andrew Solomon, "Anatomy of Melancholy," *New Yorker*, January 4, 1998; Halliwell, *Voices of Mental Health*, 212–214.

91. Franzen, "Why Bother?," 68, 58; Franzen, "Pain Won't Kill You," 9. See also Jonathan Franzen, "Capitalism in Hyperdrive," in *The End of the End of the Earth: Essays* (New York: Farrar, Straus and Giroux, 2018), 69–74.

92. Franzen, "Scavenging," 8. See Rebecca Greenfield, "Jonathan Franzen Continues to Hate Technology," *Atlantic*, January 30, 2012; James Annesley, "Market Corrections: Jonathan Franzen and the "'Novel of Globalization,'" *Modern Literature* 29 (Winter 2006): 111–128.

93. On robot ethics research, see Anouk van Maris, Nancy Zook, Sanja Dogramadzi, Matthew Studley, Alan Winfield, and Praminda Caleb-Solly, "A New Perspective on Robot Ethics through Investigating Human-Robot Interactions with Older Adults," *Applied Sciences* 11 (2021): 10136.

94. David Hyde Pierce, remarks at the White House Conference on Aging, July 13, 2015, accessed April 12, 2024, https://www.c-span.org/video/?c4544046/user-clip-2015 -white-house-conference-aging.

95. Butler, *Longevity Revolution*, 111–114.

96. Margaret Atwood, *Oryx and Crake* (New York: Anchor, 2003), 291.

97. Atwood, *Oryx and Crake* 294.

98. Atwood, *Oryx and Crake* 295.

99. Butler and Lewis, *The New Love and Sex after 60*, 119–127.

100. Butler, *Longevity Revolution*, 313–314; Andrew Kimbrell, *The Human Body Shop: The Cloning, Engineering, and Marketing of Life*, 2nd ed. (Washington, DC: Regnery, 1997), 334.

101. Butler, *Longevity Revolution*, 13, 313–314.

102. Butler, *Longevity Revolution*, 161; President's Council on Bioethics, *Beyond Therapy*, 200; Leon R. Kass, "Biotechnology and Our Human Future: Some General Reflections," in *Biotechnology: Our Future as Human Beings and Citizens*, ed. Sean D. Sutton (New York: SUNY Press, 2009), 25–26. Butler makes passing mention of Kass in the *Longevity Revolution*, 103. For a consideration of Butler and Kass on pro-longevity discourses, see Stephen G. Post, "Decelerated Aging: Should I Drink from a Fountain of Youth?," in *The Fountain of Youth: Cultural, Scientific, and Ethical Perspectives on a Biomedical Goal*, ed. Stephen G. Post and Robert H. Binstock (Oxford: Oxford University Press, 2004), 72–93.

103. Tom Junod, "No One Wants to Live Forever," *Esquire*, November 20, 2007.

104. See Nick Bostrom, "Recent Developments in the Ethics, Science, and Politics of Life-Extension," *Ageing Horizons* 3 (2005): 28–33.

105. *To Age and Not to Age*, dir. Robert Kane Pappas (2010); Aubrey de Grey with Michael Rae, *Ending Aging: The Rejuvenation Breakthroughs that Could Reverse Human Aging in Our Lifetimes* (New York: St Martin's, 2007), 11. On Butler and pundits, see Achenbaum, *Robert N. Butler*, 182–183.

106. S. Jay Olshansky, Leonard Hayflick, and Bruce A. Carnes, "Position Statement on Human Aging," *Journal of Gerontology* 57 (August 2002): B292.

107. Olshansky, Hayflick, and Carnes, "Position Statement on Human Aging," B293. See also Stephen S. Hall, *Merchants of Immortality: Chasing the Dream of Human Life Extension* (New York: Houghton Mifflin, 2003), 345–346; Kaite Moisse, "Anti-Aging Talk: Getting Old or Just Getting Started?," *Scientific American*, February 13, 2010.

108. Aubrey de Grey, "Leon Kass: Quite Substantially Right," *Rejuvenation Research* 7 (Summer 2004): 89–91; Leon R. Kass, "Ageless Bodies, Happy Souls: Biotechnology and the Pursuit of Perfection," *New Atlantis*, Spring 2003, www.thenewatlantis.com/publications/ageless-bodies-happy-souls.

109. Leon R. Kass, "L'Chaim and Its Limits: Why Not Immortality?," in *Fountain of Youth: Cultural, Scientific, and Ethical Perspectives on a Biomedical Goal*, ed. Stephen G. Post and Robert H. Binstock (Oxford: Oxford University Press, 2004), 304–320.

110. President's Council on Bioethics, *Beyond Therapy*, 161–162.

111. President's Council on Bioethics, *Beyond Therapy*, 183, 197.

112. President's Council on Bioethics, *Beyond Therapy*, 199–200.

113. President's Council on Bioethics, *Beyond Therapy*, 199.

114. President's Council on Bioethics, *Beyond Therapy*, 308.

115. Kass, "L'Chaim and Its Limits," 315.

116. President's Council on Bioethics, *Beyond Therapy*, 197.

117. Achille Mbembe, "Necropolitics," *Public Culture* 15 (Winter 2003): 11–40.

118. On social death, see Heather Laine Talley, *Saving Face: Disfigurement and the Politics of Appearance* (New York: New York University Press, 2014), 39–40.

119. Butler, *Longevity Revolution*, 211–212, 378–379.

120. Butler, *Longevity Revolution*, 303.

121. Butler, *Longevity Revolution*, 315.

122. Zoë Corbyn, "The Future of Elder Care Is Here—and It's Artificial Intelligence," *The Guardian*, June 3, 2021.

123. Butler, *Longevity Revolution*, 42.

124. Virginia Blum, *Flesh Wounds: The Culture of Cosmetic Surgery* (Berkeley: University of California Press, 2003), 4. See also Abigail T. Brooks, *The Ways Women Age: Using and Refusing Cosmetic Interventions* (New York: New York University Press, 2017), 13, 29.

125. See Beth Longware Duff, "2009 Statistics from the American Academy of Facial Plastic and Reconstructive Surgery," http://www.facialplasticsurgery.net/stats-2009.htm; and AAFPRS "2009 Statistics on Trends in Facial Plastic Surgery," International Association for Physicians in Aesthetic Medicine, accessed 11 November 2022, https://aestheticmedicinenews.com/aafprs-2009-statistics-on-trends-in-facial-plastic-surgery.htm.

126. Brooks, *The Ways Women Age*, 2–3.

127. International Longevity Center, Anti-Ageism Taskforce, *Ageism in America* (New York: International Longevity Center, 2006), 49–58. On trends in noninvasive surgery, see "Low-Impact Skin Rejuvenation," *Focus on Healthy Aging* 4 (July 2001): 4–5. Butler was on the *Focus on Healthy Aging* editorial board.

128. Dana Berkowitz, *Botox Nation: Changing the Face of America* (New York: New York University Press, 2017), 124–125.

129. Bridget Graham, "Designing 'Older' Rather than Denying Agency: Problematizing Anti-Ageing Discourse in Relation to Cosmetic Surgery Undertaken by Older People," *Journal of Aging Studies* 27 (January 2013): 45.

130. Bridget Garnham, *A New Ethic of "Older": Subjectivity, Surgery, and Self-Stylization* (London: Routledge, 2017), 4, 126.

131. Kirsten L. Ellison, "Age Transcended: A Semiotic and Rhetorical Analysis of the Discourse of Agelessness in North American Anti-Aging Skin Care Advertisements," *Journal of Aging Studies* 29 (April 2014): 30. See also Abigail T. Brooks, "Aesthetic Anti-Ageing Surgery and Technology: Women's Friend or Foe?," *Sociology of Health and Illness* 32 (February 2010): 238–257.

132. Garnham, "Designing 'Older,'" 45, 126.

133. Garnham, *A New Ethic of "Older,"* 132.

134. See David J. Castle, Roberta J. Honigman, and Katharine A. Phillips, "Does Cosmetic Surgery Improve Psychosocial Wellbeing?," *Medical Journal of Australia* 176 (June 2002): 601–604.

135. Brooks, *Ways Women Age*, 9.

136. Brooks, *Ways Women Age*, 10.

137. On analog and digital contrasts, see "Interview: Jennifer Phang on Looking at the Past to See the Future in 'Advantageous,'" *The Moveable Fest*, June 26, 2015, accessed December 1, 2022, https://moveablefest.com/jennifer-phang-advantageous.

138. See "'Advantageous' Portrays a Future Where More Things Remain the Same," *New York Times*, June 25, 2015.

139. Alvaro Jarrín and Chiara Pussetti, eds., *Remaking the Human: Cosmetic Technologies of Body Repair, Reshaping and Replacement* (New York: Berghahn, 2021), 1.

140. Neda Atanasoski and Kalindi Vora, *Surrogate Humanity: Race, Robots, and the Politics of Technological Futures* (Durham, NC: Duke University Press, 2019), 4.

141. Cited in Bill Gifford, *Spring Chicken: Stay Young Forever (or Die Trying)* (New York: Grand Central, 2015), 31.

142. Richard Powers, *Generosity* (New York: Farrar, Straus and Giroux, 2009), 57.

143. De Grey with Rae, *Ending Aging*, 4–5.

144. For a condensed version of de Grey's position, see his essay "An Engineer's Approach to Developing Anti-Aging Medicine," in *Fountain of Youth: Cultural, Scientific, and Ethical Perspectives on a Biomedical Goal*, ed. Stephen G. Post and Robert H. Binstock (Oxford: Oxford University Press, 2004), 249–267.

145. Melinda Cooper, *Life as Surplus: Biotechnology and Capitalism in the Neoliberal Era* (Seattle: University of Washington Press, 2008), 143. See also the Methuselah Foundation website: www.mfoundation.org; and the SENS Research Foundation website: www.sens.org.

146. De Grey with Rae, *Ending Aging*, 29. See also Alex Zhavoronkov, *The Ageless Generation: How Advances in Biomedicine will Transform the Global Economy* (London: Palgrave Macmillan, 2013); and Sergey Young, *The Science and Technology of Growing Young* (Dallas: BenBella, 2021).

147. SENS Research Foundation, *Annual Report 2011: Challenge Accepted*, https://www.sens.org/wp-content/uploads/2020/04/SENS-Foundation-Annual-Report-2011.pdf.

148. SENS Research Foundation, "A Reimagined Research Strategy for Aging," www.sens.org/intro-to-sens-research.

149. De Grey with Rae, *Ending Aging*, 366.

150. John K. Davis, *New Methuselahs: The Ethics of Life Extension* (Cambridge: MIT Press, 2018), 28.

151. See the Founder's Fund website: https://foundersfund.com/the-future, accessed December 1, 2022.

152. Ariana Eunjung Cha, "Peter Thiel's Quest to Find the Key to Eternal Life," *Washington Post*, April 3, 2015. Thiel's biographer Max Chafkin portrays him more as a venture capitalist than a technophile: see Max Chafkin, *The Contrarian: Peter Thiel and Silicon Valley's Pursuit of Power* (New York: Bloomsbury, 2021).

153. "Peter Thiel Wants to Inject Himself with Young People's Blood," *Vanity Fair*, August 1, 2016. For a parody of Thiel, see "The Blood Boy," *Silicon Valley*, series 4, episode 3, aired May 21, 2017, on HBO.

154. Nick Bostrom, *The Transhumanist FAQ*, version 2.1 (World Transhumanist Association, 2003), nickbostrom.com/views/transhumanist.pdf.

155. The Cryonics Institute released a short film in 2013, *We Shall Live Again*, featuring the hundredth person to be frozen there.

156. Butler, *Longevity Revolution*, 480.

157. See Tad Friend, "Silicon Valley's Quest to Live Forever," *New Yorker*, April 3, 2017.

158. Atwood, *Oryx and Crake*, 292.

159. Don DeLillo, *Zero K: A Novel* (New York: Scribner's, 2016), 3, italics in the original.

160. DeLillo, *Zero K*, 71.

161. DeLillo, *Zero K*, 35.

162. See Laura Barrett, "[R]adiance in Dailiness: The Uncanny Ordinary in Don DeLillo's *Zero K*," *Journal of Modern Literature* 42 (Fall 2018): 106–123; Lay Sion Ng, "Transhumanism and the Biological Body in Don DeLillo's *Zero K*: A Materialist Feminist Perspective," *Interdisciplinary Studies in Literature and Environment* 28 (Summer 2021): 686–708.

163. DeLillo, *Zero K*, 8–9.

164. DeLillo, *Zero K*, 47.

165. DeLillo, *Zero K*, 48.

166. DeLillo, *Zero K*, 238.

167. DeLillo, *Zero K*, 161–162. On *Zero K* as a trauma narrative, see Carmen Laguarta-Bueno, "Don DeLillo's *Zero K* (2016): Transhumanism, Trauma, and the Ethics of Premature Cryopreservation," in *Transhumanism and Posthumanism in Twenty-First Century Narrative*, ed. Sonia Baelo-Allué and Monica Calvo-Pascual (New York: Routledge, 2021), 135–150.

168. DeLillo, *Zero K*, 168, 251.

169. See Dave Asprey's website: https://daveasprey.com/about, accessed December 1, 2022.

170. Dave Asprey, *Smarter Not Harder: The Biohacker's Guide to Getting the Body and Mind You Want* (New York: HarperCollins, 2023), 12.

171. Dave Asprey, *Superhuman: The Bulletproof Plan to Age Backward and Maybe Even Live Forever* (New York: Harper, 2019), 24–40.

172. Asprey, *Superhuman*, 17–18.

173. See Lana Asprey and Dave Asprey, *The Better Baby Book: How to Have a Healthier, Smarter, Happier Baby* (New York: Wiley, 2013).

174. See Courtney Rubin, "Bulletproof Coffee, the New Power Drink of Silicon Valley," *Fast Company*, July 3, 2014; and Courtney Rubin, "The Cult of the Bulletproof Coffee Diet," *New York Times*, December 12, 2014. For a sympathetic account of Asprey, see "The Supplemented Self," *New York Times Magazine*, November 15, 2015.

175. Butler, *Longevity Revolution*, 211; Richard L. Sprott, "Reality Check: What Is Genetic Research on Aging Likely to Produce?," in *Aging, Biotechnology, and the Future,*

ed. Catherine Y. Read, Robert C. Green, and Michael A. Smyer (Baltimore, MD: Johns Hopkins University Press, 2008), 4.

176. See, for example, "The Exploding Research on a Vitamin Biohack for Repair and Renewal," Goop, accessed December 1, 2022, https://goop.com/wellness/health/supplement-to-boost-nad-levels. For Goop's influence in the wellness space, see Rina Raphael, *The Gospel of Wellness* (New York: Henry Holt, 2022).

177. "Biohacking Lonvevity with NAD+, Glutathione and Glucarate with COAST Founders Chris Roselle and Chris Picerni," *Biohacking with Brittany*, podcast, February 17, 2022: https://podcasts.apple.com/us/podcast/87-biohacking-longevity-with-nad-glutathione-and/id1466703200?i=1000551374475. For COAST's marketing claims see https://coastdrink.com/pages/the-formula.

178. See the Biohacking Brittany website: www://biohackingbrittany.com, accessed December 1, 2022. See also Robert N. Bellah, "Citizenship, Diversity and the Search for the Common Good," in *The Constitution of the People: Reflections on Citizens and Civil Society*, ed. Robert E. Calvert (Lawrence: University of Kansas Press, 1991), 47–63; and Bortolini, *A Joyfully Serious Man*, 306.

179. See Ford's review of the 9th Annual Biohacking Convention at "Biohacking Conference Honest Review: Pros, Cons and the Unexpected," *Biohacking with Brittany*, podcast, June 30, 2023: https://podcasts.apple.com/us/podcast/biohacking-conference-honest-review-pros-cons-and/id1466703200?i=1000618871074.

180. Butler and Lewis, *The New Love and Sex after 60*, 129; Butler, *Longevity Revolution*, 242–55.

181. Butler, *Longevity Revolution*, 205.

182. Bellah et al., *The Good Society*, 5.

183. Ng, "Transhumanism and the Biological Body," 702; Butler, *Longevity Revolution*, 228–229.

CHAPTER 6 — TRAVELING THROUGH

1. Julie Hirschfeld Davis and Helene Cooper, "Trump Says Transgender People Will Not Be Allowed in the Military," *New York Times*, July 26, 2017.

2. Executive Office of President Donald Trump, "Military Service by Transgender Individuals," Memorandum for the Secretary of Defense [and] the Secretary of Homeland Security, March, 28, 2018, *Federal Register*, 83, 13367–13368, https://www.federalregister.gov/documents/2018/03/28/2018-06426/military-service-by-transgender-individuals.

3. Jody L. Herman, Andrew R. Flores, and Kathryn K. O'Neill, "How Many Adults Identify as Transgender in the United States?," UCLA Law School, Williams Institute, June 2016, https://williamsinstitute.law.ucla.edu/publications/trans-adults-united-states.

4. On Trump's tweets as a proxy for White House policy, see Human Rights Campaign, *Trump's Administrative Abuse and the LGBTQ+ Community* (Washington, DC: Human Rights Campaign, 2017), 12–13.

5. American Medical Association, "Military Medical Policies Affecting Transgender Individuals H-40.966," 2015, https://policysearch.ama-assn.org/policyfinder/detail/40 .966?uri=%2FAMADoc%2FHOD.xml-0-3487.xml; James L. Madara to James N. Mattis, April 3, 2018, https://searchlf.ama-assn.org/undefined/documentDownload?uri=%2Fu nstructured%2Fbinary%2Fletter%2FLETTERS%2F2018-4-3-Letter-to-Mattis-re -Transgender-Policy.pdf.

6. Camille Beredkjick, "DSM-V to Rename Gender Identity Disorder 'Gender Dys-phoria,'" *Advocate*, July 23, 2012, https://www.advocate.com/politics/transgender/2012 /07/23/dsm-replaces-gender-identity-disorder-gender-dysphoria.

7. Francine Russo, "Is There Something Unique about the Transgender Brain?," *Scientific American*, January 1, 2016; J. Graham Theisen, Viji Sundaram, Mary S. Filchak, Lynn P. Chorich, Megan E. Sullivan, James Knight, Hyung-Goo Kim, and Lawrence C. Layman, "The Use of Whole Exome Sequencing in a Cohort of Transgender Individuals to Identify Rare Genetic Variants," *Nature Research* 9 (December 2019): article 20099; Hilleke E. Hulshoff, "Changing Your Sex Influences Your Brain: Influences of Testosterone and Estrogen on Adult Brian Structure," *European Journal of Endocrinology* 155 (November 2006): S107–S114.

8. See Alice D. Dreger, "The Controversy Surrounding *The Man Who Would Be Queen*: A Case History of the Politics of Science, Identity, and Sex in the Internet Age," *Archives of Sexual Behavior* 37 (June 2008): 366–421; Stephen B. Levine, "Reflections on the Clinician's Role with Individuals Who Self-Identify as Transgender," *Archives of Sexual Behavior* 50 (November 2021): 3527–3536; and Aviva Stahl, "Prisoners, Doctors, and the Battle Over Trans Medical Care," *Wired*, July 8, 2021.

9. Adam Rogers and Megan Molteni, "Trump's Plan to Redefine Gender Makes No Scientific Sense," *Wired*, October 24, 2018. See also Erica L. Green Katie Benner, and Robert Pear, "'Transgender' Could Be Defined Out of Existence Under Trump Administration," *New York Times*, October 21, 2018.

10. Jeremy W. Peters, Jo Becker, and Julie Hirschfeld Davis, "Trump Rescinds Rules on Bathrooms for Transgender Students," *New York Times*, February 22, 2017.

11. Bill Clinton, "Remarks in the 'CBD This Morning' Town Meeting," May, 27 1993, in *Public Papers of the Presidents: William J. Clinton, 1993*, Book 1, *January 20 to July 31, 1993* (Washington, DC: Government Printing Office, 1995), 756.

12. Christopher Anders, "Lesbian and Gay Rights during President Clinton's Second Term: A Working Paper Published by the Citizens' Commission on Civil Rights," January 15, 1999, American Civil Liberties Union, https://www.aclu.org/other/lesbian-and -gay-rights-during-president-clintons-second-term-working-paper-published-citizens.

13. U.S. Department of Defense, "Transgender Policy," 2017, https://dod.defense.gov /News/Special-Reports/0616_transgender-policy-archive/. See also Michelle Dietert and Dianne Dentice, "Transgender Military Experiences: From Obama to Trump," *Journal of Homosexuality* 14 (March 2022): 1–18.

14. Barack Obama, "Remarks at the Democratic National Committee LGBT Gala in New York City," September 27, 2015, in *Public Papers of the Presidents: Barack Obama, 2015*,

Book 2, *July 1 to December 31, 2015* (Washington, DC: Government Printing Office, 2021), 1207; Substance Abuse and Mental Health Services Administration, *Ending Conversion Therapy: Supporting and Affirming LGBT Youth* (Rockville, MD: U.S. Department of Health and Human Services, 2015), https://store.samhsa.gov/sites/default/files/sma15-4928.pdf; White House Blog, David Hudson, "Why Conversion Therapy Hurts All of Us," April 10, 2017, The White House: President Barack Obama, https://obamawhitehouse.archives.gov /blog/2015/04/10/why-conversion-therapy-hurts-all-us.

15. "Gender Revolution," special issue, *National Geographic*, January 2017.

16. On transgender awareness in the early 1990s, see Susan Stryker, *Transgender History: The Roots of Today's Revolution* (New York: Seal Press, 2017), 151–194. On the rights agenda, see Helen Joyce, *Trans: When Ideology Meets Reality* (New York: One World, 2022).

17. International Conference on Transgender Law and Employment Policy, "International Bill of Gender Rights," July 4, 1996, Phyllis Randolph Frye Collection, https://www.digitaltransgenderarchive.net/files/2z10wq28m.

18. See Amet Suess Schwend, "Trans Health Care from a Depathologization and Human Rights Perspective," *Public Health Reviews* 41 (2020), https://doi.org/10.1186 /s40985-020-0118-y.

19. National Center for Transgender Equality, *Injustice at Every Turn: A Report of the National Transgender Discrimination Survey* (2011), https://transequality.org/sites/default /files/docs/resources/NTDS_Report.pdf.

20. National Center for Transgender Equality, *The Report of the 2015 U.S. Transgender Survey* (December 2016), https://transequality.org/sites/default/files/docs/usts/USTS -Full-Report-Dec17.pdf. (The survey was conducted again in 2022).

21. International Conference on Transgender Law and Employment Policy, Shannon Minter, and Phyllis Randolph Frye, "Appendix A: GID and the Transgender Movement," July 1996, https://www.digitaltransgenderarchive.net/files/44558d38d.

22. Stryker, *Transgender History*, 139. On clinical data, see Kenneth J. Zucker and Robert L. Spitzer, "Was the Gender Identity Disorder of Childhood Diagnosis Introduced into DSM-III as a Backdoor Maneuver to Replace Homosexuality? A Historical Note," *Journal of Sex and Marital Therapy* 31 (January–February 2005): 37–38.

23. See Zowie Davy, "The DSM-5 and the Politics of Diagnosing Transpeople," *Archives of Sexual Behavior* 44 (July 2015): 1165–1176; Francine Russo, "Where Transgender Is No Longer a Diagnosis," *Scientific American*, January 6, 2017.

24. On the Zucker case, see Jesse Singal, "How the Fight over Transgender Kids Got a Leading Sex Researcher Fired," *New York*, February 7, 2016; and Tey Meadow, *Trans Kids: Being Gendered in the Twenty-First Century* (Berkeley: University of California Press, 2018), 54–93.

25. Harry Benjamin, "Transvestism and Transsexualism in the Male and Female," *Journal of Sex Research* 3 (May 1967): 110. See also Kenneth J. Zucker, "Epidemiology of Gender Dysphoria and Transgender Identity," *Sexual Health* 14 (October 2017): 404–411; Davy, "The DSM-5 and the Politics of Diagnosing Transpeople."

26. American Psychiatric Association, *Diagnostic and Statistical Manual of Mental Disorders*, 5th ed. (Washington, DC: American Psychiatric Publishing, 2013), 451.

27. Hil Malatino, *Queer Embodiment: Monstrosity, Medical Experience, and Intersex Experience* (Lincoln: University of Nebraska Press, 2019), 30.

28. See Abigail Shrier, *Irreversible Damage: The Transgender Craze Seducing Our Daughters* (Washington, DC: Regnery, 2020). For a critique of Shrier, see Jennifer Finney Boylan, "Coming Out as Trans Isn't a Teenage Fad," *New York Times*, January 8, 2019.

29. Styker, *Transgender History*, 171.

30. Human Rights Campaign, "Transgender Workers at Greater Risk for Unemployment and Poverty," September 6, 2013, https://www.hrc.org/press-releases/transgender-workers-at-greater-risk-for-unemployment-and-poverty.

31. See Toby Beauchamp, *Going Stealth: Transgender Politics and U.S. Surveillance Practices* (Durham, NC: Duke University Press, 2019).

32. Barack Obama, "Remarks at the Human Rights Campaign Annual Dinner," October 10, 2009, in *Public Papers of the Presidents of the United States: Barack Obama, 2009*, Book 2, *July 1 to December 31* (Washington, DC: Government Printing Office, 2013), 1496.

33. See U.S. Department of Health and Human Services, *Advancing LGBT Health and Well-Being: 2016 Report*, https://www.hhs.gov/sites/default/files/2016-report-with-cover.pdf.

34. The White House, "Executive Order on Advancing Equality for Lesbian, Gay, Bisexual, Transgender, Queer, and Intersex Individuals," The White House: President Joe Biden, June 15, 2022, https://www.whitehouse.gov/briefing-room/presidential-actions/2022/06/15/executive-order-on-advancing-equality-for-lesbian-gay-bisexual-transgender-queer-and-intersex-individuals. See Emily Bazelon, "The Battle over Gender Therapy," *New York Times*, June 15, 2022; "Special Series: Efforts to Restrict Rights for LGBTQ Youth," NPR: https://www.npr.org/series/1085513404/trans-rights-lgbtq-youth.

35. Bill Mears, "Chelsea Manning Sues to Get Transgender Medical Treatment," CNN, September 23, 2014; Buzz Bissinger, "Caitlyn Jenner: The Full Story," *Vanity Fair*, June 25, 2015; *I Am Cait*, dir. Andrea Metz (2016).

36. Rogers Brubaker, *Trans: Gender and Race in an Age of Unsettled Identities* (Princeton, NJ: Princeton University Press, 2016), 34–35, 43–45. See Katy Steinmetz, "The Transgender Tipping Point," *Time*, June 8, 2014; and James McDonald, "Laverne Cox Declares Transgender State of Emergency," *Out Magazine*, August 20, 2015. On the trans experience in U.S. prisons and the health impacts of policed identities, see Eric A. Stanley and Nat Smith, eds, *Captive Genders: Trans Embodiment and the Prison Industrial Complex* (AK Press, 2016); and *Where Justice Ends*, dir. George Zuber (2019).

37. Mia Fischer, *Terrorizing Gender: Transgender Visibility and the Surveillance Practices of the U.S. Security State* (Lincoln: University of Nebraska Press, 2019), 4–13, 169–184. The White House, "Fact Sheet: Biden-Harris Administration Advances Equality and Visibility for Transgender Americans," March 31, 2022, https://www.whitehouse.gov/briefing

-room/statements-releases/2022/03/31/fact-sheet-biden-harris-administration-advances
-equality-and-visibility-for-transgender-americans.

38. Fischer, *Terrorizing Gender*, 5; Mia Fischer, Sarah Slater, CeCeMcDonald, and Joshua Allen, "Transgender Visibility, Abolitionism, and Restive Organizing in an Age of Trump: A Conversation with CeCe McDonald and Joshua Allen," *QED: A Journal in GLBTQ Worldmaking* 5 (Fall 2018): 185–186.

39. Adrienne Asch and Gail Geller, "Feminism, Bioethics, and Genetics," in *Feminism and Bioethics: Beyond Reproduction*, ed. Susan M. Wolf (New York: Oxford University Press, 1996), 319; Jules Gill-Peterson, "On the Possibility of Affirmative Health Care for Transgender Children," in *Edinburgh Companion to the Politics of American Health*, ed. Martin Halliwell and Sophie A. Jones (Edinburgh: Edinburgh University Press, 2022), 236.

40. See Julia Serano, *Outspoken: A Decade of Transgender Activism and Trans Feminism* (Oakland, CA: Switch Hitter Press, 2016); Julie Bindel, "Janice Raymond: The Original Terf," *Unherd*, November 2021, https://unherd.com/2021/11/meet-the-original-terf/; Katelyn Burns, "The Rise of Anti-Trans 'Radical' Feminists, Explained," *Vox*, September 5, 2019; and Serena Bassi and Greta Lafleur, eds, *Trans-Exclusionary Feminisms and the Global New Right* (Durham, NC: Duke University Press, 2022).

41. Martine Rothblatt, *The Apartheid of Sex: A Manifesto on the Freedom of Gender* (New York: Crown, 1995), 159, 164. See also Lisa Miller, "The Trans-Everything CEO," *New York*, September 7, 2014.

42. Rothblatt, *Apartheid of Sex*, 165.

43. See Margaret O'Mara, "Why Can't Tech Fix Its Gender Problem?," *MIT Technology Review*, August 11, 2022.

44. Jules Joanne Gleeson and Elle O'Rourke, eds., *Transgender Marxism* (London: Pluton, 2021), 2.

45. Slavoj Žižek, "The Sexual Is Political," *The Philosophical Salon*, August 2016, https://thephilosophicalsalon.com/the-sexual-is-political.

46. N. Katherine Hayles, *Unthought: The Power of the Cognitive Nonconscious* (Chicago: University of Chicago Press, 2017), 170.

47. Bernice L. Hausman, *Changing Sex: Transsexualism, Technology, and the Idea of Gender* (Durham, NC: Duke University Press, 1995), 2–4.

48. Eric Plemons, *The Look of a Woman: Facial Feminization Surgery and the Aims of Trans Medicine* (Durham, NC: Duke University Press, 2017), 7; Malatino, *Queer Embodiment*, 11.

49. Hausman, *Changing Sex*, 3.

50. Plemons, *The Look of a Woman*, 17.

51. Julietta Singh, *Unthinking Mastery: Dehumanism and Decolonial Entanglements* (Durham, NC: Duke University Press, 2018), 4. See Cressida J. Heyes and J. R. Latham, "Trans Surgeries and Cosmetic Surgeries: The Politics of Analogy," *Transgender Studies Quarterly* 5 (May 2018): 174–189; Nicholas Chare and Ika Willis, "Introduction: Trans-:

Across/Beyond," *Parallax* 22 (July 2016): 267–289; Kerry Beckman, "Military Sexual Assault in Transgender Veterans: Results from a Nationwide Survey," *Journal of Trauma Stress* 31 (April 2018): 181–190.

52. See Gail Weiss, *Body Images: Embodiment as Intercorporeality* (New York: Routledge, 1999); and Hil Malatino, *Trans Care* (Minneapolis: University of Minnesota Press, 2019).

53. "Transgender Terminology," International Center for Transgender Care at the American Institute of Transgender Surgery, accessed December 1, 2022, https:// thetranscenter.com/transgender-terminology.

54. Hausman, *Changing Sex*, 9.

55. Gina Marchetti, "Transamerica: Queer Cinema in the Middle of the Road," in *Hit the Road, Jack: Essays on the Culture of the American Road*, ed. Gordon E. Slethaug and Stacilee Ford (Toronto: McGill-Queen's University Press, 2012), 198–213; Oren Gozlan, ed., *Current Critical Debates in the Field of Transsexual Studies: In Transition* (London: Routledge, 2018), 181.

56. Paul B. Preciado, *Testo Junkie: Sex, Drugs, and Biopolitics in the Pharmacopornographic Era*, trans. Bruce Benderson (New York: Feminist Press, 2008] 2016), 10.

57. Shana Goldin-Perschbacher, "Transamericana: Gender, Genre, and Journey," *New Literary History* 46 (Autumn 2015): 794. *Transamerica* was screenwriter Duncan Tucker's debut as a feature film director. On Tucker's narrative approach, see A. O. Scott, "A Complex Metamorphosis of the Most Fundamental Sort," *New York Times*, December 2, 2005.

58. Jay Prosser, *Second Skins: The Body Narratives of Transsexuality* (New York: Columbia University Press, 1998), 4.

59. Gozlan, *Current Critical Debates in the Field of Transsexual Studies*, 4.

60. Gema Perez-Sanchez, "Transnational Conversations in Migration, Queer, and Transgender Studies: Multimedia Storyspaces," *Revista Canadiense de Estudios Hispánicos* 35 (Autumn 2010): 173; Niall Richardson, *Transgressive Bodies: Representations in Film and Popular Culture* (London: Routledge, 2010), 138–140.

61. Janet Mock, *Redefining Realness: My Path to Womanhood, Identity, Love and So Much More* (New York: Atria, 2014), 11.

62. Virginia L. Blum, *Flesh Wounds: The Culture of Cosmetic Surgery* (Berkeley: University of California Press, 2003), 44.

63. Joseph K. Canner, Omar Harfouch, Lisa M. Kodadek, Danielle Pelaez, Devin Coon, Anaeze C. Offodile II, Adil H. Haider, et al., "Temporal Trends in Gender-Affirming Surgery among Transgender Patients in the United States," *JAMA Surgery* 153 (2018): 609.

64. See the World Freedom Alliance's Gender Mapping Project at https://world freedomalliance.org/au/news/the-gender-mapping-project, accessed April 14, 2024.

65. Naomi Diaz, "Big Tech Weighs in on Gender-affirming Care," *Becker's Hospital Review*, March 11, 2022, accessed July 21, 2023, https://www.beckershospitalreview.com /healthcare-information-technology/big-tech-weighs-in-on-gender-affirming-care.html.

66. Kathy Davis, *Reshaping the Female Body: The Dilemma of Cosmetic Surgery* (New York: Routledge, 1995), 113.

67. Caroline Davidge-Pitts, Todd B. Nippoldt, Ann Danoff, Lauren Radziejewski, and Neena Natt, "Transgender Health in Endocrinology: Current Status of Endocrinology Fellowship Programs and Practicing Clinicians," *Journal of Clinical Endocrinology and Metabolism* 102 (April 2017): 1286–1290; Vishnu R. Mani, "Transgender Surgery: Knowledge Gap among Physicians Impacting Patient Care," *Current Urology* 15 (March 2021): 68–70; Walter O. Bockting and Joshua M. Goldberg, eds., *Guidelines for Transgender Care* (Binghamton, NY: Haworth Medical Press, 2006).

68. See, for example, Aren Zachary Aizura, "Feminine Transformations: Gender Reassignment Surgical Tourism in Thailand," *Medical Anthropology: Cross-Cultural Studies in Health and Illness* 29 (2010): 424–443.

69. Avgi Saketopoulou, speaking on "Exposing Transphobic Legacies, Embracing Trans Life," *Couched*, June 24, 2022, https://couchedpodcast.org/exposing-transphobic -legacies-embracing-trans-life. See also Avgi Saketopoulou, *Sexuality Beyond Consent: Risk, Race, Traumatophilia* (New York: New York University Press, 2023).

70. Imogen Binnie, *Nevada* (2013; repr., New York: Farrar, Straus and Giroux, 2022), 6.

71. Stephanie Burt, "The Invention of the Trans Novel," *New Yorker*, June 20, 2022. See also Marty Fink, "It Will Feel Really Bad Unromantically Soon: Crippling Insomnia through Imogen Binnie's *Nevada*," *Transgender Studies Quarterly* 60 (February 2019): 4–19; Oliver L. Haimson, "Challenging 'Getting Better' Social Media Narratives with Intersectional Transgender Lived Experiences," *Social Media and Society* 6 (March 2020): 1–12.

72. Binnie, *Nevada*, 134.

73. Binnie, *Nevada*, 7.

74. Binnie, *Nevada*, 80.

75. On culturally congruent trans health care and research, see Victoria A. Cargill, "Valuing the Vulnerable—The Important Role of Transgender Communities in Biomedical Research," *Ethnicity and Disease* 30 (Spring 2020): 247–250.

76. Laine Hughes, "Wronging the Right-Body Narrative: On the Universality of Gender Uncertainty," in *Current Critical Debates in the Field of Transsexual Studies: In Transition*, ed. Oren Gozlan (London: Routledge, 2018), 181.

77. Malatino, *Queer Embodiment*, 10.

78. See Austin H. Johnson, "Normative Accountability: How the Medical Model Influences Transgender Identities and Experiences," *Sociology Compass* 9 (September 2015): 803–813; Sari L. Reisner, Matan Benyishay, Brooke Stott, Virginia Vedilago, and Alex S. Keuroghlian, "Gender-Affirming Mental Health Care Access and Utilization among Rural Transgender and Gender Diverse Adults in Five Northeastern U.S. States," *Transgender Health* 7 (June 2022), https://www.liebertpub.com/doi/abs/10.1089 /trgh.2021.0010.

79. Binnie, *Nevada*, 45.

80. Stanley Cavell, *Conditions Handsome and Unhandsome: The Constitution of Emersonian Perfectionism* (La Salle, IL: Open Court, 1990), 2.

81. Binnie, *Nevada*, 233–234.

82. Binnie, *Nevada*, 7.

83. Donna Haraway, *Modest_Witness@Second_Millennium.FemaleMan©_Meets_OncoMouseTM: Feminism and Technoscience* (New York: Routledge, 1997), 22, 35.

84. Malatino, *Trans Care*, 35–9; Jules Gill-Peterson, "The Technical Capacities of the Body: Assembling Race, Technology, and Transgender," *Transgender Studies Quarterly* 1 (March 2014): 403.

85. Stanley Cavell, *In Quest of the Ordinary: Lines of Skepticism and Romanticism* (Chicago: University of Chicago Press, 1988), 52–53.

86. Gozlan, *Current Critical Debates*, 7.

87. Cavell, *In Quest of the Ordinary*, 154.

88. Gozlan, ed., *Current Critical Debates*, 7.

89. Singh, *Unthinking Mastery*, 4–5.

90. Julietta Singh, *The Breaks* (London: Daunt, 2021), 187.

91. Gill-Peterson, "On the Possibility of Affirmative Health Care for Transgender Children," 236.

92. On anxiety and gender regulation, see Meadow, *Trans Kids*, 142–186.

93. *Joychild*, dir. Aurora Brachman (2020).

94. Gill-Peterson, *Histories of the Transgender Child*, 188–189.

95. Jody L. Herman, Andrew Ryan Flores, and Kathryn K. O'Neill, "A Window into the Number of Trans Teens Living in America," *The Conversation*, July 5, 2022, https://theconversation.com/a-window-into-the-number-of-trans-teens-living-in-america-185361. This analysis draws from the Youth Risk Behavior Survey conducted by the Centers for Disease Control and Prevention across schools and from state-level data in 2019.

96. Hausman, *Changing Sex*, 15; Donna Haraway, "Awash in Urine: DES and Premarin® in Multispecies Response-Ability," *Women Studies Quarterly* 40 (Spring/Summer 2012): 301; Preciado, *Testo Junkie*, 43. See also Teresa de Lauretis, *Technologies of Gender: Essays on Theory, Film, and Fiction* (Bloomington: Indiana University Press, 1987).

97. *Trans Mission: What's the Rush to Reassign Gender?*, dir. Kallie Fell and Jennifer Lahl (2021); Valeria P. Bustos Samyd S. Bustos, Andres Mascaro, Gabriel Del Corral, et al, "Regret after Gender-affirmation Surgery: A Systematic Review and Meta-Analysis of Prevalence," *Plastic and Reconstructive Surgery* 9 (March 2021): e3477.

98. Gill-Peterson, "On the Possibility of Affirmative Health Care for Transgender Children," 237–238. For the latest version of the World Professional Association for Transgender Health Standards of Care see E. Coleman, A. E. Radix, W. P. Bouman, G. R. Brown, A. L. C. de Vries, M. B. Deutsch, R. Ettner, et al., "Standards of Care for the Health of Transgender and Gender Diverse People, Version 8," *International Journal of Transgender Health* 23, supplement 1 (September 2022): S1–S259.

99. Julian Gill-Peterson, *Histories of the Transgender Child* (Minneapolis: University of Minnesota Press, 2018), 33. See also Stef H. Shuster, *Trans Medicine: The Emergence and Practice of Treating Gender* (New York: New York University Press, 2021).

100. On the history of sex differentiation and hormone treatment, see Nelly Oudshoorn, *Beyond the Natural Body: An Archaeology of Sex Hormones* (New York: Routledge, 1994).

101. Austin H. Johnson, "Rejecting, Reframing, and Reintroducing: Trans People's Strategic Engagement with the Medicalization of Gender Dysphoria," *Sociology of Health and Illness* 41 (November 2018): 517; Jules Gill-Peterson, "Exposing Transphobic Legacies, Embracing Trans Life," Couched Podcast, June 24, 2022, https://couchedpodcast .org/exposing-transphobic-legacies-embracing-trans-life/. For a challenge to teleology, see Connor Lee O'Keefe's 2022 short film *Imagine a Body* at "Rethinking Identity and Testosterone in 'Imagine a Body,'" *New Yorker*, June 1, 2022.

102. Gill-Peterson, *Histories of the Transgender Child*, ii; Gill-Peterson, "On the Possibility of Affirmative Health Care for Transgender Children," 240.

103. Gill-Peterson, "On the Possibility of Affirmative Health Care," 241–242.

104. See Johanna Olson-Kennedy, "The Impact of Early Medical Treatment for Transgender Youth: Protocol for the Longitudinal, Observational Trans Youth Care Study," *Journal of Medical Internet Research* 8 (September 2018), https://s3.ca-central-1.amazonaws .com/assets.jmir.org/assets/preprints/preprint-14434-accepted.pdf.

105. Jack L. Turban Dana King, Jeremi M. Carswell, and Alex S. Keuroghlian, "Pubertal Suppression for Transgender Youth and Risk of Suicidal Ideation," *Pediatrics* 145 (February 2020), https://www.ncbi.nlm.nih.gov/pmc/articles/PMC7073269/pdf/nihms -1554242.pdf.

106. Substance Abuse and Mental Health Services Administration, *Ending Conversion Therapy*, 2. To support this claim, the report cites E. Coleman, W. Bockting, M. Botzer, P. Cohen-Kettenis, G. DeCuypere, J. Feldman, L. Fraser, et al., "Standards of Care for the Health of Transsexual, Transgender, and Gender Nonconforming People," *International Journal of Transgenderism* 13 (August 2012): 165–232.

107. Binnie, *Nevada*, 258.

108. National Center for Transgender Equality, *Injustice at Every Turn*, 23, 82; *Report of the 2015 U.S. Transgender Survey*, 5.

109. National Center for Transgender Equality, *Report of the 2015 U.S. Transgender Survey*, 103, 35, https://transequality.org/sites/default/files/docs/usts/USTS-Full-Report -Dec17.pdf.

110. Trevor Project, *2022 National Survey on LGBTQ Youth Mental Health* (2022), https:// www.thetrevorproject.org/survey-2022. See also Dawn Ennis, "'Terrible Time for Trans Youth': New Survey Spotlights Suicide Attempts—and Hope," *Forbes*, May 19, 2021.

111. See Agnès Condat, Nicolas Mendes, Véronique Drouineau, Nouria Gründler, Chrystelle Lagrange, Colette Chiland, Jean-Philippe Wolf, et al., "Biotechnologies that Empower Transgender Persons to Self-Actualize," *Philosophy, Ethics, and Humanities in Medicine* 13 (January 2018): 2.

112. See Mayo Clinic Staff, "Pubertal Blockers for Transgender and Gender-Diverse Youth," Mayo Clinic, https://www.mayoclinic.org/diseases-conditions/gender-dysphoria/in-depth/pubertal-blockers/art-20459075; Lindsey Dawson and Jennifer Kates, Policy Tracker: Youth Access to Gender Affirming Care and State Policy Restrictions, KFF, https://www.kff.org/other/dashboard/gender-affirming-care-policy-tracker, accessed April 12, 2024.

113. American Society of Plastic Surgeons, *Plastic Surgery Statistics Report: 2020*, https://www.plasticsurgery.org/documents/News/Statistics/2020/plastic-surgery-statistics-full-report-2020.pdf; "Gender Services," Boston Children's Hospital, accessed July 15, 2022, https://www.childrenshospital.org/treatments/facial-harmonization.

114. Talley, *Saving Face*, 78.

115. Jordan Deschamps-Braly and Douglas Ousterhout, *Facial Feminization Surgery: The Journey to Gender Affirmation* (Omaha, NE: Addicus, 2021). On facial feminization surgery conducted by Deschamps-Braly, see "The Story of a Trans Woman's Face," *New Yorker*, March 12, 2018; and on bioethics of face changing, see Sharrona Pearl, *Face/On: Face Transplants and the Ethics of the Other* (Chicago: University of Chicago Press, 2017), 31–32, 46–48.

116. For a critique of normalizing pressures, see Talley, *Saving Face*, 88, 96.

117. See Janet L. Dolgin, "Unhealthy Determinations Controlling Medical Necessity," *Virginia Journal of Social Policy and the Law* 22 (2015): 475–476. See also Alex Dubov and Liana Fraenkel, "Facial Feminization Surgery: The Ethics of Gatekeeping in Transgender Health," *American Journal of Bioethics* 18 (December 2018): 3–9.

118. Eric Plemons, "Gender, Ethnicity, and Transgender Embodiment: Interrogating Classification in Facial Feminization Surgery," *Body & Society* 25 (November 2018): 6–7. See also "The Surgery Issue," ed. Eric Plemons and Chris Straayer, special issue, *Transgender Studies Quarterly* 5((May 2018).

119. See "Ethno-Specific Facial Feminization Surgery," Deschamps-Braly Clinic, accessed July 15, 2022, https://deschamps-braly.com/facial-feminization-surgery/ethno-specific-ffs.

120. See Rebecca W. Persky, Siobhan M. Gruschow, Ninet Sinaii, Claire Carlson, and Nadia L. Dowshen, "Attitudes toward Fertility Preservation among Transgender Youth and their Parents," *Journal of Adolescent Health* 67 (October 2020): 583–589; and Holly C. Cooper, Jim Long, and Tandy Aye, "Fertility Preservation in Transgender and Non-Binary Adolescents and Young Adults," *PLoS One* 17 (March 2022): e0265043.

121. Condat et al., "Biotechnologies that Empower Transgender Persons to Self-Actualize," 5.

122. Martine Rothblatt, *Unzipped Genes: Taking Charge of Baby-Making in the New Millennium* (Philadelphia: Temple University Press, 1997), xiii–xiv. See also Khadija Mitu, "Transgender Reproductive Choice and Fertility Preservation," *AMA Journal of Ethics* 18 (November 2016): 119–125.

123. Singh, *The Breaks*, 199.

124. Beatrice Adler-Bolton, "'Imagine What We'll Build for One Another': An Interview with Jules Gill-Peterson," *The New Inquiry*, June 23, 2022, https://thenewinquiry.com/imagine-what-well-build-for-one-another-an-interview-with-jules-gill-peterson.

125. Adler-Bolton, "'Imagine What We'll Build for One Another.'"

126. Gill-Peterson, *Histories of the Transgender Child*, 199, 218.

127. Jeanne Thornton, "Angels Are Here to Help You," in *Meanwhile, Elsewhere: Science Fiction and Fantasy from Transgender Writers*, ed. Cat Fitzpatrick and Casey Plett, 2nd ed. (New York: Little Puss Press, 2021), 633.

128. Kim Stanley Robinson, *2312* (New York: Orbit, 2012).

129. Malatino, *Queer Embodiment*, 13.

130. Thornton, "Angels Are Here to Help You," 635.

131. Mark Sable, *The Dark* (Milwaukie, OR: Dark Horse Comics, 2021).

132. Preciado, *Testo Junkie*, 16.

133. Thornton, "Angels Are Here to Help You," 638.

134. Thornton, "Angels Are Here to Help You," 652.

135. Thornton, "Angels Are Here to Help You," 637–638.

136. Thornton, "Angels Are Here to Help You," 642, 639.

137. Thornton, "Angels Are Here to Help You," 663. On biotech efforts to optimize assemblages, see Nikolas Rose, *The Politics of Life Itself* (Princeton, NJ: Princeton University Press, 2007), 17.

138. Thornton, "Angels Are Here to Help You," 664.

139. See Rich Larson, *Annex* (New York: Hachette, 2018).

140. Hilary Malatino, "Biohacking Gender: Cyborgs, Coloniality, and the Pharmacopornographic Era," *Angelaki* 22 (June 2017): 179.

141. Tyler Santora, "Ignored by Doctors, Transgender People Turn to DIY Treatments," *Undark*, June 29, 2020 https://undark.org/2020/06/29/transgender-diy-treatments.

142. "Underground: Why This Transgender Woman Used Black Market Drugs to Transition," ABC News, May 10, 2016); Gillian Brandstetter, "Sketchy Pharmacies Are Selling Hormones to Transgender People," *The Atlantic*, August 31, 2016.

143. Rose, *The Politics of Life Itself*, 26.

144. Mary Maggic, "Open Source Estrogen," accessed December 1, 2022, https://www.media.mit.edu/publications/open-source-estrogen. See also Mark Hay, "This Biohacker Is Trying to Help People Make Their Own Estrogen," *Vice*, March 22, 2018, https://www.vice.com/en/article/xw7z4j/hacking-diy-estrogen-hormones-trans-people.

145. Rose, *The Politics of Life Itself*, 111.

146. Binnie, *Nevada*, 28.

147. Christoph Hanssmann, "Passing Torches? Feminist Inquiries and Trans-Health Politics and Practices," *Transgender Studies Quarterly* 3 (May 2016): 123.

148. Jacob Bernstein, "Amanda Lepore, Transgender Club Diva, Tells All about Her Plastic Surgery," *New York Times*, July 19, 2017.

149. See Peg Zeglin Brand, "Bound to Beauty: An Interview with ORLAN," in *Beauty Matters*, ed. Peg Zeglin Brand (Bloomington: Indiana University Press, 2000), 289–213; and Peg Brand Weiser, "ORLAN Revisited: Disembodies Virtual Hybrid Beauty," in *Beauty Unlimited*, ed. Peg Zeglin Brand (Bloomington: Indiana University Press, 2012), 306–340.

150. Megan Molteni, "A Patient Gets the New Transgender Surgery She Helped Invent," *Wired*, September 11, 2017.

151. Adriana Knouf, *Fragments of Xenology* (Amsterdam: tranxxeno lab, 2021), 9; Christine Beaudoin, "Remaking (Post-)Human Bodies in the Anthropocene through Bioart Practices," in *Remaking the Human: Cosmetic Technologies of Body Repair, Reshaping and Replacement*, ed. Alvaro Jarrín and Chiara Pussetti (New York: Berghahn, 2021), 166. See also Alisha Harris, "Juliana Huxtable's Next Chapter," *New York Times*, August 10, 2020.

152. Judith Rudakoff, ed., *Trans(per)Forming Nina Arsenault: An Unreasonable Body of Work* (Chicago: Intellect, 2012).

153. Malatino, *Trans Care*, 39.

154. Adriana Knouf, *Xenformation 1: What Does Xen Dream of in the Theatricum?* (2022), https://tranxxenolab.net/projects/xenformation1. See also Knouf's "Xenological Entanglements" series at https://kersnikova.org/en/posts/events/all/adriana-knouf-xenological-entanglements-001a-trying-plastic-variations, both accessed July 21, 2023.

155. Singh, *The Breaks*, 192.

156. Singh, *Unthinking Mastery*, 4.

CHAPTER 7 — PANDEMIC CULTURE

1. Barack Obama, "Remarks at the National Institutes of Health in Bethesda, Maryland," December 2, 2014, in *Public Papers of the Presidents of the United States: Barack Obama, 2014, Book 2, July 1 to December 31* (Washington, DC: Government Printing Office, 2019), 1542.

2. Barack Obama, "Remarks Following a Meeting with Senior Advisors to Discuss Ebola Preparedness and Containment Efforts and an Exchange with Reporters," October 22, 2014, in *Public Papers of the Presidents of the United States: Barack Obama, 2014*, Book 2, *July 1 to December 31* (Washington, DC: Government Printing Office, 2019), 1349.

3. Obama, "Remarks at the National Institutes of Health," 1541.

4. See Mike Pence, *So Help Me God* (New York: Simon & Schuster, 2022), 100, 119.

5. Lena H. Sun, Lenny Bernstein, and Joel Achenbach, "CDC Director's Challenge: Deadly Ebola Virus and Outbreak of Criticism," *Washington Post*, October 16, 2014; Shana Kushner Gadarian, Sara Wallace Goodman, and Thomas B. Pepinsky, *Pandemic*

Politics: The Deadly Toll of Polarization in the Age of COVID (Princeton, NJ: Princeton University Press, 2022), 36–37.

6. The WHO was criticized by national governments for not responding quickly enough to the African Ebola outbreak. See Marcus Cueto, Theodore M. Brown and Elizabeth Fee, *The World Health Organization: A History* (Cambridge: Cambridge University Press, 2019), 320–340. See also Peter Daszak, "We Knew Disease X Was Coming. It's Here Now," *New York Times*, February 27, 2020.

7. For this Organisation for Economic Co-operation and Development data, see Rabah Kamal and Julie Hudman, "What Do We Know about Spending Related to Public Health in the U.S. and Comparable Countries?" Peterson-KFF Health System Tracker, September 30, 2020, https://www.healthsystemtracker.org/chart-collection /what-do-we-know-about-spending-related-to-public-health-in-the-u-s-and-comparable -countries; Centers for Disease Control and Prevention, National Center for Health Statistics, "Table HExpGDP. Gross Domestic Product, National Health Expenditures, Per Capita Amounts, Percent Distribution, and Average Annual Percent Change: United States, Selected Years 1960–2019," https://www.cdc.gov/nchs/data/hus/2020-2021/HExp GDP.pdf; and [Centers for Medicare and Medicaid Services], "National Health Expenditure Accounts: Methodology Paper, 2002," accessed November 27, 2022, https://www .cms.gov/files/document/definitions-sources-and-methods.pdf. See also Chelsea Janes and William Wan, "The Nation's Public Health Agencies Are Ailing When They're Needed the Most," *Washington Post*, August 31, 2020.

8. For this 2016–2018 Statista data on state spending on preventive medicine, see "How Much Do U.S. States Spend Per Person on Public Health?," *Forbes*, July 2, 2020.

9. "Fact Sheet—President Donald J. Trump Is Ensuring We Have the Strong National Stockpile and Industrial Base Needed to Meet Any Challenge," Trump White House Archives, May 14, 2020, https://trumpwhitehouse.archives.gov/briefings-statements /president-donald-j-trump-ensuring-strong-national-stockpile-industrial-base-needed -meet-challenge; Donald J. Trump, interview with David Muir, *World News Tonight*, ABC News, May 5, 2020.

10. Jane C. Timm, "Fact Check: Trump Falsely Claims Obama Left Him 'Nothing' in the National Stockpile," NBC, May 6, 2020; Nell Greenfieldboyce, "Inside a Secret Government Warehouse Prepped for Health Catastrophes," NPR, June 27, 2016; "Press Briefing by National Security Advisor Ambassador John Bolton and Secretary of Health and Human Services Alex Azar on the National Biodefense Strategy," September 18, 2018, The American Presidency Project, https: https://www.presidency.ucsb.edu /documents/press-briefing-national-security-advisor-ambassador-john-bolton-and -secretary-health-and.

11. Barack Obama and Richard Lugar, "Grounding a Pandemic," *New York Times*, June 6, 2005. See also Andrew Lakoff, *Unprepared: Global Health in a Time of Emergency* (Berkeley: University of California Press, 2017), 60–61, 90.

12. For critical reviews of Trump's leadership, see Eric Lipton, David E. Sanger, Maggie Haberman, Michael D. Shear, Mark Mazzetti and Julian E. Barnes, "He Could Have

Seen What Was Coming: Behind Trump's Failure on the Virus," *New York Times*, April 11, 2020; "CNN Special Report: The Pandemic and the President," CNN, May 3, 2020; Philip Rucker, Yasmeen Abutaleb, Josh Dawsey, and Robert Costa, "The Lost Days of Summer: How Trump Fell Short in Containing the Virus," *Washington Post*, August 8, 2020.

13. Transcript of Coronavirus Task Force Briefing, The White House: President Donald J. Trump, March 31, 2020: https://www.whitehouse.gov/briefing-room/press-briefings/2021/03/31/press-briefing-by-white-house-covid-19-response-team-and-public-health-officials-22/; Anthony Fauci, interview on *State of the Union*, CNN, April 12, 2020.

14. Yasmeen Abutaleb, Ashley Parker, Josh Dawsey, and Philip Rucker, "The Inside Story of How Trump's Denial, Mismanagement and Magical Thinking Led to the Pandemic's Dark Winter," *Washington Post*, December 19, 2020.

15. Gadarian, Goodman, and Pepinsky, *Pandemic Politics*, 1–3. In his 2022 memoir, former Vice President Mike Pence argued that some governors' requests for federal aid were unrealistic and exaggerated the quantity of testing and medical supplies needed from the federal government: Pence, *So Help Me God*, 396–389.

16. See Alana Abramson, "President Trump's Allies Keep Talking about the 'Deep State.' What's That?," *Time*, March 8, 2017; Sheryl Gay Stolberg and Noah Weiland, "Study Finds 'Single Largest Driver' of Coronavirus Misinformation: Trump," *New York Times*, September 30, 2020; Corey H. Basch, Charles E. Basch, Grace C. Hillyer, and Zoe C. Meleo-Erwin, "Social Media, Public Health, and Community Mitigation of COVID-19: Challenges, Risks, and Benefits," *Journal of Medical Internet Research* 24 (April 2022): e36804; Ingjerd Skafle, Anders Nordahl-Hansen, Daniel S. Quintana, Rolf Wynn, and Elia Gabarron, "Misinformation about COVID-19 Vaccines on Social Media: Rapid Review," *Journal of Medical Internet Research* 24 (August 2022): e37367; Claire Birchall and Peter Knight, ed., *Conspiracy Theories in the Time of Covid-19* (London: Routledge, 2023); and James Ball, *The Other Pandemic: How QAnon Contaminated the World* (London: Bloomsbury, 2023).

17. Talk show radio host Gary Null is a prominent conspiratorial voice targeting perceived government failure. See, for example, Richard Gale and Gary Null, "Mismanaging a Pandemic: Failures in the Covid-19 Narrative," Gary Null, August 2, 2022, https://garynull.com/mismanaging-a-pandemic-failures-in-the-covid-19-narrative.

18. Colin Kahl and Thomas Wright, *Aftershocks: Pandemic Politics and the End of the Old International Order* (New York: St. Martin's Press, 2021), 291; *NYC Epicenters 9/11 to 2021½*, documentary miniseries, aired on HBO, August 22–September 11, 2021.

19. Robert N. Bellah, "Is There a Common American Culture?" (1998), in *The Robert Bellah Reader*, ed. Steven M. Tipton (Durham, NC: Duke University Press, 2006), 320. See also Taylor Shelton, "A Post-Truth Pandemic?," *Big Data and Society* 7 (July–December 2020): 1–6.

20. Pence, *So Help Me God*, 392, 400. On health care improvisation, see Ellen Block and Cecilia Vindrola-Padros, "Making Do: COVID-19 and the Improvisation of Care in the

UK and US," in *Viral Loads: Anthropologies of Urgency in the Time of COVID-19*, ed. Lenore Manderson, Nancy J. Burker, and Ayo Wahlberg (London: UCL Press, 2023), 303–323. On competing leadership perspectives, see Jan Zielonka, "Who Should Be in Charge of Pandemics? Scientists or Politicians?," in *Pandemics, Politics, and Society*, ed. Gerard Delanty (Berlin: De Gruyter, 2021), 59–73.

21. The phrase was used by UN Secretary-General António Guterres in a spring 2020 speech on the response of the global health community to COVID-19 and was widely echoed, including by Joe Biden on the campaign trail in the fall of 2020: "We Are All in This Together: Human Rights and COVID-19 Response and Recovery," United Nations: COVID-19 Response, April 23, 2020, https://www.un.org/en/un-coronavirus -communications-team/we-are-all-together-human-rights-and-covid-19-response-and.

22. Julia Lynch, Michael Bernhard, and Daniel O'Neill, "Pandemic Politics," *Perspectives on Politics* 20 (June 2022): 389. See also Martha F. Davis, "The Human (Rights) Costs of Inequality: Snapshots from a Pandemic," in *COVID-19 and Human Rights*, ed. Morten Kjaerum, Martha F. Davis, and Amanda Lyons (London: Routledge, 2021), 67–81; and Tony Sandset, "The Necropolitics of COVID-19: Race, Class and Slow Death in an Ongoing Pandemic," *Global Public Health* 16 (August–September 2021): 1411–1423.

23. See Helga Nowotny, "In AI We Trust: How the COVID-19 Pandemic Pushes Us Deeper into Digitalization," in *Pandemics, Politics, and Society*, ed. Gerard Delanty (Berlin: De Gruyter, 2021), 115.

24. Sandra C. Melvin, "The Role of Public Health in COVID-19 Emergency Response Efforts from a Rural Health Perspective," *Preventing Chronic Disease* 17 (July 23, 2020); Elissabeth Beaunoyer, Sophie Dupere, and Matthieu J. Guitton, "COVID-19 and Digital Inequalities: Reciprocal Impacts and Mitigation Strategies," *Computers in Human Behavior* 111 (October 2020): 106424; Siqin Ye, Ian Kronish, Elaine Fleck, Peter Fleischut, Shunichi Homma, David Masini, and Nathalie Moise, "Telemedicine Expansion during the COVID-19 Pandemic and the Potential for Technology-Driven Disparities," *Journal of General Internal Medicine* 36 (January 2021): 256–258.

25. Jeremy A. Greene, *The Doctor Who Wasn't There: Technology, History, and the Limits of Telehealth* (Chicago: University of Chicago Press, 2022).

26. Department of Health and Human Services, *Protecting Youth Mental Health: The U.S. Surgeon General's Advisory* (Washington, DC: Government Printing Office, 2021); House Oversight and Reform Select Subcommittee on the Coronavirus Crisis, "Understanding and Addressing Long COVID and Its Health and Economic Consequences," hearing, July 19, 2022, YouTube video, https://www.youtube.com/watch?v=DL9Am-IqL488. See also Sheryl Gay Stolberg and Davey Alba, "Surgeon General Assails Tech Companies Over Misinformation on Covid-19," *New York Times*, July 15, 2021.

27. Gadarian, Goodman, and Pepinsky, *Pandemic Politics*, 15.

28. See Jay Bhattacharya, "Zero Covid Has Cost New Zealand Dearly," *Spiked*, August 7, 2022; and Alexandra Stevenson and Benjamin Mueller, "How Bad Is China's Covid Outbreak? It's a Scientific Guessing Game," *New York Times*, December 29, 2022.

29. Mike Pence defended Trump's decision to ban flights from China on January 31, 2020, the day health secretary Alex Azar declared COVID-19 a national public health emergency; Pence, *So Help Me God*, 376–377.

30. "WHO Transformation," accessed December 5, 2022, https://www.who.int/about /transformation; Thomas J. Bollyky and Jeremy Konyndyk, "It's Not the WHO's Fault that Trump Didn't Prepare for the Coronavirus," *Washington Post*, April 14, 2020; Andrew Restuccia, Gordon Lubold, and Drew Hinshaw "Trump Threatens to Permanently Cut Funding to World Health Organization," *Wall Street Journal*, May 19, 2020.

31. Anne Applebaum, "When the World Stumbled: COVID-19 and the Failure of the International System," in *COVID-19 and World Order: The Future of Conflict, Competition, and Cooperation*, ed. Hal Brands and Francis J. Gavin (Baltimore, MD: Johns Hopkins University Press, 2020), 223–237; World Health Organization, "Working Draft, Presented on the Basis of Progress Achieved," A/INB/2/3, July 13, 2022, 4, https://apps.who .int/gb/inb/pdf_files/inb2/A_INB2_3-en.pdf; Editorial Board, "The World is Unprepared for the Next Pandemic. Here's a Start to Fix That," *Washington Post*, April, 11, 2024; Stefan Elbe, *Pandemics, Pills, and Politics: Governing Global Health Security* (Baltimore, MD: Johns Hopkins University Press, 2018), 227.

32. Robert N. Bellah, Richard Madsen, William M. Sullivan, Ann Swidler, and Steven M. Tipton, *The Good Society* (New York: Knopf, 1991), 1, 92.

33. See Melinda Cooper, *Life as Surplus: Biotechnology and Capitalism in the Neo-Liberal Era* (Seattle: University of Washington Press, 2008), 51–52.

34. Nidhi Subbaraman, "Science Misinformation Alarms Francis Collins as He Leaves Top NIH Job," *Nature*, December 3, 2021.

35. Jeremy M. Levin, ed., *Biotechnology in the Time of COVID-19: Commentaries from the Front Line* (New York: Rosetta Books, 2020), 3.

36. See, for example, Angus Liu, "Pfizer to become $100B Behemoth Next Year Thanks to COVID-19 Drug and Vaccine," *Fierce Pharma*, November 23, 2021, https:// www.fiercepharma.com/pharma/pfizer-to-exceed-100b-revenue-2022-thanks-to-covid -19-drug-and-vaccine-analyst.

37. James Greenwood, "Will COVID-19 Transform the Political Landscape?," in *Biotechnology in the Time of COVID-19: Commentaries from the Front Line*, ed. Jeremy M. Levin (New York: Rosetta Books, 2020), 202. In this essay, Greenwood pits "the heroic men and women of biotechnology" against federal government inertia.

38. Alex Zhavoronkov, "Biotechnology in the Time of COVID-19: Past, Present, and Future," *Forbes*, June 8, 2020; Brook Byers, "Biotech to the Rescue, Again!," in *Biotechnology in the Time of COVID-19: Commentaries from the Front Line*, ed. Jeremy M. Levin (New York: Rosetta Books, 2020), 35.

39. Jeremy M. Levin, ed., *Biotechnology in the Time of COVID-19: Commentaries from the Front Line* (New York: Rosetta Books, 2020), 2. See also Alex de Waal, *New Pandemics, Old Politics* (Cambridge: Polity, 2021).

40. Proclamation No. 9787, September 14, 2018, "Prescription Opioid and Heroin Epidemic Awareness Week, 2018," 83 Fed. Reg. 182 (September 19, 2018), 47543; Donald J.

Trump, "Remarks at a White House Coronavirus Task Force Press Briefing," April 4, 2020, https://www.presidency.ucsb.edu/documents/remarks-white-house-coronavirus-task-force-press-briefing-20; Donald J. Trump, "Remarks by President Trump to the 75th Session of the United Nations General Assembly," September 22, 2020, White House Archives, https://trumpwhitehouse.archives.gov/briefings-statements/remarks-president-trump-75th-session-united-nations-general-assembly.

41. Pence, *So Help Me God*, 404.

42. Robert N. Butler, *The Longevity Revolution: The Benefits and Challenges of Living a Long Life* (New York: Public Affairs, 2008), 362–379; Tanya Lewis, "The U.S. Just Lost 26 Years' Worth of Progress on Life Expectancy," *Scientific American*, October 17, 2022; Deidre McPhillips, "Covid-19 and Drug Overdoses Drive US Life Expectancy to Lowest Level in 25 Years, CDC Reports," CNN, December 22, 2022.

43. On public-mindedness during the pandemic, see Matteo Bonotti and Steven T. Zech, *Recovering Civility during COVID-19* (London: Palgrave Macmillan, 2021).

44. Elizabeth A. Povinelli, Mathew Coleman, and Kathryn Yusoff, "Elizabeth Povinelli: Geontopower Biopolitics and the Anthropocene," *Theory, Culture and Society* 34 (Spring 2017): 173.

45. Priscilla Wald, *Contagious: Cultures, Carriers, and the Outbreak Narrative* (Durham, NC: Duke University Press, 2008); 42–43; Priscilla Wald, "Pandemics and the Politics of Planetary Health," in *The Edinburgh Companion to the Politics of American Health*, ed. Martin Halliwell and Sophie A. Jones (Edinburgh: Edinburgh University Press, 2022), 614; Brian King and Kelley A. Crews, eds., *Ecologies and Politics of Health* (London: Routledge, 2013), xix.

46. King and Kelley, *Ecologies and Politics of Health*, 1.

47. Tim Cooper, "Recycling Modernity: Waste and Environmental History," *History Compass* 8 (September 2010): 964.

48. Ling Ma, *Severance* (London: Text Publishing, 2018), 9.

49. Obama, "Remarks at the National Institutes of Health," 1542.

50. On the laboratorization of urban space, see Albena Yaneva, *Architecture after COVID* (London: Bloomsbury, 2023), 37–79.

51. Mike Chen, *The Beginning of the End* (Toronto: MIRA Books, 2020). See also Tim M. Cook, "COVID-19 Vaccines: One Step towards the Beginning of the End of the Global Impact of the Pandemic," *Anaesthesia* 76 (December 2020): 435–443; Srividya Kakulavarapu, "SARS-CoV-2 Vaccine Candidates: A Beginning of the End of COVID-19 Pandemic," *Annals of Medicine and Surgery* 62 (February 2021): 460–462.

52. United Nations, "The End of the COVID-19 Pandemic Is in Sight: WHO," *UN News*, September 14, 2022, https://news.un.org/en/story/2022/09/1126621.

53. Guobin Yang, *The Wuhan Lockdown* (New York: Columbia University Press, 2022), 10. The raccoon dog theory did not emerge until early 2023; see Katherine J. Wu, "The Strongest Evidence Yet that an Animal Started the Pandemic," *Atlantic*, March 16, 2023.

54. See Kelly McGuire, "COVID-19, *Contagion*, and Vaccine Optimism," *Journal of Medical Humanities* 42 (February 2021): 51–62.

55. Michele N. Norris, "He Wrote 'Contagion.' Here's What He Had to Say about the Response to the Coronavirus," *Washington Post*, April 1, 2020.

56. Marco Grosoli, "Ocean Doesn't Live Here Anymore: Steven Soderbergh's *Contagion* and the Stock Market Crash," in *States of Crisis and Post-Capitalist Scenarios*, ed. Heiko Feldner, Fabio Vighi, and Slavoj Žižek (Burlington, VT: Ashgate, 2014), 171.

57. Sari Altschuler, "After the Outbreak: Narrative, Infrastructure, and Pandemic Time," *Resilience: A Journal of the Environmental Humanities* 8 (Fall 2021): 128–129.

58. Altschuler, "After the Outbreak," 129. On the persistence of outbreak narratives, see David Willman and Joby Warrick, "Research with Exotic Viruses Risks a Deadly Outbreak, Scientists Warn," *Washington Post*, April 10, 2023.

59. See David J. Rothkopf, "When the Buzz Bites Back," *Washington Post*, May 11, 2003; Jon D. Lee, *An Epidemic of Rumors: How Stories Shape Our Perception of Disease* (Boulder: University Press of Colorado, 2014); and "The Infodemic Metaphor," Infodemic, April 8, 2021), infodemic.eu/2021/04/08/infodemic-metaphor.html.

60. For the wet-market theory, see Michael Worobey, "Dissecting the Early COVID-19 Cases in Wuhan," *Science* 374, November 18, 2021.

61. U.S. Senate Committee on Health, Education, Labor, and Pensions, "The Path Forward: A Federal Perspective on the COVID-19 Response," transcripts of hearing of July 21, 2021, https://www.help.senate.gov/hearings/the-path-forward-a-federal-perspective -on-the-covid-19-response. Rand Paul was quoting the molecular biologist Richard E. Bright at this point in his opening statement. For the paper Rand referred to, see Ben Hu, Lei-Ping Zeng, Xing-Lou Yang, Xing-Yi Ge, Wei Zhang, Bei Li, Jia-Zheng Xie, et al., "Discovery of a Rich Gene Pool of Bat SARS-Related Coronaviruses Provides New Insights into the Origin of SARS Coronavirus," *PLOS Pathogens* 13 (November 30, 2017): 29190287. For right-wing media coverage, see "Sen. Rand Paul, MD: NIH Lied and Continues to Lie about 'Gain of Function' Research and COVID," Fox News, November 4, 2021; and Emma Colton "Rand Paul Pins Blame for Thousands of Monthly COVID Deaths on Fauci over Longstanding Biases," Fox News, December 28, 2021.

62. See Anthony S. Fauci, "The Role of the National Institute of Allergy and Infectious Diseases in Research to Address the COVID-19 Pandemic: Testimony before the United States Senate Committee on Health, Education, Labor, and Pensions Hearing Titled: The Path Forward: A Federal Perspective on the COVID-19 Response," July 20, 2021, accessed August 20, 2021, https://www.help.senate.gov/imo/media/doc/Fauci10.pdf. For differing media accounts of the exchange, see Josh Rogin, "What the Fight between Anthony Fauci and Rand Paul Is Really About," *Washington Post*, July 22, 2021; Editorial Board, "Anthony Fauci, Rand Paul and Wuhan," *Wall Street Journal*, July 25, 2021. For Lawrence Tabak's testimony, see the report of the House Energy and Commerce Committee hearing "The Federal Response to COVID-19," held on February 8, 2023, in Sheryl Gay Stolberg, "N.I.H. Leader Rebuts Covid Lab Leak Theory at House Hearing," *New York Times*, February 8, 2023. On the classified Department of Energy report, see

Michael R. Gordon and Warren P. Strobel, "Lab Leak Most Likely Origin of Covid-19 Pandemic, Energy Department Now Says," *Wall Street Journal*, February 26, 2023; and Sheryl Gay Stolberg and Benjamin Mueller, "Lab Leak or Not? How Politics Shaped the Battle of Covid's Origin," *New York Times*, March 19, 2023. See also Alison Young, *Pandora's Gamble: Lab Leaks, Pandemics, and a World at Risk* (New York: Hachette, 2023).

63. Donald J. Trump, Coronavirus Task Force Press Briefing, the White House, April 15, 2020, video, UVA Miller Center, accessed September 16, 2022, https://millercenter.org/the-presidency/presidential-speeches/april-15-2020-press-briefing-coronavirus-task-force. The second season of *Biohackers* had concluded on Netflix twelve days before this Senate hearing and the viral zombie series *Black Summer* had concluded the previous month.

64. Rand Paul, *Government Bullies: How Everyday Americans Are Being Harassed, Abused, and Imprisoned by the Feds* (New York: Center Street, 2012); untitled press release about letter Rand Paul sent to Lawrence A. Tabak on July 27, 2022, Dr. Rand Paul website, accessed December 5, 2022, https://www.paul.senate.gov/news-dr-rand-paul-sends-letter-acting-nih-director-tabak-demanding-transparency-origins-covid-19.

65. Untitled press release about letter Rand Paul sent to Lawrence Tabak.

66. Isaac Stanley-Becker, "Rand Paul Discloses 16 Months Late that His Wife Bought Stock in Company Behind Covid Treatment," *Washington Post*, August 12, 2021; Berkeley Lovelace Jr., "Dr. Anthony Fauci Says Gilead's Remdesivir Will Set a New 'Standard of Care' for Coronavirus Treatment," CNBC, April 29, 2020.

67. US Coronavirus Vaccine Tracker, USAFacts, accessed December 1, 2022, https://usafacts.org/visualizations/covid-vaccine-tracker-states.

68. Rand Paul speaking on GrowUp Live, July 16, 2020, accessed December 1, 2022, https://twitter.com/robbystarbuck/status/1283778218193850369.

69. Rand Paul with Kelly Ashby Paul, *The Case against Socialism* (New York: Broadside, 2019).

70. April Siese, "Rand Paul Says He Won't Get Vaccinated Because He's Already Had COVID-19," ABC News, May 23, 2021.

71. Amitai Etzioni, *The Spirt of Community: Rights, Responsibilities, and the Communitarian Agenda* (New York: Crown, 1993), 166.

72. Arguably, the board's January 2023 report on regulating gain-of-function research was belated. See U.S. National Science Advisory Board for Biosecurity, *Proposed Biosecurity Oversight Framework for the Future of Science*, accessed February 1, 2023, https://osp.od.nih.gov/wp-content/uploads/2023/01/DRAFT-NSABB-WG-Report.pdf.

73. Lori Rozsa, "De Santis Forms Panel to Counter CDC, a Move Decried by Health Professionals," *Washington Post*, December 13, 2022. For an autobiographical account of challenging the biomedical consensus, see Ron De Santis, *The Courage to Be Free: Florida's Blueprint for America's Revival* (New York: HarperCollins, 2023).

74. Lauren Boebert, CPAC-Texas, Dallas, August 6, 2022, YouTube video, accessed April 12, 2024, https://www.youtube.com/watch?v=K88pvKZbOio.

75. *Rise of the Zombies: The Unauthorized and Unaccountable Government You Pay For: Hearing before the Subcommittee on Federal Spending Oversight and Emergency Management of the Committee on Homeland Security and Governmental Affairs, U.S. Senate, One Hundred Fifteenth Congress, Second Session, October 30, 2019* (Washington, DC: Government Printing Office, 2020), 4–5, https://www.govinfo.gov/content/pkg/CHRG-116shrg38897/pdf/CHRG-116shrg38897.pdf.

76. The zombie discourse backfired on Paul and stuck to him because of his obfuscations. For example, economist Paul Krugman called him out for "zombie lies" based on comments Paul made about the veracity of official employment figures at the end of Obama's first term. See Paul Krugman, "The Zombie that Ate Rand Paul's Brain," *New York Times*, September 9, 2012.

77. See, for example, Jack Butler, "Zombies in the Age of COVID-19," *National Review*, March 21, 2020.

78. Max Brooks, *The Zombie Survival Guide* (New York: Three Rivers, 2003), 2.

79. Brooks, *The Zombie Survival Guide*, xiii; Max Brooks, *World War Z: An Oral History of the Zombie War* (New York: Three Rivers, 2006), 7–8.

80. Comic-Con@Home 2020, "Zombies and the Coronavirus: Planning for the Next Big Outbreak," June 24, 2020, YouTube video, accessed December 1, 2022, https://youtu.be/GK7bCi52-vo.

81. Melissa Bell, "CDC Prepares for Zombie Apocalypse: Tips on How to Survive," *Washington Post*, May 19, 2011; Melissa Bell, "Zombie Apocalypse a Coup for CDC Emergency Team," *New York Times*, May 20, 2011.

82. Ma, *Severance*, 158.

83. Jiayang Fan, "Ling Ma's 'Severance' Captures the Bleak, Fatalistic Mood of 2018," *New Yorker*, December 19, 2018.

84. Ma, *Severance*, 29.

85. Ma, *Severance*, 29.

86. Ma, *Severance*, 4.

87. Ma, *Severance*, 19.

88. Ma, *Severance*, 149.

89. Ma, *Severance*, 31. On Candace's possible depression, see Courtney Vinopal, "Author Ling Ma Answers Your Questions about 'Severance,'" PBS, December 30, 2020, https://www.pbs.org/newshour/arts/author-ling-ma-answers-your-questions-about-severance.

90. Alison Bashford, "Epilogue: Panic's Past and Global Futures," in *Empires of Panic: Epidemics and Colonial Anxieties*, ed. Robert Peckham (Hong Kong: Hong Kong University Press, 2015), 204.

91. Yoram Lass, "Nothing Can Justify This Destruction of People's Lives"(interview with Fraser Myers), *Spiked*, May 20, 2020, https://www.spiked-online.com/2020/05/22/nothing-can-justify-this-destruction-of-peoples-lives.

92. Anthony Fauci, CNN, December 15, 2022, https://edition.cnn.com/audio/podcasts/axe-files/episodes/7a6f5b84-e344-44e7-9b1f-af6c00202c31. See also Anthony Fauci, *On Call: A Doctor's Journey in Public Service* (New York: Viking, 2024).

93. See Brendan Borrell, *The First Shots: The Epic Rivalries and Heroic Science behind the Race to the Coronavirus Vaccine* (Boston: Mariner, 2021), 127; Sandy Cohen, "The Fastest Vaccine in History," UCLA Health, December 10, 2020, https://www.uclahealth.org/news/the-fastest-vaccine-in-history; Brendan Borrell, "Inside the Messy Race to Develop a COVID Vaccine," *Esquire*, October 19, 2021.

94. Meagan C. Fitzpatrick, Seyed M. Moghadas, Abhishek Pandey, and Alison P. Galvaney, "Two Years of U.S. COVID-19 Vaccines Have Prevented Millions of Hospitalizations and Deaths," Commonwealth Fund, December 13, 2022, https://www.commonwealthfund.org/blog/2022/two-years-covid-vaccines-prevented-millions-deaths-hospitalizations.

95. Clinton, "Remarks at the California Institute of Technology in Pasadena, California," January 21, 2000, in *Public Papers of the Presidents of the United States: William J. Clinton, 2000, Book 1, January 1 to June 26, 2000* (Washington, DC: Government Printing Office, 2001), 100; Al Gore, *The Future: Six Drivers of Global Change* (New York: Random House, 2013), 208–211.

96. Edward H. Livingston, "Necessity of 2 Doses of the Pfizer and Moderna COVID-19 Vaccines," *JAMA* 325 (February 2021): 898.

97. Noam Barda, Noa Dagan, Yatir Ben-Shlomo, Eldad Kepten, Jacob Waxman, Reut Ohana, and Miguel A. Hernán, et al., "Safety of the BNT162b2 mRNA Covid-19 Vaccine in a Nationwide Setting," *New England Journal of Medicine* 385 (September 2021): 1078–1090.

98. CDC director Rochelle Walensky, speaking at "Press Briefing by White House COVID-19 Response Team and Public Health Officials," The White House, November 22, 2021, https://www.whitehouse.gov/briefing-room/press-briefings/2021/11/22/press-briefing-by-white-house-covid-19-response-team-and-public-health-officials-69.

99. On the liberal side of public health conspiracies, see Robert F. Kennedy Jr., *A Letter to Liberals: Censorship and COVID: An Attack on Science and American Ideals* (New York: Simon & Schuster, 2022).

100. Dan Diamond, "The Coronavirus Vaccine Skeptics Who Changed Their Minds," *Washington Post*, May 3, 2021; Savannah Walsh, "Anti-Vaxxer Fears Immunization Will Make Her a Zombie, Like *I Am Legend*," *Vanity Fair*, August 9, 2021.

101. Carlo Caduff, *The Pandemic Perhaps: Dramatic Events in a Public Culture of Danger* (Berkeley: University of California Press, 2015), 19.

102. Jonathan Lemire, Amanda Seitz, and Jill Colvin, "Trump Admin Tries to Narrow Stockpile's Role for States," PBS, April 3, 2022; Aaron Blake, "Trump Finds Someone to Blame for Coronavirus: Andrew Cuomo," *Washington Post*, March 24, 2020; Josh Dawsey and Michael Sherer, "How Cuomo's Flexing of Political Power Became His Undoing," *Washington Post* August 10, 2021.

103. *California Smarter: The Next Phase of California's COVID-19 Response*, February 2022, https://files.covid19.ca.gov/pdf/smarterplan.pdf.

104. Nik Brown, *Immunitary Life: A Biopolitics of Immunity* (London: Palgrave Macmillan, 2018), 5. See also Daniele Lorenzini, "Biopolitics in the Time of Coronavirus," *Critical Inquiry* 47 (Winter 2021): S40–S45.

105. Brown, *Immunitary Life*, 169.

106. Quotations from Roberto Esposito, *Bios: Biopolitics and Philosophy*, trans. Timothy Campbell (Minneapolis: University of Minnesota Press, 2008), 104. See also "The Biopolitics of Immunity in Times of COVID-19: An Interview with Roberto Esposito," Antipode Online, June 16, 2020, accessed December 1, 2022, https://antipodeonline.org /2020/06/16/interview-with-roberto-esposito/. See also Bithaj Ajana, "Immunitarianism: Defence and Sacrifice in the Politics of Covid-19," *History and Philosophy of the Life Sciences* 43 (February 2021), https//doi.org/10.1007/s40656-021-00384-9.

107. Roberto Esposito, *Immunitas: The Protection and Negation of Life*, trans. Zakiya Hanafi (2002; repr., Cambridge: Polity, 2011), 7.

108. Esposito, *Bios*, 104.

109. "The Biopolitics of Immunity in Times of COVID-19."

110. "The Biopolitics of Immunity in Times of COVID-19."

111. Esposito, *Immunitas*, 16.

112. Roberto Esposito, "Community, Immunity, Biopolitics," trans. Zakiya Hanafi, *Angelaki* 18 (September 2013): 85.

113. Esposito, "Community, Immunity, Biopolitics," 86.

114. Esposito, *Bios*, 44.

115. Roberto Esposito, *Terms of the Political: Community, Immunity, Biopolitics*, trans. Rhiannon Noel Welch (New York: Fordham University Press, 2013), 188. On the value and limitations of Esposito's ecological view of health, see Cary Wolfe, "(Auto)Immunity in Esposito and Derrida," in *Roberto Esposito: New Directions in Biophilosophy*, ed. Tilottama Rajan and Antonio Calcagno (Edinburgh: Edinburgh University Press, 2021), 153–173.

116. Roberto Esposito, *Persons and Things: From the Body's Point of View*, trans. Zakiya Hanafi (Cambridge: Polity, 2015), 142–144.

117. Roberto Esposito, *Communitas: The Origin and Destiny of Community*, trans. Timothy Campbell (1998; repr., Stanford, CA: Stanford University Press, 2013), 134; Esposito, *Bios*, 157; Esposito, "Community, Immunity, Biopolitics," 89.

118. Esposito, *Bios*, 159, 194; Esposito, "Community, Immunity, Biopolitics," 89.

119. Esposito, *Bios*, 194; Robert N. Bellah, Richard Madsen, William M. Sullivan, Ann Swidler, and Steven M. Tipson, *Habits of the Heart: Individualism and Commitment in American Life*, updated ed. (Berkeley: University of California Press, 1996), 218.

120. Bellah et al., *Habits of the Heart*, 218; Bellah et al., *The Good Society*, 279, 26.

121. Bellah et al., *The Good Society*, 278.

122. Steven Taylor and Caeleigh A. Landry, "COVID Stress Syndrome: Concept, Structure, and Correlates," *Depression and Anxiety* 37 (August 2020): 706–714.

123. Esposito, *Immunitas*, 147.

124. See Nikolas Rose, *Powers of Freedom: Reframing Political Thought* (Cambridge: Cambridge University Press, 1999), 188–191.

125. Esposito, "Community, Immunity, Biopolitics," 88; Esposito, *Immunitas*, 147 (quotation).

126. Alexander Gelfand, "COVID-19's Lasting Toll on Mental Health," *Hopkins Bloomberg Public Health*, November 2, 2020, https://magazine.jhsph.edu/2020/covid-19s-lasting-toll-mental-health; Alison Abbott, "COVID's Mental-Health Toll: How Scientists Are Tracking a Surge in Depression," *Nature* 590 (February 3, 2021); Josh Keller, "How Long Covid Exhausts the Body," *New York Times*, February 19, 2022.

127. Bruno Latour, *After Lockdown: A Metamorphosis*, trans. Julie Rose (Cambridge: Polity, 2021), 3, 7.

128. Elizabeth Povinelli, *Economies of Abandonment: Social Belonging and Endurance in Late Liberalism* (Durham, NC: Duke University Press, 2011), 133.

129. Noah Weiland, Maggie Haberman, Mark Mazzetti and Annie Karni, "Trump Was Sicker than Acknowledged with Covid-19," *New York Times*, February 11, 2021.

130. "Regeneron's REGN-COV2 Antibody Cocktail Reduced Viral Levels and Improved Symptoms in Non-Hospitalized COVID-19 Patients," PR Newswire, September 29, 2020, https://investor.regeneron.com/news-release-details/regenerons-regn-cov2-antibody-cocktail-reduced-viral-levels-and.

131. "Donald Trump Rally Johnstown, PA," October 13, 2020, https://www.rev.com/blog/transcripts/donald-trump-rally-johnstown-pa-transcript-october-13, accessed April 12, 2024.

132. "Donald Trump Rally Johnstown, PA."

133. Donald J. Trump, "Remarks at a White House Coronavirus Task Force Press Briefing," April 23, 2020, The American Presidency Project: https://www.presidency.ucsb.edu/documents/remarks-white-house-coronavirus-task-force-press-briefing-36. See also Meredith McGraw and Sam Stein, "It's Been Exactly One Year since Trump Suggested Injecting Bleach. We've Never Been the Same," *Politico*, April 23, 2021, https://www.politico.com/news/2021/04/23/trump-bleach-one-year-484399.

134. "Remarks by President Trump in Announcement on Remdesivir," May 1, 2020, White House Archives, https://trumpwhitehouse.archives.gov/briefings-statements/remarks-president-trump-announcement-remdesivir.

135. Julie Carrie Wong, "Hydroxychloroquine: How an Unproven Drug became Trump's Coronavirus "Miracle Cure,'" *Guardian*, April 7, 2020.

136. See Paige Williams, "Trump's Dangerous Messaging about a Possible Coronavirus Treatment," *New Yorker*, March 27, 2020; Kacper Niburski and Oskar Niburski, "Impact of Trump's Promotion of Unproven COVID-19 Treatments and Subsequent Internet Trends: Observational Study," *Journal of Medical Internet Research*, 22 (2020): e20044.

137. Dan Diamond, "Colleagues Paint a Mixed Picture of Ousted Vaccine Chief," *Politico*, May 13, 2020, https://www.politico.com/news/2020/05/13/rick-bright-vaccine-chief-coronavirus-254127.

138. See the People's CDC website: https://peoplescdc.org; and Emma Green, "The Case for Wearing Masks Forever," *New Yorker*, December 28, 2022. See also Peter J. Hotez, "The Antiscience Movement Is Escalating, Going Global and Killing Thousands," *Scientific American*, March 29, 2021; Tom Inglesby and J. Stephen Morrison, "How to Overhaul the C.D.C.," *New York Times*, May 7, 2023. The U.S. House's Committee on Energy and C'ommerce held a hearing on "Unmasking Challenges DCD Faces in Rebuilding Trust Amid Respiratory Illness Season," November 30, 2023, https://democrats-energycommerce.house.gov/committee-activity/hearings/hearing-unmasking-challenges-cdc-faces-rebuilding-public-trust-amid.

139. Open Letter from faculty members of Stanford University's Department of Medicine, September 9, 2020, https://int.nyt.com/data/documenttools/read-the-open-letter-from-stanford-doctors-on-scott-atlas/813b50f72b6543b4/full.pdf, accessed April 12, 2024.

140. "Open Letter from Stanford University's Department of Medicine"; "Dr. Scott Atlas: There Is No Risk to Children from Covid-19," Fox News Radio, July 9, 2020, https://radio.foxnews.com/2020/07/09/dr-scott-atlas-there-is-no-risk-to-children-from-covid-19-i-dont-know-why-people-deny-this.

141. Valerie Richardson, "Hydroxychloroquine Uproar Shows 'Objective Science Is Nearly Dead': Dr. Scott Atlas," *Washington Times*, August 29, 2020; Kelly Hooper, "Deborah Birx: 'Parallel Set of Data' on Covid-19 Was Delivered to Trump," *Politico*, January 24, 2021, https://www.politico.com/news/2021/0124/birx-trump-parallel-covid-data-461928. In 2023, Scott Atlas invited Rand Paul onto his Independent Institute podcast to discuss Rand's critiques of Fauci and the medical establishment: The Independent with Scott Atlas podcast, "Rand Paul: Unraveling Government Lies and Cover-Ups during the COVID Pandemic," October 12, 2023, https://www.independent.org/multimedia/detail.asp?id=7390.

142. On the dubious prescription practices of the Trump White House physician Ronny Jackson and his medical team see "'No Prescription Needed': Inside a White House Clinic's 'Systemic Problems,'" *Washington Post*, February 16, 2024.

143. Department of Health and Human Services, Food and Drug Administration, "Compliance Policy Guide Sec. 400.400 Conditions under Which Homeopathic Drugs May Be Marketed; Withdrawal of Guidance," 84 Fed. Reg. 207 (October 25, 2019), 57439–57441.

144. Letters from Anne Bressler to Ira Magaziner and Hillary Clinton, n.d. [1993], "Homeopaths/Chiropractors [Loose]," OA/ID 576, Box 22, Clinton Presidential Records Health Care Task Force General Files, Clinton Presidential Library, Little Rock, Arkansas.

145. U.S. Department of Health and Human Resources, *White House Commission on Complementary and Alternative Medicine Policy Final Report*, March 2002, https://govinfo.library.unt.edu/whccamp/pdfs/fr2002_document.pdf.

146. "FDA Warns Manufacturers of Products Labeled as Homeopathic for Putting Consumers at Risk with Significant Violations of Manufacturing Quality Standards," FDA news release, May 14, 2019, https://www.fda.gov/news-events/press-announcements/fda-warns-manufacturers-products-labeled-homeopathic-putting-consumers-risk-significant-violations.

147. Ashley Laderer, "Forsythia Is an Herbal Remedy that May Have Antibacterial and Antiviral Properties," *Business Insider India*, accessed December 1, 2022, https://www.insider.com/guides/health/forsythia-medicine.

148. See Jackson Oliver Webster, "The Forsythia-Industrial Complex," Medium, May 22, 2020, https://medium.com/wonk-bridge/the-forsythia-industrial-complex-abcb2cee678d.

149. Hannah E. Davis, Lisa McCorkell, Julia Moore Vogel, and Eric J. Topol, "Long COVID: Major Findings, Mechanisms and Recommendations," *Nature Reviews Microbiology*, January 2023, https://doi.org/10.1038/s41579-022-00846-2.

150. House Oversight and Reform Select Subcommittee on the Coronavirus Crisis, "Understanding and Addressing Long COVID and Its Health and Economic Consequences," 17, 20.

151. Pam Belluck, "'I Feel Like I Have Dementia': Brain Fog Plagues Covid Survivors," *New York Times*, July 20, 2021.

152. Arman Fesharaki-Zadeh, Naomi Lowe, and Amy F. T. Arnsten, "Clinical Experience with the α2A-Adrenoceptor Agonist, Guanfacine, and N-acetylcysteine for the Treatment of Cognitive Deficits in 'LongCOVID19,'" *Neuroimmunology Reports* 3 (November 2022): 100154; Department of Health and Human Services, "HHS Announces the Formation of the Office of Long COVID Research and Practice and Long COVID Trials through the Recover Initiative," July 31, 2023, https://www.hhs.gov/about/news/2023/07/31/hhs-announces-formation-office-long-covid-research-practice-launch-long-covid-clinical-trials-through-recover-initiative.html.

153. "Day 4: Microdosing with THCV, NMN for Longevity and More with Valhalla Vitality," *Biohacking Brittany*, podcast, December 4, 2022, https://biohackingbrittany.com/blogs/podcast/day4; "Hacking Brain Fog," *The Human Upgrade with Dave Asprey*, podcast, September 27, 2022, https://podcasts.apple.com/us/podcast/hacking-brain-fog-interventions-with-dave-keri/id451295014?i=1000580819671; "How to Hack Zombie Cells and Maximize Your Lifespan," Dave Asprey, n.d., accessed December 1, 2022, https://daveasprey.com/how-to-hack-your-lifespan. In June 2020, Asprey was warned by the FTC for "unlawfully advertising that certain products prevent or treat" COVID; "Warning Letter to Dave Asprey," June 19, 2020, FTC, accessed December 1, 2022, https://www.ftc.gov/legal-library/browse/warning-letters/warning-letter-dave-asprey.

154. Casey Schwartz, "The Age of Distracti-pression," *New York Times,* July 9, 2022.

155. "When WTF Means Your Freedom's at Stake," *The Human Upgrade with Dave Asprey*, podcast, January 31, 2022, https://daveasprey.com/dave-solo-freedom-898.

CHAPTER 8 — INVISIBLE TOXICITIES

1. Cambridge Institute for Applied Research, Inc., "Black Americans," briefing document for Domestic Policy Council, Box 1, John Bridgeland Subject Files, Domestic Policy Council, George W. Bush Presidential Library, Dallas, Texas.

2. Paul Crutzen and Eugene Stoermer, "The Anthropocene," *IGBP Global Change Newsletter* 41 (May 2000): 17–18; Sverker Sorlin and Paul Warde, eds., *The Future of Nature: Documents of Global Change* (New Haven, CT: Yale University Press, 2013).

3. Jessica Fanzo, "No Food Security, No World Order," in *COVID-19 and World Order: The Future of Conflict, Competition, and Cooperation*, ed. Hal Brands and Francis J. Gavin (Baltimore, MD: Johns Hopkins University Press, 2020), 148–168.

4. Jennifer Thomson, *The Wild and the Toxic: American Environmentalism and the Politics of Health* (Chapel Hill: University of North Carolina Press, 2019), 1.

5. "Recent Positive Environmental Action by Administration," March 2001, Earth Work, Box 6, John Bridgeland Subject Files, Domestic Policy Council, George W. Bush Presidential Library.

6. George W. Bush, "Remarks on Global Climate Change," June 11, 2001, in *Public Papers of the Presidents of the United States: George W. Bush, 2001, Book 1, January 20 to June 30, 2001* (Washington, DC: Government Printing Office, 2003), 634.

7. Bush, "Remarks on Global Climate Change," 634.

8. Jane M. Orient, president of Doctors for Disaster Preparedness, to Andrew Card, March 30, 2001, "Global Climate Change [Folder 3]: Doctors for Disaster Preparedness [1]," Box 11, John Bridgeland, Domestic Policy Council, George W. Bush Presidential Library.

9. Tim Dickinson, "The Secret Campaign of President Bush's Administration to Deny Global Warming," *Rolling Stone*, June 20, 2007.

10. Bush, "Remarks on Global Climate Change," 635–636.

11. Bush, "Remarks on Global Climate Change," 634, 637. See also Geof Rayner and Tim Lang, *Ecological Public Health: Reshaping the Conditions for Good Health* (London: Routledge, 2012), 213–218; and David B. Resnik, *Environmental Health Ethics* (Cambridge: Cambridge University Press, 2012), 56–79.

12. Barack Obama, "Remarks to the Detroit Economic Club," May 7, 2007, American Presidency Project, https://www.presidency.ucsb.edu/documents/remarks-the-detroit-economic-club-0.

13. Barack Obama, "Remarks Following a Roundtable Discussion on Climate Change and Public Health at Howard University," April 7, 2015, in *Public Papers of the Presidents of the United States: Barack Obama, 2015, Book 1, January 1 to June 30, 2015* (Washington, DC: Government Printing Office, 2020), 394–6. See also Judith Rodin, "Climate Action Is a Health Priority," *Time*, September 25, 2014.

14. White House Public Health and Climate Change Summit, June 23, 2015, YouTube video, accessed November 15, 2022, https://youtu.be/5OTeoMHZkrI.

15. Bruno Latour, *After Lockdown: A Metamorphosis*, trans. Julie Rose (Cambridge: Polity, 2021), 3, 30; Exec. Order no. 13855, "Promoting Active Management of America's Forests, Rangelands, and Other Federal Lands to Improve Conditions and Reduce Wildfire Risks," December 21, 2018, 84 Fed. Reg. 4 (January 7, 2019), 45–48; Joseph R. Biden, "Statement by the President-Elect Joe Biden on the 50th Anniversary of the Environmental Protection Agency," December 2, 2020, American Presidency Project, https://www.presidency.ucsb.edu/documents/statement-president-elect-joe-biden-the-50th-anniversary-the-environmental-protection.

16. Justin Worland, "Taking Climate Seriously," *Time*, November 23, 2020.

17. Latour, *After Lockdown*, 115.

18. John Kerry, "Implementation Plus: Global Climate Action in 2022," remarks at American University Cairo, February 21, 2022, U.S. Department of State, https://www.state.gov/special-presidential-envoy-for-climate-john-kerry-implementation-plus-global-climate-action-in-2022.

19. US Senate, Committee on Environment and Public Works, *Examining the Human Health Impacts of Global Warming: Hearing Before the Committee on Environment and Public Works, United States Senate, One Hundred Tenth Congress, First Session, October 23, 200*, (Washington, DC: Government Printing Office, 2013), 23.

20. Thomson, *The Wild and the Toxic*, 132.

21. Nik Brown, "Containing Contradictions: Debating Nature, Controversy and Biotechnology," in *Reconfiguring Nature: Issues and Debates in the New Genetics*, ed. Peter Glasner (London: Ashgate, 2004), 260.

22. "National Biotechnology Week," Proclamation 7438, May 16, 2001, 37 Fed. Reg. 20 (May 21, 2001), 755.

23. Declassified Documents Concerning Agricultural Biotechnology, Clinton Digital Library, https://clinton.presidentiallibraries.us/items/show/100502; US Senate, Committee on Agriculture, Nutrition, and Forestry, "Agriculture Biotechnology: A Look at Federal Regulation and Stakeholder Perspectives," October 21, 2015, accessed November 10, 2022, https://www.agriculture.senate.gov/hearings/agriculture-biotechnology-a-look-at-federal-regulation-and-stakeholder-perspectives; U.S. Department of Agriculture, "Biotechnology FAQs," accessed November 10, 2022, https://www.usda.gov/topics/biotechnology/biotechnology-frequently-asked-questions-faqs.

24. On the health impacts of PCBs in Anniston, see the CBS film *Toxic Town* (2003) and Jane Kay and Cheryl Katz, "Pollution, Poverty and People of Color: Living with Industry," *Scientific American*, June 2012.

25. Ruth Ozeki, *All Over Creation* (New York: Canongate, 2013); *Seeding Fear*, dir. Craig Jackson (2015).

26. See Donald L. Barlett and James B. Steele, "Monsanto's Harvest of Fear," *Vanity Fair*, May 2008; Carey Gillam, *Whitewash: The Story of a Weed Killer, Cancer, and the Corruption of Science* (New York: Island Press, 2017).

27. See Henry I. Miller and George Conko, *The Frankenfood Myth: How Protest and Politics Threaten the Biotech Revolution* (New York: Praeger, 2004).

28. Robert N. Butler, *The Longevity Revolution: The Benefits and Challenges of Living a Long Life* (New York: Public Affairs, 2008), 365.

29. Butler, *The Longevity Revolution*, 363.

30. Butler, *The Longevity Revolution*, 374.

31. "An Ecomodernist Manifesto," accessed July 1, 2023, http://www.ecomodernism .org/manifesto-english.

32. World Economic Forum, "Biosolutions: A Clear Path to Fighting Climate Change," May 23, 2022, https://www.weforum.org/agenda/2022/05/biosolutions-clear -path-to-fight-climate-change; Organisation for Economic Co-operation and Development, *Industrial Biotechnology and Climate Change: Opportunities and Challenges* (Organisation for Economic Co-operation and Development, 2011); George Monbiot, "Meet the Ecomodernists: Ignorant of History and Paradoxically Old-Fashioned," *Guardian*, September 24, 2015.

33. George H. W. Bush, "Remarks to the National Academy of Sciences," April 23, 1990, *Public Papers of the Presidents of the United States, George H. W. Bush: Book 1, January 1 to June 30, 1990* (Washington, DC: Government Printing Office, 1991), 545. For Bush-era environmental and biotech studies, see Committee on Earth Sciences, *Our Changing Planet: A U.S. Strategy for Global Change Research* (Washington, DC: National Academies Press, 1988); and "Fact Sheet on FDA Biotechnology Food Policy," May 26, 1992, "Bio Tech Food Products," Box 18, Council on Competitiveness Files, Office of Vice President Dan Quayle, George H. W. Bush Presidential Library, College Station, Texas.

34. Bush, "Remarks to the National Academy of Sciences," 545.

35. Bill McKibben, *The End of Nature* (1989; repr., New York: Doubleday, 1999), 204; Bill McKibben, *Enough: Staying Human in an Engineered Age* (New York: Henry Holt, 2003), 65.

36. Bill McKibben, *Eaarth: Making a Life on a Tough New Planet* (New York: St Martin's, 2011), 2–3; Ursula K. Heise, *Imagining Extinction: The Cultural Meanings of Endangered Species* (Chicago: University of Chicago Press, 2016), 8–9.

37. Thomson, *The Wild and the Toxic*, 124–127, 134.

38. "Bill McKibben: The Trump Presidency Comes When the Warming World Can Least Afford It," *Democracy Now*, December 10, 2016, https://www.democracynow.org /2016/11/10/bill_mckibben_trumps_presidency_comes_when; Bill McKibben, "Barack Obama, the Carbon President," *Guardian*, June 3, 2011; "McKibben to Clinton: Now It's Really Time to Get Serious about Climate Change," *Grist*, June 12, 2015, https://grist.org /politics/mckibben-to-clinton-here-are-7-things-you-need-to-do-to-clean-up-your -climate-act; Bill McKibben, "The Biden Administration's Landmark Day in the Flight for the Climate," *New Yorker*, January 28, 2021; Bill McKibben, "Joe Biden Just Did the Rarest Thing in US Politics: He Stood Up To The Oil Industry," *The Guardian*, February 7, 2024.

39. Timothy Clark, "Scale. Derangements of Scale," in *Telemorphosis: Theory in the Era of Climate Change*, vol. 1, ed. Tom Cohen (Open Humanities Press, 2012), 148–166.

40. Latour, *After Lockdown*, 125.

41. See Artemis Dona and Ioannis S. Arvanitoyannis, "Health Risks of Genetically Modified Foods," *Critical Review of Food Science and Nutrition* 49, no. 2 (February 2009): 164–175.

42. Naomi Wilson and Keith Rae, *Climate Change and Mental Health: Report from a COP-26 Public Participation Event* (World Health Foundation, April 2022), https://www .mentalhealth.org.uk/sites/default/files/2022-07/MHF-Scotland-Climate-Change -COP26-report_0.pdf; World Health Organization, *Mental Health and Climate Change: Policy Brief* (2022), https://www.who.int/publications/i/item/9789240045125; Maya K. Gislason, Angel M. Kennedy and Stephanie M. Witham, "The Interplay between Social and Ecological Determinants of Mental Health for Children and Youth in the Climate Crisis," *International Journal of Environmental Research and Public Health* 18, no. 9 (April 2021): 4573, https://doi.org/10.3390/ijerph18094573.

43. See Robert Carton, "Fluoridation: Scientific Fraud Alleged," *Health Freedom News*, August 1993.

44. Heather Houser, *Ecosickness in Contemporary U.S. Fiction* (New York: Columbia University Press, 2014), 2–3.

45. Houser, *Ecosickness in Contemporary U.S. Fiction*, 1.

46. Houser, *Ecosickness in Contemporary U.S. Fiction*, 224. On toxicity in *Safe*, see Lawrence Buell, "Toxic Discourse," *Critical Inquiry* 24 (Spring 1998): 639–665; and Sara Hosey, "Canaries and Coalmines: Toxic Discourse in 'The Incredible Shrinking Woman' and 'Safe,'" *Feminist Formations* 23, no. 2 (Summer 2011): 77–97.

47. Jeff VanderMeer, *Borne: A Novel* (New York: HarperCollins, 2017), 145.

48. Environmental Defense Fund, *Toxic Ignorance: The Continuing Absence of Basic Health Testing for Top-Selling Chemicals in the United States* (New York: Environmental Defense Fund, 1997).

49. See Atif Khan, Oleguer Plana-Ripoll, Sussie Antonsen, Jørgen Brandt, Camilla Geels, Hannah Landecker, Patrick F. Sullivan, et al., "Environmental Pollution Is Associated with Increased Risk of Psychiatric Disorders in the US and Denmark," *PLOS Biology* 17, no. 10 (October 2019): e3000513.

50. Susan L. Prescott and Jeffrey S. Bland, "Spaceship Earth Revisited: The Co-Benefits of Overcoming Biological Extinction of Experience at the Level of Person, Place and Planet," *Environmental Research and Public Health* 17, no. 4 (February 2020), 10.3390/ijerph17041407.

51. Dorceta E. Taylor, *Toxic Communities: Environmental Racism, Industrial Pollution, and Residential Mobility* (New York: New York University Press, 2014), 22–24; Emma Marris, "First Tests Show Flood Waters High in Bacteria and Lead," *Nature* 427 (September 15, 2005).

52. National Research Council, *Oil in the Sea III: Inputs, Fates, and Effects* (Washington, DC: National Academies Press, 2003), 119–158; Joy D. Osofsky and Howard J. Osofsky, "Hurricane Katrina and the Gulf Oil Spill: Lessons Learned about Short-Term and

Long-Term Effects," *International Journal of Psychology* 56, no. 1 (February 2021): 56–63; Danielle Buttke, Sara Vagi, Tesfaye Bayleyegn, Kanta Sircar, Tara Strine, Melissa Morrison, Mardi Allen, et al., "Mental Health Needs Assessment after the Gulf Coast Oil Spill—Alabama and Mississippi, 2010," *Prehospital and Disaster Medicine* 27, no. 5 (October 2012): 401–408.

53. George H. W. Bush, "The President's News Conference," April 10, 1992, in *Public Papers of the Presidents of the United States: George H. W. Bush, 1992, Book 1, January 1 to July 31, 1992* (Washington, DC: Government Printing Office, 1993), 587.

54. David Biello, "How Microbes Helped Clean BP's Oil Spill," *Scientific American*, April 28, 2015; Ronald M. Atlas and Terry C. Hazen, "Oil Biodegradation and Bioremediation," *Environmental Science and Technology* 45, no. 16 (August 2015): 6709–6715; Catherine Kilduff and Jaclyn Lopez, "Dispersants: The Lesser of Two Evils or a Cure Worse than the Disease?," *Ocean and Coastal Law Journal* 16, no. 2 (2010): 375–394.

55. Barack Obama, "Foreword," in in *Public Papers of the Presidents of the United States: Barack Obama, 2010, Book 1, January 1 to June 30, 2010* (Washington, DC: Government Printing Office, 2013), v.

56. Barack Obama, "Remarks on the Oil Spill in the Gulf of Mexico," May 14, 2010 and "The President's Weekly Address," May 22, 2010, in *Public Papers of the Presidents: Barack Obama, 2010,* Book 1, 658, 691, respectively.

57. US House of Representatives, *The BP Oil Spill: Human Exposure and Environmental Fate: Hearing before the Subcommittee on Energy and Environment of the Committee on Energy and Commerce, House of Representatives, One Hundred Eleventh Congress, Second Session, June 10, 2010* (Washington, DC: Government Printing Office, 2013); Lynn M. Grattan, Sparkle Roberts, William T. Mahan Jr., Patrick K. McLaughlin, W. Steven Otwell, and J. Glenn Morris Jr., "The Early Psychological Impacts of the Deepwater Horizon Oil Spill on Florida and Alabama Communities," *Environmental Health Perspectives* 119, no. 6 (June 2011): 838–843; Howard Osofsky, Joy D. Osofsky, and Tonya C. Hansel, "Deepwater Horizon Oil Spill: Mental Health Effects on Residents in Heavily Affected Areas," *Disaster Medicine and Public Health Preparedness* 5, no. 4 (December 2011): 280–286; Mark A. D'Andrea and G. Kesava Reddy, "The Development of Long-Term Adverse Health Effects in Oil Spill Cleanup Workers of the Deepwater Horizon Offshore Drilling Rig Disaster," *Frontiers of Public Health* 6, no. 117 (April 2018), https://doi.org/10.3389/fpubh.2018.00117.

58. Barack Obama "Remarks Following a Meeting with the Cochairs of the National Commission on the BP Deepwater Horizon Oil Spill and Offshore Drilling," June 1, 2010, in *Public Papers of the Presidents of the United States: Barack Obama, 2010, Book 1, January 1 to June 30, 2010* (Washington, DC: Government Printing Office, 2010), 747.

59. Kyle Purdy, "The Long-Term Health Effects of the BP Deepwater Horizon Oil Disaster," intern blog, Mobile Baykeeper, April 17, 2020, accessed March 1, 2023, https://facultystaff.richmond.edu/~sabrash/110/Chem%20110%2001%20Spring%202021%20Homework%20Articles/B00_Long_Term_Health_Effects.pdf.

60. Hannah B. Vander Zanden, Alan B Bolten, Anton D Tucker, Kristen M. Hart, Margaret M. Lamont, Ikuko Fujisaki, Kimberly J. Reich, et al., "Biomarkers Reveal Sea

Turtles Remained in Oiled Areas Following the Deepwater Horizon Oil Spill," *Ecological Applications* 26, no. 7 (October 2016): 2145–2155; Connie May Fowler, *A Million Fragile Bones* (Tallahassee, FL: Twisted Road, 2017), 13.

61. "Interview: Paolo Bacigalupi Talks about *The Windup Girl*," *Boston Phoenix*, August 6, 2010.

62. *The Big Fix*, dir. Joshua Tickell (2011); *Pretty Slick*, dir. James Fox (2015); Fowler, *A Million Fragile Bones*, 300–301.

63. Fowler, *A Million Fragile Bones*, 242. See also Craig J. McGowan, Richard K. Kwok, Lawrence S. Engel, Mark R. Stenzel, Patricia A. Stewart, and Dale P. Sandler, "Respiratory, Dermal, and Eye Irritation Symptoms Associated with Corexit™," *Environmental Health Perspectives* 125, no. 9 (September 2017), https://doi.org/10.1289/EHP1677.

64. Zane Grey, *Tales of Southern Rivers* (1924; repr., New York: Derrydale Press, 2000), 82.

65. Rob Nixon, *Slow Violence and the Environmentalism of the Poor* (Cambridge, MA: Harvard University Press, 2011), 2–3.

66. Harry S. Truman, "Address on Conservation at the Dedication of Everglades National Park," December 6, 1947, in *Public Papers of the Presidents of the United States: Harry S. Truman, 1947* (Washington, DC: Government Printing Office, 1963), 505.

67. Michael Grunwald, *The Swamp: The Everglades, Florida, and the Politics of Paradise* (New York: Simon & Schuster, 2007), 1–3.

68. Bill Clinton, "Remarks at a Democratic National Committee Dinner," August 7, 1997, in *Public Papers of the Presidents of the United States: William J. Clinton, 1997*, Book 2, *July 1 to December 31, 1997* (Washington, DC: Government Printing Office, 1999), 1078; Clinton, "The President's Radio Address," May 29, 1999, in *Public Papers of the Presidents of the United States: William J. Clinton, 1999*, Book 1, *July 1 to December 31, 1999* (Washington, DC: Government Printing Office, 2001), 856; Truman, "Address on Conservation at the Dedication of Everglades National Park," 505–506.

69. Bill Clinton, "Opening Remarks at the White House Conference on Climate Change," October 6, 1997, in *Public Papers of the Presidents of the United States: William J. Clinton, 1997*, Book 2, *January 1 to June 30, 1997* (Washington, DC: Government Printing Office, 1999), 1294.

70. Bill Clinton, "Interview with Leonardo DiCaprio for ABC News' 'Planet Earth 2000,'" March 31, 2000, in *Public Papers of the Presidents of the United States: William J. Clinton, 2000*, Book 1, *January 1 to June 26, 2000* (Washington, DC: Government Printing Office, 2002), 761.

71. Clinton, "The President's Radio Address," 856.

72. "Florida Trip," "Everglades [1]," Box 8, John Bridgeland Subject Files, Domestic Policy Council, George W. Bush Library.

73. George W. Bush, "Everglades National Park," June 4, 2001, in *Public Papers of the Presidents of the United States: George W. Bush, 2001*, Book 1, *January 20 to June 30, 2001* (Washington, DC: Government Printing Office, 2003), 607–608.

74. Bush, "Everglades National Park," 608.

75. Donavyn Coffey, "First Genetically Modified Mosquitos Released in U.S. Are Hatching Now," *Scientific American*, May 14, 2021.

76. Brigit Katz, "'Staggering' Damage to Florida's Everglades Remains in the Wake of Hurricane Irma," *Smithsonian Magazine*, April 20, 2018.

77. US House of Representatives, *Florida Everglades Restoration: What Are the Priorities? Oversight Hearing before the Subcommittee on Fisheries, Wildlife, Oceans, and Insular Affairs of the Committee on Natural Resources, U.S. House of Representatives, One Hundred Twelfth Congress, First Session, Thursday, November 3, 2011* (Washington, DC: Government Printing Office, 2012); Barack Obama, "Remarks at Everglades National Park in Homestead, Florida," April 22, 2015, in *Public Papers of the Presidents of the United States: Barack Obama, 2015, Book 1, January 1 to June 30, 2015* (Washington, DC: Government Printing Office, 2020), 491–493.

78. Houser, *Ecosickness in Contemporary U.S. Fiction*, 219.

79. Everglades Ecosystem Assessment Program, *Everglades Ecosystem Assessment: Water Management and Quality, Eutrophication, Mercury Contamination, Soils and Habitat* (Washington, DC: US Environmental Protection Agency, 2007), 16.

80. Steven M. Davis and John C. Ogden, *Everglades: The Ecosystem and Its Restoration* (Delray Beach, FL: St. Lucie Press, 1994); Benis N. Egoh, Charity Nyelele, Karen D. Holl, James M. Bullock, Steve Carver, and Christopher J. Sandom, "Rewilding and Restoring Nature in a Changing World," *PLOS ONE* 16, no. 7 (July 2021): e0254249.

81. Taylor, *Toxic Communities*, 103–104. On increasing tourism, see Barack Obama, "Remarks at Walt Disney World Resort in Lake Buena Vista, Florida," January 19, 2012, in *Public Papers of the Presidents of the United States: Barack Obama, 2012, Book 1, January 1 to June 30, 2012* (Washington, DC: Government Printing Office, 2016), 50–52.

82. Jeff VanderMeer, "The Annihilation of Florida: An Overlooked National Tragedy," *Current Affairs*, May 18, 2022, https://www.currentaffairs.org/2022/05/the-annihilation -of-florida-an-overlooked-national-tragedy. On VanderMeer's response to the BP oil spill, see "Nature, the Oil Spill, and Interdependence," Jeff VanderMeer, May 19, 2010, accessed March 1, 2023, https://www.jeffvandermeer.com/2010/05/19/nature-the-oil-spill -and-interdependence.

83. VanderMeer published *Absolution*, a fourth book in the Southern Reach series, in October 2024.

84. Jeff VanderMeer, "From Annihilation to Acceptance: A Writer's Surreal Journey," *Atlantic*, January 28, 2015.

85. Jeff VanderMeer, "Hauntings in the Anthropocene: An Initial Exploration," *Environmental Critique*, July 7, 2016, accessed November 1, 2022, https://environmentalcritique .wordpress.com/2016/07/07/hauntings-in-the-anthropocene; Timothy Morton, *Hyperobjects: Philosophy and Ecology after the End of the World* (Minneapolis: University of Minnesota Press, 2013), 28.

86. Morton, *Hyperobjects*, 39.

87. Morton, *Hyperobjects*, 33; Brian Bethune "How Annihilation Author Jeff Vander-Meer Became King of the 'New Weird,'" *McLean's* 131, no. 2 (March 2018).

88. VanderMeer, "Hauntings in the Anthropocene"; Steve Lerner, *Sacrifice Zones: The Front Lines of Toxic Chemical Exposure in the United States* (Cambridge, MA: MIT Press, 2010).

89. Jeff VanderMeer, *Authority* (New York: HarperCollins, 2014), 8.

90. Taylor, *Toxic Communities*, 33–46.

91. Jeff VanderMeer, *Annihilation* (New York: HarperCollins, 2014), 94; VanderMeer, *Authority*, 35, 29.

92. VanderMeer, *Authority*, 28.

93. VanderMeer, "From Annihilation to Acceptance"; Louise Econimides and Laura Shackleford, eds., *Surreal Entanglements: Essays on Jeff VanderMeer's Fiction* (New York: Routledge, 2021), 6–7. The Southern Reach books suggest that the phrase "pristine wilderness" might be part of the government cover-up.

94. VanderMeer, "Hauntings in the Anthropocene."

95. Jeff VanderMeer, *Acceptance* (New York: HarperCollins, 2014), 178. See also Georgie Newson-Errey, "Weird Horizons and the Mysticism of the Unhuman in Jeff Vander-Meer's *Southern Reach* Trilogy," *Cambridge Quarterly* 50, no. 4 (December 2021): 368–388. On planetary eccentricity, see Frédéric Neyrat, *The Unconstructable Earth: An Ecology of Separation*, trans. Drew S. Burk (New York: Fordham University Press, 2019), 172–174.

96. "Working Definition of New Weird," Jeff VanderMeer, September 27, 2007, accessed November 1, 2022, https://www.jeffvandermeer.com/2007/09/27/working-definition-of-new-weird.

97. VanderMeer, *Authority*, 113.

98. Clark, "Scale," 148–149; VanderMeer, *Annihilation*, 174.

99. VanderMeer, *Annihilation*, 178.

100. VanderMeer, *Annihilation*, 175.

101. VanderMeer, *Annihilation*, 82, 34.

102. VanderMeer, *Annihilation*, 30.

103. Morton, *Hyperobjects*, 43.

104. VanderMeer, *Authority*, 89–96.

105. VanderMeer, *Annihilation*, 133, 171.

106. Jon Hegglund, "Unnatural Narratology and Weird Realism in Jeff VanderMeer's *Annihilation*," in *Environment and Narrative: New Directions in Econarratology*, ed. Erin James and Eric Morel (Columbus: Ohio State University Press, 2020), 30.

107. VanderMeer, *Annihilation*, 69.

108. Andrew Strombeck, "Inhuman Writing in Jeff VanderMeer's Southern Reach Trilogy," *Textual Practice* 34, no. 8 (August 2020): 1366.

109. Strombeck, "Inhuman Writing in Jeff VanderMeer's Southern Reach Trilogy," 1367.

110. VanderMeer, *Annihilation*, 97–98.

111. VanderMeer, *Annihilation*, 170.

112. VanderMeer, *Annihilation*, 193.

113. VanderMeer, *Annihilation*, 74.

114. VanderMeer, *Authority*, 17.

115. VanderMeer, *Acceptance*, 185, 162–163.

116. VanderMeer, *Acceptance*, 168. See also Lara Choksey, *Narrative in the Age of the Genome* (London: Bloomsbury, 2021), 180–181.

117. VanderMeer, *Acceptance*, 178.

118. VanderMeer, *Authority*, 55–7.

119. Fowler, *A Million Fragile Bones*, 292.

120. Beatriz da Costa and Kavita Philip, eds., *Tactical Biopolitics: Art, Activism, and Technoscience* (Cambridge, MA: MIT Press, 2008), xix.

121. VanderMeer, *Borne*, 21–2.

122. See Monica Sousa, "'Am I a Person?': Biotech Animals and Posthumanist Empathy in Jeff VanderMeer's *Borne*," in *Transhumanism and Posthumanism in Twenty-First Century Narrative*, ed. Sonia Baelo-Allué and Monica Calvo-Pascual (New York: Routledge, 2021), 191.

123. Jeff VanderMeer, "It's 2071, and We Have Bioengineered Our Own Extinction," *New York Times*, December 9, 2019.

124. Jeffrey Kluger, "Earth at the Tipping Point: Global Warming Heats Up," *Time*, April 3, 2006.

125. Eugene Linden/Churchill, "The Big Meltdown," *Time*, September 4, 2000.

126. Finis Dunaway, *Seeing Green: The Use and Abuse of American Environmental Images* (Chicago: University of Chicago Press, 2015), 260.

127. Annie Leibovitz, "Leo and the Bear," *Vanity Fair*, May 2007; Bryan Walsh, "It's Very, Very Alarming. It's a Warning Signal," *Time*, October 15, 2007.

128. See Dunaway, *Seeing Green*, 264, 268.

129. The book of the documentary sequel was published as Al Gore, *An Inconvenient Sequel: Truth to Power* (New York: Rodale, 2017).

130. Tom Simonite, "Drowning Polar Bears Worry Researchers," *Nature*, December 20, 2005; Stephen Leahy, "Polar Bears Really Are Starving Because of Global Warming, Study Shows," *National Geographic*, February 1, 2018.

131. Al Gore, *An Inconvenient Truth* (New York: Rodale, 2006), 11, 166–169; Dunaway, *Seeing Green*, 260.

132. Bill McKibben, President's Medal Speech, Geological Society of America, November 4, 2012, YouTube video, accessed March 1, 2023, https://www.youtube.com /watch?v=go2TxNZOB4w.

133. Sharon Bushell and Stan Jones, *The Spill: Personal Stories from the Exxon Valdez Disaster* (Kenmore, WA: Epicenter Press, 2009), 242–255.

134. Al Gore, *The Future: Six Drivers of Global Change* (New York: Random House, 2013), 317–318.

135. Jeff Richardson, "'Frozen Gore' Sculpture Returns in Fairbanks to Fuel Climate Change Debate," *Fairbanks Daily News-Miner,* January 5, 2010.

136. Gore, *The Future,* 280–281; Al Gore, *The Assault on Reason* (New York: Penguin, 2007), 25.

137. Gore, *The Future,* 281.

138. Ursula K. Heise, *Sense of Place and Sense of Planet: The Environmental Imagination of the Global* (Oxford: Oxford University Press, 2008), 209. See also James Lyons, "'Gore Is the World': Embodying Environmental Risk in *An Inconvenient Truth,*" *Journal of Risk Research* 22, no. 9 (February 2019): 1156–1170.

139. Al Gore, Nobel Lecture, Oslo, Norway, December 10, 2007, https://www .nobelprize.org/prizes/peace/2007/gore/lecture.

140. Dan McDougall, "Life on Thin Ice," *Guardian,* August 12, 2019.

141. Subhankar Banerjee, "Why Polar Bears? Seeing the Arctic Anew," in *Living in the Anthropocene: Earth in the Age of Humans,* ed. W. John Kress and Jeffrey K. Stine (Washington, DC: Smithsonian Institute, 2017), 120.

142. Lerner, *Sacrifice Zones,* 221.

143. Lerner, *Sacrifice Zones,* 222–225.

144. Sheila Watt-Cloutier, *The Right to Be Cold: One Woman's Fight to Protect the Arctic and Save the Planet from Climate Change* (Minneapolis: University of Minnesota Press, 2015), xix, 247, 307–310.

145. "Fact Sheet: President Obama Announces New Investments to Combat Climate Change and Assist Remote Alaskan Communities," September 2, 2015, American Presidency Project, https://www.presidency.ucsb.edu/documents/fact-sheet-president-obama -announces-new-investments-combat-climate-change-and-assist.

146. Watt-Cloutier, *The Right to Be Cold,* 99–100, 193.

147. Jennifer Redvers, Peter Bjerregaard, Heidi Eriksen, Sahar Fanian, Gwen Healey, Vanessa Hiratsuka, Michael Jong, et al., "A Scoping Review of Indigenous Suicide Prevention in Circumpolar Regions," *International Journal of Circumpolar Health* 74, no. 1 (March 2015): 10.3402/ijch.v74.27509.

148. Watt-Cloutier, *The Right to Be Cold,* 134–136; Sheila Watt-Cloutier, "The Inuit Journey toward a POPs-Free World," in *Northern Lights against POPs: Combatting Toxic Threats in the Arctic,* ed. David Leonard Downie and Terry Fenge (Montreal: McGill-Queen's University Press, 2003), 256–267. See also Stephen Bocking, "Toxic Surprises: Contaminants and Knowledge in the Northern Environment," in *Ice Blink: Navigating Northern Environmental History,* ed. Stephen Bocking and Brad Martin (Calgary: University of Calgary Press, 2017), 421–464.

149. Debra F. Horwitz, "Mental Health in Animals: A Veterinary Behaviorist's View," in *Mental Health and Well-being in Animals*, ed. Franklin D. McMillan, 2nd ed. (Boston: CABI, 2020), 3.

150. David Sherpedson, Karen D. Lewis, Kathy Carlstead, Joan Bauman, and Nancy Perrin, "Individual and Environmental Factor Associated with Stereotypic Behavior and Fecal Glucocorticoid Metabolite Levels in Zoo Housed Polar Bears," *Applied Animal Behaviour Science* 147, no. 3–4 (August 2013): 268–277; "Confined, Hot and Lonely, No Wonder Arturo the Depressed Polar Bear Is Shaking His Head," *The Conversation*, July 17, 2014.

151. Leendert Vergeynst, Susse Wegeberg Jens Aamand, Pia Lassen, Ulrich Gosewinkel, Janne Fritt-Rasmussen, Kim Gustavson, et al., "Biodegradation of Marine Oil Spills in the Arctic with a Greenland Perspective," *Science of the Total Environment* 626 (June 2018): 1243–1258.

152. Claire Palmer, "Should We Provide the Bear Necessities? Climate Change, Polar Bears and the Ethics of Supplemental Feeding," in *Animals in Our Midst: The Challenges of Co-Existing with Animals in the Anthropocene*, ed. Bernice Bovenkerk and Jozef Keulartz (Cham, Switzerland: Springer, 2021), 377–398.

153. Kristin L. Laidre, Megan A. Supple, Erik W. Born, Eric V. Regehr, Øystein Wiig, Fernando Ugarte, Jon Aars, et al., "Glacial Ice Supports a Distinct and Undocumented Polar Bear Subpopulation Persisting in Late 21st-Century Sea-Ice Conditions," *Science* 376 (June 16, 2022): 1333–1338; Andreanna J. Welch, "Polar Bears Exhibit Genome-Wide Signatures of Bioenergetic Adaptation to Life in the Arctic Environment," *Genome Biology and Evolution* 6, no. 3 (February 2014): 443–450.

154. Else M. Poulsen, V. Honeyman, P. A. Valentine, and G. C. Teskey, "Use of Fluoxetine for the Treatment of Stereotypic Pacing Behavior in a Captive Polar Bear," *Journal of the American Veterinary Medical Association* 209, no. 8 (October 1996): 1470–1474; David Leary, *Bioprospecting in the Arctic* (Tokyo: United Nations University Press, 2008).

155. Richard Grusin, ed., *After Extinction* (Minneapolis: University of Minnesota Press, 2018), x.

156. International Union for the Conservation of Nature, *IUCN SSC Guiding Principles on Creating Proxies of Extinct Species for Conservation Benefit* (Gland, Switzerland: IUCN Species Survival Commission, 2016). On Tasmanian tigers, see Ben A. Minteer, *The Fall of the Wild: Extinction, De-Extinction, and the Ethics of Conservation* (New York: Columbia University Press, 2019), 109–118.

157. TEDx DeExtinction event, March 15, 2013, National Geographic Headquarters, Washington, DC, https://reviverestore.org/events/tedxdeextinction. See also Amy Lynn Fletcher, *De-Extinction and the Genomics Revolution: Life on Demand* (London: Palgrave Macmillan, 2020), 17–20.

158. Britt Wray, *Rise of the Necrofauna: The Science, Ethics, and Risks of De-Extinction* (London: Greystone, 2019), 95, 103–107; Heise, *Imagining Extinction*, 24.

159. Beth Shapiro, *How to Clone a Mammoth: The Science of De-Extinction* (Princeton, NJ: Princeton University Press, 2015), 191.

160. Wray, *Rise of the Necrofauna*, 10–13, 42; George Church and Ed Regis, *Regenesis: How Synthetic Biology Will Reinvent Nature and Ourselves* (New York: Basic Books, 2012), 11. See also artist Richard Pell's satirical Mermaid De-Extinction Project, *Art's Work in the Age of Biotechnology: Shaping Our Genetic Future* (Chapel Hill: University of North Carolina Press, 2019), 99–107.

161. Bernice Bovenkerk and Jozef Keulartz, "Animals in Our Midst: An Introduction," *Animals in Our Midst: The Challenges of Co-Existing with Animals in the Anthropocene*, ed. Bernice Bovenkerk and Jozef Keulartz (Cham, Switzerland: Springer, 2021), 10.

162. Ben Mezrich, *Woolly: The True Story of the Quest to Revive One of History's Most Iconic Extinct Creatures* (New York: Atria, 2017); Laura DeFrancesco, "Church to De-Extinct Woolly Mammoths," *Nature Biotechnology* 39 (October 2021): 1171.

163. George Church, quoted in Wray, *Rise of the Necrofauna*, 147; Church and Regis, *Regenesis*, 252.

164. "Genetics Company Wants to Bring Iconic Tasmanian Tiger Back from Extinction," *Newsweek*, August 16, 2022, https://www.newsweek.com/tasmanian-tiger-thylacine-extinction-colossal-biosciences-woolly-mammoth-1733900. For the focus of Colossal Biosciences on reviving the wooly mammoth see "The Mammoth," https://colossal.com/mammoth, accessed April, 14, 2024.

165. Harry Baker, "World's First Wolf Clone Born of Surrogate Dog, Chinese Company Reveals," *Live Science*, September 26, 2022.

166. Juanita Sundberg, "Researching Resistance in a Time of Neoliberal Entanglements," in *Neoliberal Environments: False Promises and Unnatural Consequences*, ed. Nik Heynen, James McCarthy, Scott Prudham, and Paul Robbins (London: Routledge, 2007), 269; Ashley Dawson, "Biocapitalism and De-Extinction," in *After Extinction*, ed. Richard Grusin (Minneapolis: University of Minnesota Press, 2018), 176.

167. "The Yard," Jeff Vandermeer, n.d., accessed October 15, 2022, https://www.jeffvandermeer.com/yard; Michael Pollan, "Why Bother?," *New York Times*, April 20, 2008. See also "Jeff VanderMeer on the Beauty and Weirdness of Florida," *Los Angeles Times*, July 22, 2016; and Alexandra Kleeman, "His Novels of Planetary Devastation Will Make You Want to Survive," *New York Times*, December 12, 2019.

168. E. Dinerstein, C. Vynne, E. Sala, A. R. Joshi, S. Fernando, T. E. Lovejoy, J. Mayorga, et al., "A Global Deal for Nature: Guiding Principles, Milestones, and Targets," *Science Advances* 5, no. 4 (April 2019), https://doi.org/10.1126/sciadv.aaw2869; Carlos Carroll and Reed F. Noss, "Rewilding in the Face of Climate Change," *Conservation Biology* 35, no. 1 (June 2020): 155–167; Jeff VanderMeer, *Hummingbird Salamander* (New York: Fourth Estate, 2019).

169. Elizabeth Pennisi, "'Rewilding' Landscapes with Rhinos and Reindeer Could Prevent Fires and Keep Arctic Cool," *Science*, October 23, 2018; Sabrina Imler, "Meet Elizabeth Ann, the First Cloned Black-Footed Ferret," *New York Times*, February 18, 2021.

170. Wray, *Rise of the Necrofauna*, 197. See also VanderMeer, "How to Rewild Your Balcony, One Native Plant at a Time," *Esquire*, April 22, 2021.

171. Wildfed website: https://www.wild-fed.com/about, accessed October 15, 2022.

172. Minteer, *Fall of the Wild*, 119.

CONCLUSION

1. "Advancing Biotechnology and Biomanufacturing Innovation for a Sustainable, Safe, and Secure American Bioeconomy," Executive Order 14081, September 12, 2022, 87 Fed. Reg. 178 (September 15, 2022), 56849.

2. "Fact Sheet: President Biden to Launch a Biomanufacturing and Biotechnology Initiative," The White House, September 12, 2022, https://www.whitehouse.gov/briefing-room/statements-releases/2022/09/12/fact-sheet-president-biden-to-launch-a-national-biotechnology-and-biomanufacturing-initiative.

3. "White House Summit on Biotechnology and Biomanufacturing," September 14, 2022, YouTube video, accessed March 3, 2023, https://youtu.be/LcP9zPNuUh4.

4. Stephen M. Walt, "America Is Too Scared of the Multipolar World," *Foreign Policy*, March 7, 2023; "Modernizing the Regulatory Framework for Agricultural Biotechnology Products," Executive Order 13874, June 11, 2019, 84 Fed. Reg. 115 (June 14, 2019), 27899.

5. White House Office of Science and Technology Policy, "The White House Advances Biotechnology and Biomanufacturing Leadership with the Launch of the National Bioeconomy Board," March, 24, 2024, https://www.whitehouse.gov/ostp/news-updates/2024/03/22/the-white-house-advances-biotechnology-and-biomanufacturing-leadership-with-the-launch-of-the-national-bioeconomy-board.

6. US Department of Health, Education, and Welfare, *Healthy People: The Surgeon General's Report on Health Promotion and Disease Prevention* (Washington, DC: Government Printing Office, 1979).

7. Julius B. Richmond, *Currents in American Medicine: A Developmental View of Medical Care and Education* (Cambridge, MA: Harvard University Press, 1969), 70–74.

8. Office of the U.S. Surgeon General, *Our Epidemic of Loneliness and Isolation* (Washington, DC: Government Printing Office, 2023).

9. US Department of Health and Human Services, *Healthy People 2020: An End of Decade Snapshot* (Washington, DC: Government Printing Office, 2021), https://health.gov/sites/default/files/2020-12/HP2020EndofDecadeSnapshot.pdf; Office of Disease Prevention and Health Promotion, "Healthy People 2030," accessed February 1, 2023, https://health.gov/healthypeople.

10. "Fact Sheet: HHS Takes Action on Executive Order Launching a National Biotechnology and Biomanufacturing Initiative," US Department of Health and Human Services, September 14, 2022, https://www.hhs.gov/about/news/2022/09/14/fact-sheet-hhs-takes-action-executive-order-launching-national-biotechnology-biomanufacturing-initiative.html.

11. White House Office of Science and Technology Policy, *Bold Goals for U.S. Biotechnology and Biomanufacturing: Harnessing Research and Development to Further Societal Goals* (Washington, DC: Office of the President, 2023). On the age statistic, see National

Institute on Aging, *Strategic Directions for Research, 2020–2025* (National Institute on Aging, 2020), 1, https://www.nia.nih.gov/sites/default/files/2020-05/nia-strategic-directions -2020-2025.pdf.

12. Joe Biden, "Address Before a Joint Session of the Congress on the State of the Union," March 1, 2022, American Presidency Project, https://www.presidency.ucsb.edu /documents/address-before-joint-session-the-congress-the-state-the-union-28.

13. See Jennifer Egan, *The Candy House* (New York: Scribner, 2022).

14. "Fact Sheet: President Biden to Announce Strategy to Address Our National Mental Health Crisis, As Part of Unity Agenda in His First State of the Union," The White House, March 1, 2022, https://www.whitehouse.gov/briefing-room/statements -releases/2022/03/01/fact-sheet-president-biden-to-announce-strategy-to-address-our -national-mental-health-crisis-as-part-of-unity-agenda-in-his-first-state-of-the-union.

15. Patricio V. Marque and Shekhar Saxena, "Making Mental Health a Global Priority," *Cerebrum*, July/August 2016, 28058091.

16. George Church and Ed Regis, *Regenesis: How Synthetic Biology Will Reinvent Nature and Ourselves* (New York: Basic Books, 2012), 243.

17. For a conservative reimagining of the federal government's role in health care governance see Roger Severino, "Department of Health and Human Services", in Project 2025, *Mandate for Leadership: The Conservative Promise* (Washington, DC: The Heritage Foundation, 2023), 449–502.

18. "The Age of Inclusive Intelligence," Dentsu Global, n.d., accessed February 15, 2023, https://brands.dentsu.com/consumer-vision-2030.

19. "The Age of Inclusive Intelligence."

20. Notably, in 2022, the Office of Science and Technology Policy released a blueprint for an AI Bill of Rights; see Office of Science and Technology Policy, "Blueprint for an AI Bill of Rights: Making Automated Systems Work for the American People," The White House, n.d., https://www.whitehouse.gov/ostp/ai-bill-of-rights.

21. Joel Achenbach, "Human Blueprint Breakthrough: Scientists Publish 'Gapless' Human Genome," *Washington Post*, March 31, 2022.

22. OECD International Futures Project, *The Bioeconomy to 2030: Designing a Policy Agenda* (OECD, 2009), http://biotech2030.ru/wp-content/uploads/docs/int/The%20 Bioeconomy%20to%202030_OECD.pdf.

23. Robert N. Bellah, Richard Madsen, William M. Sullivan, Ann Swidler, and Steven M. Tipton, *The Good Society* (New York: Vintage, 1991), 278.

24. For example, sociologist Catherine Bliss credits the development of race-positive paradigms in genetic science but also critiques the persistent tendency to biologize race within the postgenomic landscape. See Catherine Bliss, *Race Decoded: The Genomic Fight for Social Justice* (Stanford, CA: Stanford University Press, 2012); and Catherine Bliss "Conceptualizing Race in the Genomic Age," *Hastings Center Report* 50 (May 2020): S15–S22.

25. Richard Rorty, *Achieving Our Country: Leftist Thought in Twentieth-Century America* (Cambridge, MA: Harvard University Press, 1998), 23.

26. Richard Rorty, "Heidegger, Contingency, and Pragmatism," in *Essays on Heidegger and Others: Philosophical Papers*, vol. 2 (New York: Cambridge University Press, 1991), 27, 47.

27. Rorty, *Achieving Our Country*, 29.

28. Francis Fukuyama, *The Great Disruption: Human Nature and the Reconstitution of Social Order* (New York: Profile, 1999), 282.

29. Franco Furger and Francis Fukuyama, "Beyond Bioethics A Proposal for Modernizing the Regulation of Human Biotechnologies," *Innovations: Technology, Governance, Globalization* 2, no. 4 (October 2007):124, 127.

30. Nikolas Rose, *The Politics of Life Itself: Biomedicine, Power, and Subjectivity in the Twenty-First Century* (Chicago: Chicago University Press, 2007), 5.

31. Rose, *The Politics of Life Itself*, 5, 252.

32. Rose, *The Politics of Life Itself*, 252.

33. Rose, *The Politics of Life Itself*, 252.

34. Paul Rabinow and Nikolas Rose, "Biopower Today," *BioSocieties* 1 (June 2006): 215.

35. Nikolas Rose, *Our Psychiatric Future: The Politics of Mental Health* (London: Polity, 2019), 193–194.

36. Nikolas Rose, Rasmus Birk, and Nick Manning, "Towards Neuroecosociality: Mental Health in Adversity," *Theory, Culture and Society* 39, no. 3 (May 2022): 121–144.

Index

Abbott, Greg, 163
Abi-Rached, Joelle, 5, 74, 90
abortion, 47–51, 56, 59, 67, 244, 250n13,
    270n11, 272n30, 276n73, 279n127
abortion rights, 47–48
Achenbaum, W. Andrew, 132
Adelman, Richard, 136
Advantageous (2015), 135, 145–147, 150
adventurism, 4, 8, 12, 15, 65, 135, 140, 147,
    149–150, 233, 237
Affordable Care Act. *See* Patient Protection
    and Affordable Care Act (2010)
Afghanistan War (2001–2021), 103, 111, 115,
    120, 197
Agamben, Giorgio, 6, 198–199
Age Discrimination Act (1975), 127
age tech. *See* technology
aging, 10, 13, 77, 95, 103, 127–144, 148–149,
    151–152. *See also* anti-aging; gerontology
A. I. Artificial Intelligence (2001), 103, 108, 117
AIDS. *See* HIV/AIDS
alcohol use, 132, 200, 228
Alcor Life Extension Foundation, 149–150
Alt, Jane Fulton, 217
Altschuler, Sari, 189
Alzheimer's Association, 96, 128, 133, 137, 140
Alzheimer's disease, 1, 29, 58, 76–77, 92–97,
    128, 132–140, 148, 151, 195
American Academy of Facial Plastic and
    Reconstructive Surgery, 143
American Association for the Advancement
    of Science, 33, 241
American Medical Association, 154
American Psychiatric Association, 5, 38,
    76, 154
American Psychological Association, 57
American Society for Cell Biology, 58
American Society of Plastic Surgeons, 171
Amgen, 4
ancestral practice, 11, 206, 233, 237
Aniston, Jennifer, 151
anthrax, 197
anti-aging, 140–143, 147. *See also* aging
anti-vaxxers, 192, 196, 198. *See also*
    vaccination
anxiety disorders, xiii, 80, 84, 131
apocalyptic thinking, xiv, 8, 42, 101, 192–194,
    199, 210, 212, 215, 223, 226, 232

Appleyard, Brian, 11
Army, U.S., 112, 115, 155, 158
Army Corps of Engineers, U.S., 217
Arrowsmith-Young, Barbara, 75, 89–92
Arsenault, Nina, 177–178
artificial intelligence, 75, 80, 98–104, 108,
    112, 117, 120
Asian American health care, 137, 145
Asimov, Isaac, 102, 117
Asprey, Dave, 151–152, 206, 335n153
assemblage, 10, 104, 161, 166–168, 177
AstraZeneca, 195–196
Atanasoski, Neda, 101, 103
Atlas, Scott, 202–203
Atwood, Margaret, 13, 18, 27, 39, 42–44, 119,
    135, 140, 149, 226
authenticity, xiii, 15–16, 45, 107, 121–122,
    160–161, 166, 178
Avatar (2009), 18, 104, 116–123, 174
Azar, Alex M., 182

Bacigalupi, Paolo, 210, 216
Bailey, J. Michael, 155
Ball, Philip, 74
Baltimore, 23–24
Banco Bilbao Vizcaya Foundation, 31–32
Barabino, Gilda, 241
Baudrillard, Jean, 12
Bear, Greg, 40
Becerra, Xavier, 236–237
Becker, Gay, 50–51
Bellah, Robert N., xiv, 17–18, 24–25, 39, 45,
    128, 152, 178, 184, 186, 194, 199, 239–241
Benjamin, Harry, 157
Benjamin, Ruha, 70
BetterUp, 4
Biden, Joe, xi, 4, 157–158, 183, 190, 201,
    208–209, 212, 218, 235–237, 325n21
Biden administration, xii, 17, 157, 170, 205,
    212, 218, 235–236, 243
Bigelow, Kathryn, 115–116
Big Pharma, 25, 66, 163, 186
Big Science, 34, 55, 225
Big Tech, 4, 11, 18, 163, 184, 206, 238
Billington, James H., 84
Binnie, Imogen, 160, 164–166, 170, 172
bioart, 13, 43, 144, 150, 177
biodiversity, 45, 217–218, 225, 232–233

About the Author

MARTIN HALLIWELL is a professor of American thought and culture at the University of Leicester in the United Kingdom. His published work encompasses American cultural and intellectual history, the medical humanities, public and mental health, twentieth-century American literature, American film since 1945, and popular music. He is the author and editor of fifteen books, most recently *American Health Crisis: One Hundred Years of Panic, Planning, and Politics* and *The Edinburgh Companion to the Politics of American Health*. He was the chair of the British Association for American Studies (2010–2013) and president and chair of the English Association (2014–2021).